OXFORD MEDICAL PUBLICATIONS

Varicose veins, venous disorders, and lymphatic problems in the lower limbs

Dose schedules are being continually revised and new side effects recognized. Oxford University Press makes no representation, express or implied, that the drug dosages in this book are correct. For these reasons the reader is strongly urged to consult the pharmaceutical company's printed instructions before administering any of the drugs recommended in this book.

Varicose veins, venous disorders, and lymphatic problems in the lower limbs

David J. Tibbs,
David C. Sabiston Jr., Mark G. Davies,
Peter S. Mortimer, and John H. Scurr

Oxford   New York   Tokyo
Oxford University Press
1997

Oxford University Press, Great Clarendon Street, Oxford OX2 6DP

Oxford   New York
Athens   Auckland   Bangkok   Bogota   Bombay   Buenos Aires
Calcutta   Cape Town   Dar es Salaam   Delhi   Florence   Hong Kong
Instanbul   Karachi   Kuala Lumpur   Madras   Madrid   Melbourne
Mexico City   Nairobi   Paris   Singapore   Taipei   Tokyo   Toronto   Warsaw

and associated companies in
Berlin   Ibadan

Oxford is a trade mark of Oxford University Press

Published in the United States by Oxford University Press Inc., New York
© D.J. Tibbs and the contributors listed on p. vi, 1997

A catalogue record for this book is available from the British Library

Library of Congress Cataloging in Publication Data
Varicose veins, venous disorders, and lymphatic problems in the lower
limbs / edited by David Tibbs.
(Oxford medical publications)
Includes bibliographical references and index.
1. Extremities, Lower—Blood-vessels—Diseases. 2. Varicose
veins. 3. Extremities, Lower—Lymphatics—Diseases. I. Tibbs,
David J. II. Series.
[DNLM: 1. Vascular Diseases. 2. Leg—blood supply. 3. Lymphatic
Diseases—complications. 4. Lymphatic System—physiopathology. WG
600 V287 1997]
RC951.V36   1997   616.1′4—dc21   96–39274
ISBN 0 19 262762 7

Typeset by EXPO Holdings, Malaysia

Printed in Hong Kong, China

Foreword

It is now quite evident that the incidence and prevalence of venous diseases is much higher than was first thought. When the high cost of these diseases, and more particularly of their complications in terms of morbidity and socio-economics began to be assessed, interest in this sytem developed rapidly.

It was soon realized that patients suffering from a venous disease were often under-investigated and poorly managed. This led to the development of phlebology as a special interest on its own which drew specialists from many fields. Until recently in Great Britain, the practice of phlebology was almost exclusively in the hands of surgeons. Now, however, this discipline is enriched by the input from dermatologists, physicians/angiologists, radiologists, specialists in the field of the new investigative techniques which have developed, as well as from surgeons and gynaecologists.

As a result, great advances are being made in the understanding and management of these conditions from which, it is hoped, better prevention will result. The complications of venous diseases are, to a large extent, preventable and thus much of the morbidity and socio-economic cost can be reduced.

David Tibbs and his co-authors are to be congratulated on producing what is essentially a clinical textbook on this subject. It is very pleasing that a whole Part is concerned with abnormalities of the lymphatic system in the context of venous diseases as the two systems are so closely inter-related, particularly at the capillary end of the circulation. It is only when more knowledge of what goes on at the capillary level is acquired that we shall understand why venous ulcers occur and their pathophysiology — essential elements in their prevention.

The pattern of the book, which is based on producing a text 'for all readers' together with 'panels for specialist readers', should help to overcome the problem of producing a book too detailed for the general reader but too basic for the 'phlebologist'.

This well-written book, richly illustrated, and with copious references will be of value to all those interested in the veno-lymphatic return circulation.

Georges Jantet
President
Union Internationale de Phlébologie

Authors

Part I
John H. Scurr FRCS
Consultant Surgeon at Middlesex and University College Hospitals
London W1
UK

David J. Tibbs MS, FRCS
Honorary Consulting Surgeon
John Radcliffe Hospital
Oxford
UK

Part II
Mark G. Davies MD, PhD
Research Fellow
Department of Surgery
Duke University Medical Center
Durham NC 27710
USA

David C. Sabiston, Jr. MD
James B. Duke Professor of Surgery and Chief of Staff
Department of Surgery
Duke University Medical Center
Durham NC 27710
USA

Part III
Peter S. Mortimer MD, FRCP
Consultant Skin Physician and Reader in Dermatology
St. Georges Hospital, the Royal Marsden Hospital, and the University of London
London
UK

Preface

The understanding of venous disorders, particularly varicose veins, has improved dramatically over the last 10 years. This has been made possible by the development of methods identifying venous flow patterns in the exercising upright patient—the position in which venous problems arise. The X-ray image intensifier, which allowed more prolonged viewing, opened the way for functional phlebographic studies, soon followed by ultrasonic Doppler directional flowmetry; more recently, ultrasonic imaging, combining the ability to display vessels and the direction and velocity of flow within them, has provided a sophisticated instrument that is non-invasive and permits repetition of examination as often as required to ensure accurate identification of flow. These techniques have unravelled the characteristic flow patterns of the various categories of venous disorder and have proved of outstanding value in the practical management of clinical problems. Other methods, such as phlethysmography, can provide additional information, and there is also a range of electronic and radioactive methods that can be used in unusual problems or for research purposes. With such a variety of new methods there is a need for a practical guide to identify those most effective for everyday use, and this is the intention of our book.

The importance of the new diagnostic instruments is that they allow a precise diagnosis to be made so that rational treatment can be based on this rather than a clinical guess. In the management of venous disorders, the starting point must be an accurate identification of the distinctive flow patterns. The electronic instruments provide an easily applicable non-invasive means for this. In varicose veins, for instance, it should be routine to demonstrate beyond doubt the pathway of incompetence that is to be removed; it is no longer a matter of blindly taking out a superficial vein likely to be at fault, but one that has been *proved* to be incompetent. This book is concerned with describing the basic patterns of venous disorder in the lower limbs, how to recognize them, and the appropriate action to be taken. It is intended to be a concise guide to the best of modern methods to meet the need for established surgeons to revise old ideas and update their methodology, for surgeons in training to develop their skill through the new knowledge, and for non-surgical phlebologists to ensure that their treatment is properly directed. Nurses, who play such a valuable role, will welcome the explanation of a rational basis for treatment. All forms of treatment by surgery, sclerotherapy, and conservative means are described for the appropriate circumstances.

To meet the varied requirements of such a broad readership the text is arranged as a basic narrative running throughout the book, intermingled with which are a number of boxed sections giving more detailed accounts of specialized aspects. These boxes also provide a means of quick reference to key information.

Acute deep vein thrombosis not only creates the threat of thromboembolism but is also likely to cause irreparable damage to the mechanisms of venous return against gravity with all the long-term disability that this entails. Venous specialists will often see the latter chronic state but must also be prepared to meet the acute state in their own practices or that of colleagues. Thus it is important to know how to minimize its occurrence and, when necessary, how to treat it. Present-day understanding of deep vein thrombosis and pulmonary embolism is described in Part II, and a firm policy towards this much debated subject is given which should be of interest to all physicians and surgeons.

The venous disorders are a range of widely differing states and so there is no standard approach; each case must be assessed on its own merits and the treatment for one may be unsuitable for another. Moreover, there is considerable overlap with other vascular disorders, both arterial and lymphatic, that may present with misleading features. None of these is more treacherous than the ulcerated ischaemic limb, the treatment of which conflicts directly with that required by a venous disorder. Although many readers will be primarily concerned with the treatment of varicose veins, this cannot be considered in isolation and for this reason other conditions in the lower limb that may cause confusion are described. Oedema, so often attributed to the veins, deserves special consideration and Part III is devoted to the swollen limb and lymphatic disorders.

The modern concept of the venous disorders is explained in this book, and in each case a course of action based on the combined experience of the authors is given. Scholarly debate upon the alternatives has been avoided, but the most effective approach which is in accord not only with our own beliefs but with international expert opinion is presented.

We should particularly like to express our gratitude to E.W. Fletcher for the many functional phlebograms that are reproduced in this book. We are also indebted to Georges Jantet, who has enlivened so many meetings and has been outstanding in promoting international discussion on venous topics, for the Foreword to this book.

With five authors of this book it is not possible to thank individually all those associated with each of us for their help in so many ways, but we would like them to know their support has been fully appreciated and highly valued. We are very conscious of the numerous kindred spirits all over the world who have done so much to advance understanding and treatment of venous and lymphatic problems in recent years. It has been a great pleasure to meet so many of you at international meetings. We hope that this book expresses adequately the best of all our collective efforts.

Oxford, UK   D.J.T.
Durham, USA   D.C.S. Jr
Durham, USA   M.G.D.
London, UK   P.S.M.
London, UK   J.H.S.
March 1997

About the cover

Front cover

A composite functional phlebogram and explanatory drawing of the flow patterns. It shows superficial vein incompetence in the right lower limb being filled from the opposite side through a cross-over collateral circulation caused by longstanding left iliac occlusion.

The patient had sustained left ilio-femoral thrombosis 30 years previously, with residual oedema and venostatic changes on that side. Recently, varicose veins and early skin changes at the ankle had appeared on the right side. In this functional phlebogram, with the patient in near-vertical position, opaque medium injected into superficial veins on the left calf travelled upwards and across to the opposite right femoral vein by pubic collateral veins. With exercise by rising up and down on the toes three times, the cross-over flow increased and is seen here immediately afterwards descending down the right long saphenous vein and into varicose veins arising from it (and see Figs 4.13(b) (page 54), 6.4 (e) and (f) (page 116)).

Surgery to the incompetent right sapheno-femoral junction was avoided because it might interfere with the collateral circulation from the left, to the detriment of that limb. The patient responded well to simple knee length elastic support.

Back cover

For further details about the illustration a free-floating thrombus in the superficial femoral vein displayed by duplex ultrasonography, see Fig. 10.5(b) (ii) and (iii).

Contents

Part I

Varicose veins and venous disorders

John H. Scurr and David J. Tibbs

1 Normal anatomy and physiology

The veins of the lower limb must not be viewed as a series of inert venous conduits but rather as a complex pumping mechanism capable of returning venous blood to the heart against the force of gravity in the upright position. If active thrombosis is excluded, it is some form of failure in this mechanism that underlies nearly all venous disorders in the lower limb. The essentials of normal anatomy and physiology will be described first, particularly those aspects that may undergo change and cause venous problems.

Essential properties of veins

Structure of the veins

Unlike arteries, the veins are specifically designed to allow flow in one direction only, i.e. towards the heart, and this is achieved by the presence of numerous valves arranged along their length (Fig. 1.1).

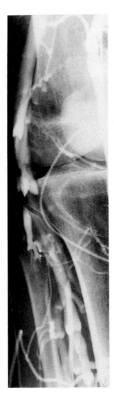

Fig. 1.1 Normal competent valves in a popliteal vein and its branches shown by phlebography. Such valves are essential for normal function in both superficial and deep veins.

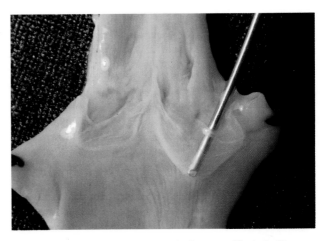

Fig. 1.2 A vein opened to show a pair of valve cusps. The probe lifts one cusp to display its delicate structure.

Only in the common iliac veins, the vena cava, the portal system, and the cranial sinuses are these valves absent. They form an essential part of the venous pumping mechanisms returning blood from the lower limbs against gravity and act to protect the peripheral tissues from the back pressure set up by columns of blood when the patient is upright. Each valve is made up of two gossamer-thin cusps which, despite their delicate appearance, are surprisingly strong (Fig. 1.2). The cusps are supported by the vein walls, and their integrity as functioning valves depends on this supports having sufficient strength to resist the forces dilating the veins and tending to separate the cusps. The vein walls are thin but are capable of considerable distension or contraction; these qualities are provided by circumferential rings of elastic tissue and smooth muscle. When the patient is upright and standing still, the veins are maximally distended and the diameter may be several times greater than in the horizontal limb at rest. The veins are very flexible; if the limb is elevated so that all blood leaves the veins, not only do they contract down to minimal size, but they also collapse into a thin ribbon-like shape. Such a highly flexible thin-walled structure which collapses easily does not allow suction to be transmitted along its length, and siphonage plays virtually no part in the movement of venous blood. It is incorrect to think of blood ever being sucked from one part of the venous system to another in the limbs.

As with arteries, the interior of the veins is lined with endothelium, providing a non-thrombogenic surface, but in the case of veins, where slow flow and long periods of stasis might encourage thrombosis more easily than arteries, there is an enhanced protective mechanism providing prostacyclins, to prevent aggregation of platelets, and actively forming fibrinolysins (plasmin) capable of dissolving thrombus and clot (a detailed account of this is given in Part II).

Box 1.1   Properties and structure of veins

Contain valves—an essential component
Allow flow only towards heart
Thin, elastic, highly flexible contractile walls
Endothelium—non-thrombogenic and releases anticlotting factors (plasmin)

Arrangement of deep veins in the lower limbs

The deep veins lie beneath the deep fascia but do not all serve the same function, merely varying in size. They can be divided into two major categories.

The veins as conduits

The major veins in the limbs and the numerous branches joining them serve as conduits, taking blood back from the tissues towards the heart. These are the veins shown in most anatomical diagrams starting as plantar veins running to tibial veins, through popliteal and superficial femoral veins to common femoral and iliac veins, and so into the inferior vena cava (Fig. 1.3). However, these veins make only a limited contribution to the active pumping of blood upwards against gravity which is so essential in the lower limbs, and this function is largely dependent on the venous sinuses within muscle that act as highly efficient pumping chambers.

Veins as pumping chambers

The lower limbs have powerful muscles capable of great effort. During activity these require a copious flow of blood. Numerous venous sinuses are distributed throughout these muscles (Fig. 1.4). Their shape varies considerably in different muscles, with some being long and thin, for example in the peroneal muscles, and others being broad and bulky, as found in the soleal and gastrocnemius muscles. The greater the effort required of the muscle, the larger the venous sinuses will be. Because the sinuses are surrounded by the muscle fibres, they are strongly compressed when the muscle contracts and blood within them is driven out through connecting veins to join the main conduit veins (Fig. 1.5); the connecting veins are valved and situated at the heartward end of each sinus. Blood that has crossed the capillary beds of muscle passes through numerous small vessels into each sinus which fills to capacity from this source or until it is emptied by the next muscle contraction. In addition, veins communicating with superficial veins perforate the deep fascia and enter many sinuses near their distal ends (Fig. 1.6). The valves of these perforating veins allow flow inwards to the sinuses but prevent outward flow from them; in this way, blood accumulated in superficial veins can enter the muscle sinuses when they are slack. Each sinus, together with the surrounding muscle fibres, forms an elegant and effective pumping chamber emptied at each contraction and propelling blood towards the heart. The valve arrangement in the conduit veins ensures that blood only moves in this direction and protects the sinus from unwanted reflux once contraction has ceased and the sinus is empty. Thus the sinus can only

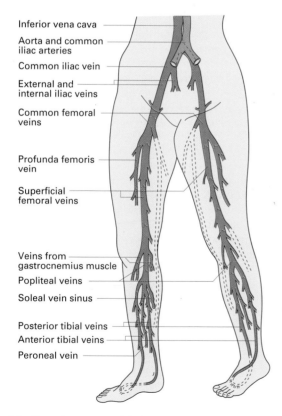

Inferior vena cava

Aorta and common iliac arteries

Common iliac vein

External and internal iliac veins

Common femoral veins

Profunda femoris vein

Superficial femoral veins

Veins from gastrocnemius muscle

Popliteal veins

Soleal vein sinus

Posterior tibial veins

Anterior tibial veins

Peroneal vein

Fig. 1.3   The main venous conduits formed by the deep veins of the lower limbs; numerous branch veins join these.

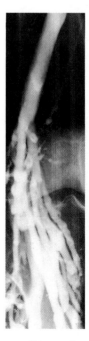

Fig. 1.4   Multiple venous sinuses within a gastrocnemius muscle. These are valved and act as pumping chambers for returning blood from muscle back to the heart against gravity. The soleus also has notably large venous sinuses but all muscles have similar provision for pumping although varying greatly in size, distribution, and number.

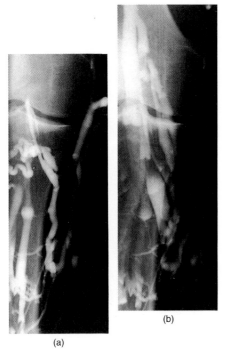

(b)

(a)

Fig. 1.5 Functional phlebograms demonstrating the pumping action of venous sinuses in gastrocnemius muscle: (a) during contraction, the sinuses are emptied; (b) after contraction, with muscle relaxed, the sinuses fall slack and allow easy refilling with blood ready to be expelled upwards with the next contraction.

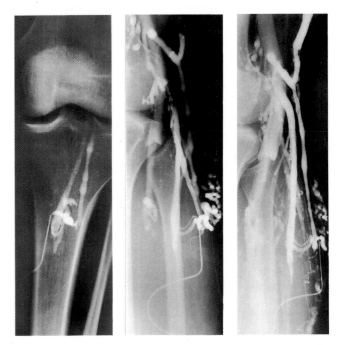

Fig. 1.6 Filling of a venous sinus in muscle from overlying superficial (varicose) veins. Phases of filling are viewed in two different rotations. A pair of perforating veins take flow directly from the superficial veins into a gastrocnemius sinus. Such inward flow is normal and often seen at all levels. A gastrocnemius sinus outlined in this fashion is easily mistaken for the neighbouring short saphenous vein, also shown here with an upward extension from it (Giacomini vein).

fill from the intended sources, the capillary beds in muscle, perforating veins, and interconnecting veins running between sinuses. All the muscles in the lower limbs, ranging from diminutive muscles such as the plantar to the massive muscles of the calf, contribute to this widespread pumping system which is often collectively termed the musculovenous pump. Sometimes this is referred to, for convenience, as the 'calf muscle pump'; however, this implies that the muscles of the calf are the only ones that matter when, in fact, all muscle groups in the leg* and foot play an important part and are also implicated in any disorders that may arise.

Box 1.2   Deep veins—two categories

Conduits—convey blood passively but are capable of some pumping

Pumping chambers within muscles—emptied by muscle contraction; highly effective and can match blood supply required by working muscle

---

Additional pumping mechanisms

Because of their valves, all veins are capable of contributing to venous return against gravity in response to pressure by surrounding muscles or by any form of external pressure.

---

*In Part I of this book the term 'leg' is used in the anatomical sense, referring to the portion of lower limb below the knee.

Changing the position of the limb from dependency to elevation will cause blood trapped between valves to empty proximally so that a form of pumping can be provided by repeatedly changing the position of the limb.

The underside of the foot provides a substantial pumping mechanism, partly because of the muscles within it, but perhaps even more so because the bodyweight compresses the underside of the foot against the ground at each footstep. The pool of blood in the capacious venous plexus under the foot is emptied upwards and, in the normal state, prevented from returning by valves in the superficial and deep veins of the lower leg. Loss of effective valves here plays a significant part in venous disease.

Conclusion

Proper venous return from the lower limb depends upon an intricate pumping mechanism requiring numerous effective valves. Failure of the valves for any reason will reduce the effectiveness of venous return in the upright posture and may lead to an undesirable state of sustained venous pressure unrelieved by exercise, which is known as venous hypertension (venotension).

Superficial veins and perforating veins

Superficial veins

In addition to the deep vein system of conduits and pumping chambers described above, there is a system of superficial veins lying outside the deep fascia subcutaneously. This commences as a

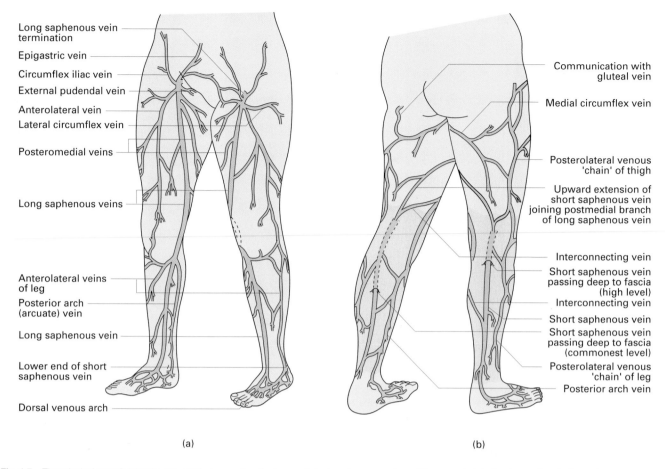

Long saphenous vein termination
Epigastric vein
Circumflex iliac vein
External pudendal vein
Anterolateral vein
Lateral circumflex vein
Posteromedial veins
Long saphenous veins
Anterolateral veins of leg
Posterior arch (arcuate) vein
Long saphenous vein
Lower end of short saphenous vein
Dorsal venous arch

Communication with gluteal vein
Medial circumflex vein
Posterolateral venous 'chain' of thigh
Upward extension of short saphenous vein joining postmedial branch of long saphenous vein
Interconnecting vein
Short saphenous vein passing deep to fascia (high level)
Interconnecting vein
Short saphenous vein
Short saphenous vein passing deep to fascia (commonest level)
Posterolateral venous 'chain' of leg
Posterior arch vein

(a)   (b)

Fig. 1.7 The principal superficial veins are mainly arranged as the long and short saphenous systems. These empty into the deep veins via the saphenous terminations but also by numerous perforating veins. (a) Anterior aspect. (b) Posterior aspect.

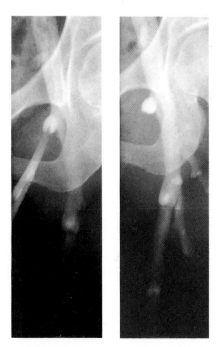

Fig. 1.8 A normal saphenous termination shown in two phases of filling at phlebography. Note the valve guarding its uppermost part and preventing reflux down it.

network of fine veins, mainly from the skin itself, that merge into branch veins running into two principal superficial veins, the long and the short saphenous veins (synonyms: greater or internal, and lesser or external). These, together with their branches, form two clearly identifiable systems but there is free interconnection between them. Figure 1.7 shows a typical arrangement of the superficial veins, including those branches commonly involved in venous disorders. There is much individual variation in the details, and some of these variants will be discussed later. The long saphenous vein runs subcutaneously up the inner leg and thigh to the groin, where it passes through the fossa ovalis to join the common femoral vein (Fig. 1.8). The short saphenous vein passes through the deep fascia somewhere between midcalf and knee and runs for a short distance beneath the fascia to end by joining the popliteal vein at a variable level but usually opposite the femoral condyles (Fig. 1.9); here it commonly gives off an upward extension (sometimes called the Giacomini vein) which may run deeply, in continuity with the profunda femoris vein, or superficially, curving round to join the long saphenous vein by its posteromedial branch in the upper thigh. Both saphenous systems have valves at intervals along their length, and these become more numerous in the lower part of the leg, in keeping with the progressive increase in pressure to be resisted down the length of the limb when upright (Fig. 1.10).

The superficial veins, draining skin and subcutaneous tissues, play a major role in the regulation of body temperature. In hot conditions, greatly increased blood flow through the skin causes it to act as a radiator which, aided by evaporation of sweat, very effectively

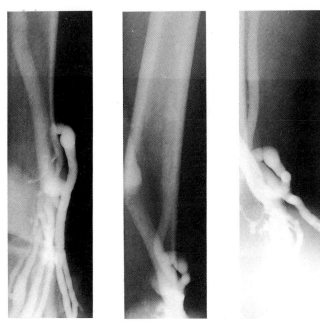

removes body heat. The superficial veins dilate to remove the rapid flow of blood; in warm conditions or during exercise these veins are maximally dilated, but in cold and inactive circumstances they are constricted and inconspicuous. In venous disorders, enlarged or varicose veins will reflect these changes and thus the venous defects are most obvious in the very conditions in which patients wish to uncover their limbs.

Box 1.3 Superficial veins

Mainly from skin which provides an important temperature-regulating mechanism

Drain inwardly to deep veins via perforators (immediately after muscle contraction) and/or via saphenous vein terminations (by passive upflow when standing still, or when limb is horizontal or elevated)

Have little true pumping capability

Fig. 1.9 A short saphenous termination shown in differing rotations at phlebography. In this example, the main junction with popliteal vein is at the most common level, opposite to the femoral condyles, and a substantial branch continues upwards (Giacomini vein) to join the profunda femoris vein. This upward extension commonly occurs and many variations are possible; for example, it may follow a superficial course to join the long saphenous vein posteromedially.

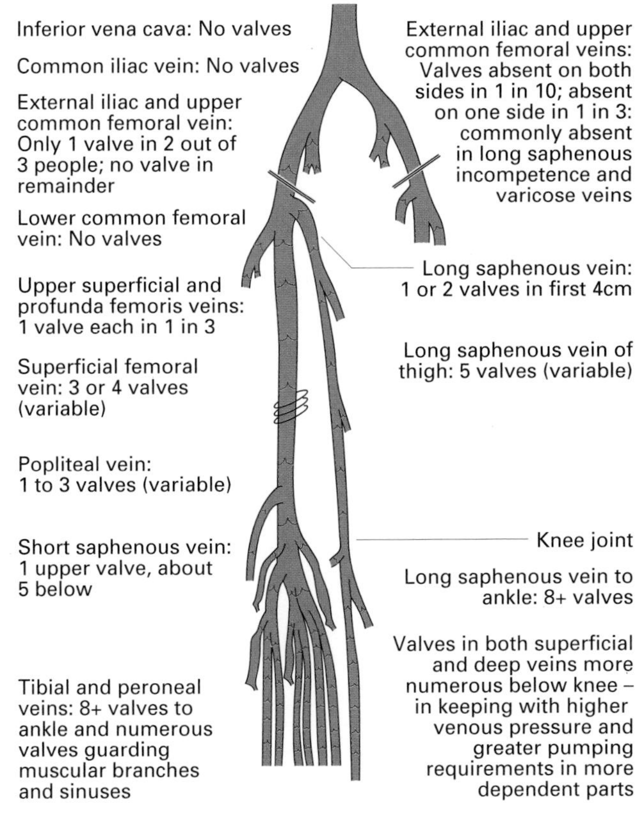

Inferior vena cava: No valves

Common iliac vein: No valves

External iliac and upper common femoral vein: Only 1 valve in 2 out of 3 people; no valve in remainder

Lower common femoral vein: No valves

Upper superficial and profunda femoris veins: 1 valve each in 1 in 3

Superficial femoral vein: 3 or 4 valves (variable)

Popliteal vein: 1 to 3 valves (variable)

Short saphenous vein: 1 upper valve, about 5 below

Tibial and peroneal veins: 8+ valves to ankle and numerous valves guarding muscular branches and sinuses

External iliac and upper common femoral veins: Valves absent on both sides in 1 in 10; absent on one side in 1 in 3: commonly absent in long saphenous incompetence and varicose veins

Long saphenous vein: 1 or 2 valves in first 4cm

Long saphenous vein of thigh: 5 valves (variable)

Knee joint

Long saphenous vein to ankle: 8+ valves

Valves in both superficial and deep veins more numerous below knee – in keeping with higher venous pressure and greater pumping requirements in more dependent parts

Fig. 1.10 Diagram of the distribution of valves usually present in superficial and deep veins.

Perforating veins

At their terminations the saphenous veins empty blood into the popliteal and common femoral veins, but they can also empty by numerous perforating veins running from the superficial veins through the deep fascia to join deep veins (Fig. 1.11). It has been estimated that there are over 60 such perforating veins distributed over all aspects of a lower limb. These perforators are often paired, and many run directly into the deep conduit veins but, as previously stated, others communicate with the venous sinuses (the pumping chambers) in muscles (Fig. 1.6). Some perforators are more liable than others to be involved in venous disorders and have been given eponyms after the authority first drawing attention to them, but this is an oversimplification because other perforators, found extensively over the lower limbs, are often implicated in venous disorders.

Most perforators are valved to allow only inward flow from superficial to deep veins, but it is probable that the arrangement of fibres at the fascial apertures also plays a part in preventing outward flow when muscle contraction causes a sharp rise of pressure within the sinuses. Small perforators (less than 2 mm in diameter) tend not to be valved and presumably are responsible for equalization of pressure by outflow from deep to superficial veins.

When the limb is horizontal, superficial drainage is partly through the saphenous terminations and partly by the perforators to the deep veins. However, when upright, there is normally very little pumping action sending blood up the saphenous veins and the perforators play a major role in venous return from the superficial veins. When standing still, the saphenous veins tend to fill steadily, but after muscular contraction, the resulting fall in deep venous pressure attracts flow from superficial to deep veins through the perforators in the direction allowed by valves. Thus, in an upright and actively moving person most superficial drainage is by multiple perforators up the length of the limb rather than following each saphenous vein to its termination. When upright but motionless, both superficial and deep pressures remain equal, rising slowly in parallel fashion to maximum, and there is a slow drift of passive flow up both sets of veins; in this state, even a single movement causing muscle contraction to empty the deep veins will be followed immediately by flow from superficial veins, via perforators, into the deep veins. Because the saphenous veins and their branches have numerous

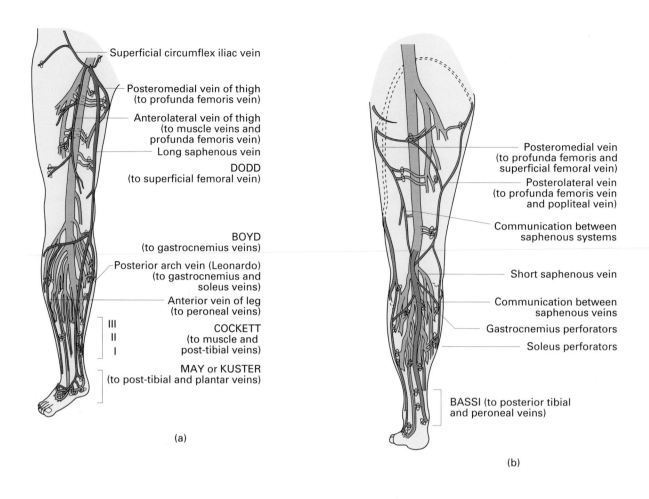

Superficial circumflex iliac vein

Posteromedial vein of thigh
(to profunda femoris vein)

Anterolateral vein of thigh
(to muscle veins and
profunda femoris vein)

Long saphenous vein

DODD
(to superficial femoral vein)

BOYD
(to gastrocnemius veins)

Posterior arch vein (Leonardo)
(to gastrocnemius and
soleus veins)

Anterior vein of leg
(to peroneal veins)

III
II
I

COCKETT
(to muscle and
post-tibial veins)

MAY or KUSTER
(to post-tibial and plantar veins)

(a)

Posteromedial vein
(to profunda femoris and
superficial femoral vein)

Posterolateral vein
(to profunda femoris vein
and popliteal vein)

Communication between
saphenous systems

Short saphenous vein

Communication between
saphenous veins

Gastrocnemius perforators

Soleus perforators

BASSI (to posterior tibial
and peroneal veins)

(b)

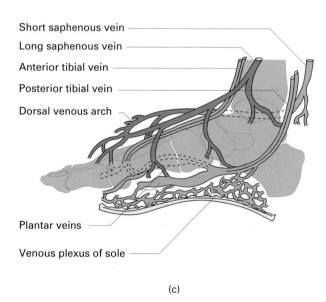

Short saphenous vein

Long saphenous vein

Anterior tibial vein

Posterior tibial vein

Dorsal venous arch

Plantar veins

Venous plexus of sole

(c)

Fig. 1.11 Diagram of the principal perforator veins communicating between superficial and deep veins. Many have been named eponymously after the authorities describing their importance in venous disorders. In addition to those shown here, there are many more present at all levels, any of which may participate in venous problems. (a) Anterior aspect. (b) Posterior aspect. (c) The foot.

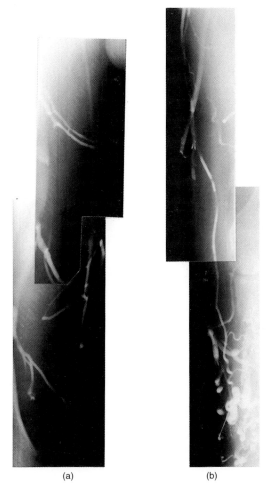

Fig. 1.12 Perforating veins in the thigh and their role in emptying the long saphenous vein in the upright position. Phlebograms from two limbs are shown. (a) Three sets of normal perforating veins are outlined. The upper pair run posteriorly to join the profunda femoris; the lower ones run obliquely to the femoral vein in the mid and lower thigh. (b) Segmentation of blood into columns between valves in the thigh after repositioning the limb has partially emptied the saphenous vein.

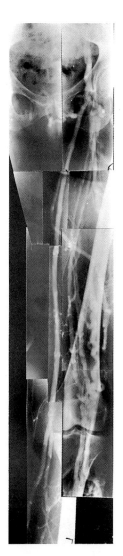

Fig. 1.13 Composite phlebogram of a limb with extensive obstruction of the deep veins following thrombosis some years previously. The long saphenous vein is shown acting as an important collateral channel past the deficient deep veins; although somewhat enlarged, it is well valved and providing an excellent substitute. In the pubic region, branch veins are enlarged and tortuous because they are acting as collaterals across to the opposite side, compensating for left iliac vein occlusion.

valves the continuous column of blood in these veins becomes segmented between the valves as each part empties inwardly through its own group of perforators (Fig. 1.12). In this way, a continuous column of blood up a saphenous vein becomes a series of cascades between the valves.

Box 1.4 Perforators

Numerous connections between superfical and deep conduit veins and pumping chambers

All except the smallest are valved to prevent outflow and allow only inflow

The small valveless perforators may allow equalization of pressure between deep and superficial veins

Reversed flow via a perforator can be part of an important collateral mechanism if normal outlet to deep vein is obstructed

---

Collateral flow

Reversed flow through perforators in a leg, i.e. outwardly from the deep veins, can often be demonstrated in apparently normal limbs when the popliteal vein is compressed so that surface veins are artificially caused to take on the temporary role of collaterals. This phenomenon becomes a permanent feature in post-thrombotic deep vein obstruction where the perforators and superficial veins become part of a regular collateral system allowing continuous outflow up the superficial veins and past the underlying obstructed deep veins (Fig. 1.13). Such collateral veins may become greatly enlarged by forceful flow through them. In other circumstances, primary failure of the valve mechanism in a perforating vein may allow it to become the source of downflow in superficial veins with incompetent valves, and this will be discussed later. Occasionally, failure of perforator valves allows forceful ejection from intramuscular venous sinuses on contraction and causes enlarged tortuous veins in the vicinity (Chapter 7, p. 138).

Creation of flow within veins

The main forces that create movement of venous blood in the limbs are arterial pressure across the capillary beds, the musculovenous pumps, and gravity. However, external pressure and abdominothoracic pressure can also influence flow.

1. In the arteries, pressure created at each heartbeat pumps the blood towards the peripheral capillary beds and is only slightly assisted or impeded by gravity, depending on the position of the limb. When standing upright and motionless, venous blood derived from peripheral capillary beds starts back towards the heart at a low pressure and slow delivery. This transcapillary flow leads to a slow build-up of pressure sufficient to give a drift of bloodback to the heart. Eventually, this process causes a prolonged rise of capillary and venous pressure to 100 mmHg or more, in the foot and ankle region which has undesirable consequences if maintained too long. This aspect is discussed further in Chapter 2.

2. By far the most powerful force creating venous return flow is the musculovenous pumping mechanism which can handle large volumes rapidly and generate a force well in excess of that required for venous return against gravity. Operation of the 'pump' (Fig. 1.14) is followed by a sharp fall in venous pressure in the lower part of the limb; as will be seen later, extensive damage to this pumping system by thrombosis can seriously impair the well-being of the limb.

3. The third force causing venous flow is gravity itself. If the limb is elevated above the horizontal, flow towards the heart occurs by simple gravitational downflow without any need for assistance by transcapillary pressure or the musculovenous pump. Elevating the limb to promote venous flow is an important principle in the treatment of conditions where venous return is impeded for any reason. When the limb is in a dependent position, a normal set of valves in deep and superficial veins will prevent reflux of blood against the normal direction of venous flow. However, a failure of competence in the valves will lead to retrograde flow down the limb when the patient first stands or after an exercise movement has created slack veins in the lower part of the leg. In the superficial veins, this is the basis of the most common venous disorder of all – simple varicose veins.

4. Movement of venous blood is also influenced by external pressure which can give a purposeful pumping movement if the valves are effective.

5. Abdominothoracic pressure can influence venous movement in the limb. A raised pressure will cause a brief downward shift as far as is allowed by valves, and on inspiration the thorax can create a negative pressure that will briefly encourage venous return. Of course, phasic ebb and flow in the movement of venous blood with respiration is normal in the lower limbs; this is most marked when the subject is supine and can be used as evidence of unobstructed veins. Forced inspiration against a closed glottis exerts a brief but powerful suction effect towards the heart.

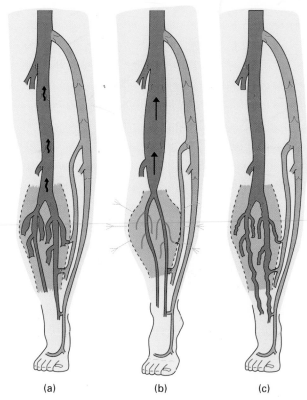

Fig. 1.14   Normal venous return against gravity in the upright position: (a) when standing still the veins fill to capacity in about 30 s; (b) with contraction of leg muscles, the deep veins are compressed and empty upwards, the only direction permitted by valves; (c) with relaxation of muscle, the veins, protected from reflux by valves, are slack and refill slowly by arterial flow across capillary beds.

Box 1.5   Flow in veins

By arterial inflow across capillary beds
By musculovenous pumping mechanism (muscle contraction and external pressure)
By gravity
  • elevation of limb gives easy flow to heart
  • downflow is prevented by valves when upright but gravity becomes a potent force if valves are incompetent
By abdominothoracic pressure which can exert a brief but powerful downward thrust normally resisted by valves; a negative thoracic pressure will draw blood towards the heart; phasic respiratory ebb and flow in venous return is normally present.

Venous pressure changes within the lower limbs

When a person with normal veins rises from the horizontal to the upright position and the veins steadily fill by arterial inflow, the venous pressure in superficial and deep veins in the foot and ankle gradually rise over the next 30 to 60 s to that exerted by the column

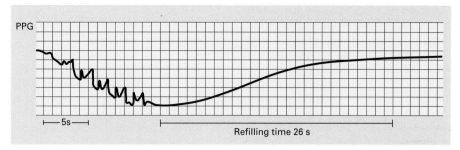

Fig. 1.15 A normal photoplethysmogram from the lower leg during and after five exercise movements in an upright position. This records the change in skin capillary filling, which in turn runs parallel with venous filling and venous pressure in that part of the limb. A substantial drop in filling accompanies exercise and recovers over the next 26 s. This recovery or refiling time is due to arterial inflow, but will be unnaturally shortened if a venous disorder allowing reflux is present.

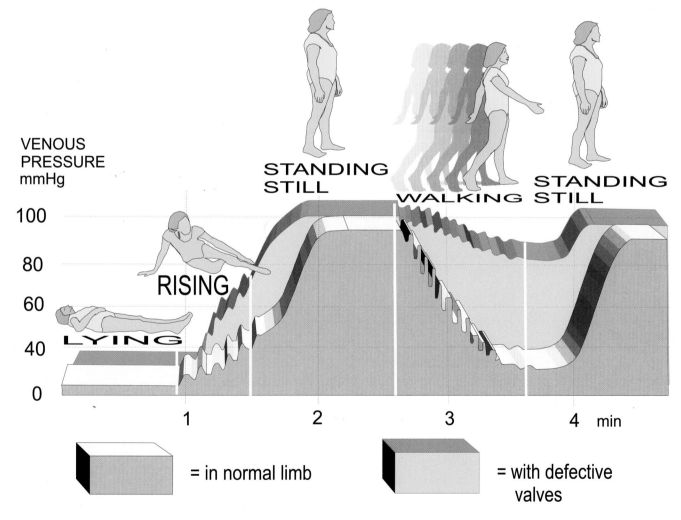

THE EFFECT OF POSTURE AND EXERCISE ON VENOUS PRESSURE AT ANKLE

Fig. 1.16 Changes in venous pressure with varying position and exercise, comparing normal behaviour with venous disorder. Changes in limb volume and degree of capillary filling run parallel with this, so that various forms of phlethysmography can be used to indicate the rate and extent of pressure changes in response to exercise and posture. Note how venous pressure in venous disorder is lowered inadequately with exercise and rapidly returns to high level. High venous pressure, unrelieved by movement when upright, is damaging and causes the harmful effects of venous disorder; this is maximal on standing and minimal or absent when the patient is recumbent.

of blood from foot to heart level, which is about 100 mmHg, depending upon overall height. This assumes that the subject stands still without movement, because as soon as movement occurs blood is pumped upwards and the pressure within the veins drops. A series of movements, such as walking, will empty the veins in the lower leg very effectively (Fig. 1.14) so that the pressure within them drops to around 20 mmHg where it remains whilst movement continues (Fig. 1.15). On ceasing to walk and standing still the venous pressure again climbs steadily over the next minute to its previous level, but even a small single movement of the lower limb will cause a significant drop for many seconds. When capillary flow is greatly enhanced by muscular activity, each muscle contraction creates a corresponding increase in venous return and a fall in the venous pressure. Without effective musculovenous pumping, removing the large flow of blood through contracting muscle, a most damaging rise in venous pressure occurs, giving severe venous hypertension (Fig. 1.16). The characteristic changes and harmful effects caused by this are discussed in Chapters 4, 5, and 6, but the causes of ineffective pumping are summarized in the next chapter.

Box 1.6   Venous pressure changes with position and movement (see Fig. 1.16)

When horizontal, pressure is near zero

On rising to standing position pressure rises steadily to 100 mmHg (or more in a tall person) over 30 to 60 s

On walking, by action of musculovenous pump, pressure falls within a few steps to 20 mmHg and remains there whilst walking continues.

On ceasing walking and standing still pressure rises again to 100 mmHg over 30 s or more

Defective valves may prevent response to exercise so that pressure remains high (potentially damaging) and quickly reverts to maximal.

2 Disordered venous function

When a patient is lying with the lower limbs elevated, blood will flow from them by gravity to the heart without the need for any pump (assuming that there is no deep vein obstruction). However, when the patient rises to an upright position, the return of blood is progressively opposed by gravity and a pumping mechanism becomes essential for proper venous return. It is only in the upright position that venous problems become evident and can be effectively demonstrated.

Causes of inadequate venous return and resulting venous hypertension

Venous insufficiency, which is a state of inadequate venous return in the upright position accompanied by venous hypertension, may occur in the following circumstances.

1. Overwhelming of the pumping mechanism by massive downflow in superficial veins with deficient or defective valves, as often occurs in simple varicose veins.

2. Widespread impairment of the musculovenous pumping mechanism during and after active venous thrombosis, for example acute deep vein thrombosis in which adherent clot disables numerous pumping units and may cause permanent fibrotic damage to them (see Part II).

3. Obstruction or deformity in the main venous conduits as a consequence of venous thrombosis (post-thrombotic syndrome).

4. Obstruction of deep veins by external pressure (e.g. a tumour).

5. Loss of deep vein valve competence, or replacement of the deep veins by enlarged valveless collateral veins, as occurs in post-thrombotic states.

6. Inborn deficiency of deep vein valves or inherent weakness in the vein walls with consequent valve failure (valveless and weak vein syndromes).

7. Prolonged inactivity of the muscles with the limbs in a dependent position, as in paralysis or disease states, such as arthritis, which inhibit use of muscles. However, the blood flow through muscles will be correspondingly reduced and venous hypertension may not be too severe.

It should be noted that arteriovenous fistula, by direct arterial inflow to the venous side, can cause venous hypertension and the characteristic venotensive changes resulting from this (see Chapter 8).

Symptoms are described at the end of this chapter because they are so often based upon the visible manifestations of venous disorder and, rightly or wrongly, any discomforts are attributed, to these. The signs are defined first.

Box 2.1 Causes of failure in adequate venous return against gravity

Venous pump overwhelmed by downflow in incompetent superficial veins (varicose veins)
Deep vein thrombosis—active or late consequences causing:
- damage to pumping units
- obstruction to deep veins
- reflux from damaged valves in conduit deep veins
- reflux in over-expanded veins acting as collaterals

Deep veins obstructed by external pressure
Inborn deficiency of valves
Inactivity of muscles (paralysis or arthritis) in a dependent limb

---

Signs of venous abnormality in the lower limb

There is much variation between individuals in the prominence of normal superficial veins when standing. Not only may the calibre of veins be very different between one person and another, but the ease with which they are seen will differ greatly according to the depth of subcutaneous tissue and general skin texture. The superficial veins of a lean athletic person will appear large and easily seen, but they will be far less obvious in the amply covered subject, perhaps with equally large veins. Superficial veins may vary from one hour to the next in changing conditions of heat or cold. In women, the size of veins is greatly affected by the hormonal state; for example there is obvious enlargement just before menstruation, and in pregnancy there is substantial prolonged enlargement which may be an important factor in the development of varicose veins. Other variations are related to vasomotor control; for instance the tone of superficial veins in the lower part of the leg increases considerably on standing as part of a vasomotor reflex, adjusting veins to meet the increased pressure. For these reasons size alone is not a satisfactory indication of abnormality in a superficial vein unless the enlargement is gross. However, certain other signs may be present that allow immediate recognition of abnormality in the superficial veins.

The deep veins are not easily accessible and abnormality in them can only be implied indirectly from changes found at clinical examination. Direct evidence of the state of the deep veins is obtained by special investigation or imaging techniques.

Visible and palpable signs of venous abnormality

Patient standing

Tortuosity

This change in the veins has been recognized since antiquity and is the most significant visible sign of abnormality. The Latin *varix* (pleural *varices*), possibly derived from *varus*, meaning bent, specifically refers to tortuous dilatation of a vein. The word varicose is defined in medical dictionaries as describing veins that are tortuous, twisted, knotted, or lengthened. It may be seen in greatly varying forms in small-calibre veins running over a considerable distance, in a convoluted mass of enormously enlarged veins (Fig. 2.1), or, at the other extreme, in a single bulge. This change is almost always associated, intermittently or continuously, with substantial flow in the reverse direction to that natural for the vein. By far the most common example is seen in superficial vein incompetence, where strong gravitational downflow occurs repeatedly in varicose veins when upright and exercising, with progressive enlargement and increasing tortuosity in the affected veins. Conversely, high flow in the normal direction at increased pressure, either intermittently or continuously, will cause enlargement but is seldom accompanied by tortuosity.

Saccules on the veins

A saphenous vein, as opposed to its branches, seldom becomes tortuous, perhaps because it is too robust. However, one or more saccules may often be seen or palpated along its length (Fig. 2.2(a)). The term 'saphena varix' is given to a saccule which commonly develops close to the long saphenous termination (Fig. 2.2(b)). Usually a saccule is immediately below valve cusps (Figs 2.2(c) and 2.2(d)) which are leaking heavily. The gross turbulence that this causes on coughing gives rise to a characteristic palpable thrill, readily confirmed by Doppler flowmetry and functional phlebography. It is possible that this turbulent jet of blood beneath the

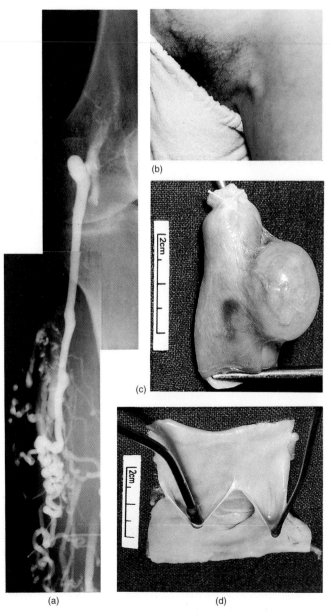

(a)

(b)

(c)

(d)

Fig. 2.2 Saphenous veins seldom show tortuosity but may develop a saccule below an incompetent valve: (a) a large saccule shown by phlebography on a short saphenous vein which is the source of extensive varicose veins; (b) clinical appearance of a saphena varix, i.e. a saccule arising immediately below the upper valve of the long saphenous vein in the groin; (c) a saphena varix distended with saline after surgical removal; (d) the same vein opened to display the mouth of the saccule immediately beneath the cusps.

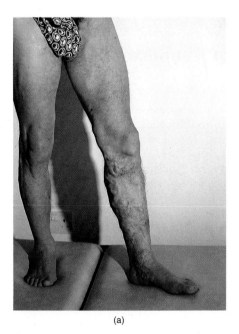

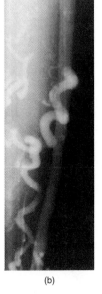

(a)

(b)

Fig. 2.1 Massive varicose veins arising from the long saphenous vein. (a) As seen clinically, running from the lower thigh to the foot. (b) As seen on phlebography, with a tortuous enlarged posterior arcuate branch arising in the lower thigh. The long saphenous vein itself is enlarged but not tortuous.

cusps creates a phenomenon similar to the post-stenotic dilatation in arteries described by Holman; occasionally a saccule arises within a cusp, but again this can be attributed to turbulence in malaligned cusps. However, this assumes that the initiating defect is the leaking valve, but the primary fault could be weakening of the vein wall causing separation of the cusps and a resulting valvular incompetence, with the saccule as obvious evidence of structural failure in the wall. Perhaps it is most likely that the two processes combine, each aggravating the other. However derived, the presence of a saccule is a clear indication of an incompetent valve and therefore reversed flow down the vein when upright and exercising. Saccules are occasionally seen separately from valves, but usually this will be part of a more extensive process, with a grossly enlarged and sacculated vein due to generalized weakening of its walls.

Inky blue-black veins

Varicose veins commonly become adherent to overlying skin and may stretch it so much that the dark blue venous blood shows through very clearly. This fragile covering will be vulnerable to minor trauma which may cause heavy haemorrhage.

Distended subdermal and intradermal venules

Extensive patterns of radiating venules are commonly seen around the ankle and on the foot (corona phlebectatica). These flares of veins (Fig. 2.3(a)) indicate venous congestion with increased venous pressure. They occur more readily in the weakened tissues of the elderly and are not necessarily the precursors of ulceration. These veins must be distinguished from small clusters of intradermal venules (thread or spider veins) increasingly seen on the thigh or upper leg as middle age approaches; these may signify underlying venous disorder (Fig. 2.3(b)) but often occur without any evidence of this.

Cough impulse

Varicose veins commonly give a palpable impulse when the patient coughs. This is because there is no functioning valve between the abdomen and the vein, and it confirms incompetence in the valves of deep and superficial veins leading down to this point. A large proportion of patients with incompetence in the long saphenous system lack any valves in the deep veins above the saphenous termination so that abdominal pressure is easily transmitted to varicosities in the limb.

Increased warmth in veins

Normally a superficial vein does not feel warm to the touch when compared with the neighbouring skin. Veins carrying a strong reversed flow of blood that has just emerged from a deep vein at true body temperature, as in simple varicose veins, often show obvious warmth to the touch compared with skin alongside. This is valuable confirmation of the vein's abnormal state. Similarly, enlarged veins caused by arteriovenous fistula will feel warm to the touch.

Patient lying

Hollows and grooves in the elevated limb

When the limb is elevated the veins will empty and the space occupied by large varicose veins becomes a hollow or a groove readily palpable or even visible. This is particularly marked when the surrounding tissues have become fibrotic in response to venous hypertension. Such hollows are often incorrectly diagnosed as fascial apertures enlarged by abnormal perforating veins. In fact, the hollow signifies no more than a large vein, but such a vein may have special significance, possibly related to surge from an underlying perforator.

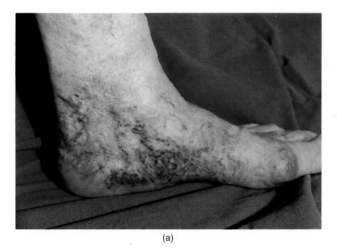

(a)

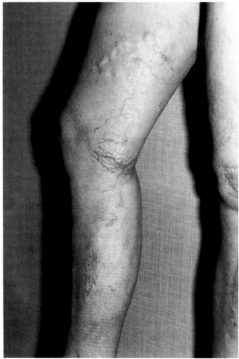

(b)

Fig. 2.3 Intradermal venules caused by venous stress. (a) A flare of grossly overdistended venules on the ankle and foot in long saphenous incompetence. This may develop as a result of raised venous pressure from any cause, particularly in elderly people. (b) Venules behind the knee in a young woman overlying varicose veins running down the inner thigh and leg.

Box 2.2   Signs of venous abnormality in superficial veins

Tortuosity (varicose veins)
Bulges on saphenous veins caused by saccules beneath leaking valves
Blue-black veins seen through thinned stretched skin
Subdermal and intradermal venules, often indicating an underlying vein problem
Cough impulse in varicose veins
Increased warmth over varicose veins
Hollows and grooves, visible and palpable, when limb is elevated

---

The nature of varicose veins

Enlarged tortuous veins, i.e. varicose veins, arise in three circumstances of unnatural flow.

1. *Simple (or primary) varicose veins.* These occur only in the superficial veins of the lower limbs and are by far the most common type of varicose veins. Such veins have no competent valves and are subject to substantial gravitational downflow when the patient is upright and moving (see Fig. 4.1). This retrograde flow is opposite to the natural direction allowed by valves, and it is plausible to say that varicose veins are caused by the turbulent reversed flow beneath inadequate valves. However, it is equally plausible to argue that veins with inherently weak walls expand in width and length so that valve cusps separate and allow reverse flow to occur. In this case, as with the saphenous saccules, discussed earlier, varicose veins could be the result of a vicious circle of weak walls and valve failure, causing turbulent reversed flow expanding the walls still further. Certainly there are many light and electron microscopy studies confirming degenerative changes in the wall structure in these circumstances, but the question is whether this is a primary process or secondary to undue stress on the walls. This debate is unresolved and both circumstances may play a part, each aggravating the other. Whatever initiates the retrograde flow, it is a useful rule to regard tortuous veins as veins with intermittent or continuous reverse (retrograde) flow in them. Certainly this is true in commonplace simple varicose veins, which are the expression of a dynamic phenomenon and not merely static distension.

2. *Secondary varicose veins.* Tortuosity is often seen in superficial veins carrying reversed flow as part of a collateral mechanism compensating for obstruction in a neighbouring deep vein. This is an acquired response, and it seems that enforced reversed flow against the natural direction will cause enlargement and tortuosity in previously normal veins, for example, suprapubic veins acting as collaterals to iliac vein obstruction (see Fig. 6.4(d)), or in oesophageal varices in portal hypertension. In contrast, veins acting as collaterals but taking flow in their natural direction enlarge but seldom show tortuosity, for example long saphenous branches overlying obstructed popliteal or femoral deep veins. The determining factor seems to be enforced reversed flow. (Note that clinical observation is often

---

Box 2.3   Characteristics of varicose veins

Enlarged and tortuous, with incompetent valves
Incompetence of valves allows:
- turbulent downflow which exerts significant dynamic 'thrust'
- a column of blood, not interrupted by effective valves, giving sustained high pressure and exposed to surges of abdominal pressure (cough impulse)

These factors, dynamic and static, contribute to expanding the veins.
Enlargement is in both width and length, hence tortuosity but which comes first, the incompetent valves or the enlarged veins?
- Do leaking valves (deficient in number and quality) give turbulent reversed flow which causes stress and stretching of vein walls?
  or
- Are the vein walls are inherently weak (inborn or degenerative change) so that they expand and separate valve cusps to cause their incompetence?

It is likely that there is no single initiating process and not all varicose veins have the same origin. However, once established, leaking valves and weak walls combine to accentuate the changes caused by each other.

---

confused by the coexistence of deep vein obstruction and simple superficial vein incompetence in the same limb (see Fig. 4.13(a) (i)).

3. *Arteriovenous fistula.* Tortuosity is often present in lesser veins in the vicinity of an arteriovenous fistula, but the major veins leading from it enlarge without tortuosity.

Box 2.4   Tortuosity—a working rule

Tortuosity (varicosity) in veins gives a strong indication of reversed flow which may be due to either gravitational downflow in incompetent superficial veins (as in simple varicose veins) or enforced reversed flow; the latter occurs most commonly in collateral branch veins past deep vein obstruction but is also seen in veins near an arteriovenous fistula. It is possible for both states to be present in the same limb.

Signs of venous hypertension (venotensive changes)

Tissue damage caused by venotension

As explained above, venous hypertension of varying severity is a common consequence of venous disorder. Raised venous pressure will cause a corresponding increase in capillary pressure and, if sustained over long periods with inadequate relief, will cause characteristic changes in the skin and subcutaneous tissues. These are mainly

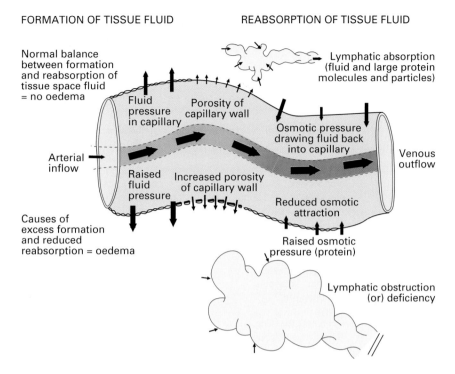

FORMATION OF TISSUE FLUID   REABSORPTION OF TISSUE FLUID

Fig. 2.4 Diagram of factors influencing formation and reabsorption of tissue fluid. The lymphatic system is responsible for removal of any large protein molecules that pass out of the capillaries, and failure of this is a potent cause of oedema.

the result of excess capillary transudation carrying with it protein molecules (Fig. 2.4) and leading to the deposition of fibrin which forms a barrier to nutritional exchange between capillaries and the surrounding tissues. This is caused, at least in part, by local trapping of white cells which slow the microvascular circulation and release of injurious products which harm the capillary walls (see also the section on Venous ulceration in Chapter 9). Other substances are also extravasated, including haemosiderin which eventually gives the characteristic brown skin pigmentation of venous hypertension. The venotensive changes listed below take many months, or even years, to develop fully. They occur in varying combinations of severity and extent, and are to be found where the venous pressure is greatest. In this respect their position in the lower leg is gravitationally determined, but an exception is seen with arteriovenous fistula where the high venous pressure is related to the arterial inflow in that vicinity. A number of conditions can cause venous hypertension, and the following changes may be seen in varying degree in any of them as a direct result of the raised venous pressure.

Venotensive changes

Swelling

Swelling is mainly due to oedema which may be localized or found extensively over the limb, according to the nature of the venous abnormality causing it. The volume of overdistended veins can also make a significant contribution to the bulk of a limb, particularly in the foot and leg, when the patient is standing. It must be remembered that there are a number of other causes for oedema in a limb, and these are summarized in Table 2.1 and Fig. 2.4. Inadequate lymphatic drainage causing oedema can be an added component to

venous disorders, particularly in congenital states (and see section on 'venous' oedema in Part III). Oedema always represents a degree of inadequate lymphatic drainage, whether it is simply overwhelmed or impaired by repeated inflammatory episodes or, at its most severe, is grossly defective as in many of the congenital states.

Induration

A characteristic diffuse fibrosis develops in the subcutaneous tissues. This may vary from a slight thickening at an early stage through to extensive areas of hard tissue in which the veins form large hollows and grooves that are evident when the leg is elevated. These changes may be accentuated by fat necrosis and chronic inflammatory changes. The terms 'lipodermatosclerosis' or 'liposclerosis' are often used to describe induration due to venous disorder.

Pigmentation

This is one of the most characteristic signs of venotension and is due to the accumulation of haemosiderin in the skin. It is often the earliest change to be seen and should immediately arouse suspicion of a venous disorder. If accompanied by the other changes given here, it is diagnostic of venous hypertension (see Fig. 4.17(a) (iii)).

Ulceration

If venous hypertension and the changes it causes remain untreated, progressive deterioration in skin nutrition leads to small areas of tissue death which coalesce to form an ulcer. A venous ulcer will always be surrounded by pigmented skin and at least some induration (see Figs 4.18(a), 5.3(a), and 6.3(g)), but there is great variation in the severity and extent of these accompanying features; in long-standing ulcers the neighbouring skin may also show a characteristic

Table 2.1   Causes of oedema in lower limbs

Features	Diagnosis
Long-standing severe oedema of whole limb or moderate oedema up to knee level: unilaterally or bilaterally	
History of deep vein thrombosis Pigmentation Ulceration Enlarged superficial veins	Venous cause likely. Confirm with Doppler, phlethysmography, phlebography, ultrasonography.
Brawny and non-pitting Peau d'orange Crevices in skin	Lymphoedema. Photoplethysmography is normal. Radioactive uptake and gamma-camera can prove diagnosis. Lymphangiogram only if essential

Painful unilateral pitting oedema (but may be bilateral)

Painful
Recent onset
Acute process

May be due to one of the following:
  Deep vein thrombosis
  Superficial phlebitis
  Cellulitis, ?diabetes
  Lymphangiitis
  Injury
  Ischaemia (swelling due to hanging leg out of bed to relieve rest pain)
  Arteriovenous fistula of acute onset

Painless unilateral pitting oedema (but some discomfort when oedema is maximal)

May be due to one of the following:
  Venous causes
    Superficial incompetence (varicosities)
    Deficiency or absence of deep vein valves
    Previous deep vein thrombosis (post-thrombotic limb)
    Subacute deep vein thrombosis
  Venous obstruction (tumour or cyst)
  Bilateral state with oedema suppressed on one side by ischaemia
  Early lymphoedema
  Combined states (e.g. lymphatic and venous disease both present)
  Arteriovenous fistula
  Tight bandaging in mid or upper limb
  Hysterical manifestation (*oedeme bleu*) due to prolonged dependency or constricting band;
  see section on factitial lymphoedema in Part III
  Paralysed limb with prolonged dependency

Painless bilateral pitting oedema (but some discomfort when oedema is maximal)

May be due to one or more of the following:
  Central cause, including heart failure, renal disease, liver disease, protein deficiency
  Malnutrition
  Unsuitable drug administration or undesirable response
  Excessive intravenous fluid and electrolyte therapy
  Obstruction to inferior vena cava or iliac veins by thrombosis, tumour, or ascites
  Overt or hidden malignancy
  Arteriovenous (aortovenacaval or iliac) fistula
  Lymphatic disorder.
  Symmetrical 'unilateral' state, i.e. bilateral localized defects in lower limbs
  Ill-defined hormonal inbalance
  Prolonged dependency (e.g. air travel, habitual sleeping in chair, or paralysis)
  Inborn or acquired (e.g. menopausal) tissue changes with increased capillary permeability

See discussion of the swollen limb and lymphatic problems in Part III.

white scarring known as *atrophie blanche*. The changes given above are typical of venous ulceration and distinguish it from other forms of ulcer which often require completely different treatment. Correct diagnosis of the various ulcers that may be seen on the leg and foot is of considerable importance and is discussed in Chapter 9.

Eczema and dermatitis

In venous hypertension the skin is particularly prone to eczema and is excessively vulnerable to any sensitizing agents or allergens applied to it. Pigmented areas are most affected, but small patches of eczema can often be seen overlying varicosities and clearly related to their distribution (see Fig. 4.17(a) (ii)). In these circumstances, pruritus will be a prominent symptom and scratching will damage the skin further. Once eczema has become established, it may appear on distant parts of the body as a more general sensitization. The appearance of eczema in the vicinity of varicose veins should always be a warning that progressive skin changes are likely. All too often eczema is aggravated by sensitization to medical products applied to the skin, or materials in the fabric of elastic stockings. Antibiotic creams are particular offenders in causing skin reactions.

Box 2.5   Signs of venous hypertension

Swelling	(Has many possible causes, see Table 2.1 and Part III) Due to excess capillary exudate (fluid and proteins) with inability of lymphatics to cope. Pericapillary cuff of fibrin limits nutritional exchange.
Induration	Due to fibrosis from reduced nutrition, chronic inflammation and fat necrosis (lipo dermatosclerosis).
Pigmentation	Due to accumulation of excess haemosiderin from extravasated red cells and increasing failure of lymphatic scavenging.
Ulceration	Due to necrosis of skin by failing nutritional exchange with capillaries; is always accompanied by skin pigmentation. (See Chapter 9 for other causes of ulceration on the leg.)
Eczema	Commonly seen with venous disorder but other causes possible.
Dermatitis	Often caused by medical applications (see Chapter 9).

Symptoms of venous disorder

Now that the physical consequences of venous disorder have been considered, the symptoms arising from this can be viewed in better perspective. Many of these symptoms are not unique to veins; other conditions may account for them, even when enlarged veins are present. The symptoms should match the manifestations, and the likelihood of a relationship between them should be assessed. Even more importantly, in the absence of at least some of the clinical signs described above, the symptoms should not be attributed to 'the veins' but an open mind should be kept and other causes considered.

When venotensive changes are not present

The symptoms accompanying abnormally enlarged or varicose veins without obvious venotensive changes are as follows.

- Distress caused by their unsightly and displeasing appearance.

- Aching in the vicinity of abnormal veins, particularly after prolonged standing.

- A feeling of heaviness towards the end of the day.

- In women, discomfort associated with varicose veins is most marked over a few days before menstruation. This is often described as aching, stinging, or burning, and the veins become more prominent.

- Nocturnal cramps often appear to be related to varicose veins. This is particularly evident when the cramps occur only on the side affected by varicose veins. Moreover, attacks of cramp may cease following successful surgery to the veins. This association with varicosities is well established but ill understood. However, nocturnal cramp is a common condition in older people, so that it is difficult to predict when elimination of varicosities will relieve it and no promise upon this should be given to patients before treatment. In the elderly, care must be taken to distinguish between simple cramp and ischaemic nocturnal rest pain; both are relieved by standing out of bed, but in ischaemia the ankle pulses will be reduced or absent on palpation or Doppler flowmeter examination.

There is little relationship between the size of varicose veins and the discomforts complained of. Large long-standing varicose veins may cause no admitted discomfort; indeed, in these patients it may be difficult to persuade them to have treatment. Relatively small varicosities lying directly under the skin or intradermally, particularly if they have appeared recently, often seem to cause most discomfort, especially premenstrually in women.

Additional symptoms when venotensive changes are present

If venous disorder is accompanied by venotensive changes, one or more of the following symptoms is also likely to be present.

1. *Pruritus.* This is commonly an early sign of venotensive skin change, and repeated scratching by the patient may break the skin, possibly initiating an ulcer.

2. *Increased discomfort.* The sense of general discomfort and heaviness or actual pain is increased. If an ulcer is present, this certainly causes discomfort and often real pain if the ulcer is infected with *Staphyloccus aureus* or *Streptococcus viridans*. An ulcer will produce discharge varying from watery fluid through to frank pus and may be accompanied by unpleasant odour. Such manifestations cause the patient distress and a feeling of social insecurity, which is accentuated by the bandages or strong stockings used in treatment. Venous ulcers are a significant cause of disability, which is often underrated, and absence from work.

3. *Venous claudication.* Extensive post-thrombotic venous obstruction in the popliteal and femoral veins may so impede venous return that a few minutes of exercise cause considerable increase in venous pressure, well above the normal maximum.

This is accompanied by a bursting sensation in the calf which quickly becomes unbearable and forces the patient to stop walking. (The term claudication, derived from the name of the Emperor Claudius, means 'limping'. It is most commonly used in connection with states of arterial insufficiency, but is also used by neurologists for symptoms caused by compression of the cauda equina.) In venous claudication, the clinical features of venous obstruction will always be present and fully confirmed by the special investigations. Care must be taken to ensure that the claudication is not due to arterial insufficiency coincidentally present with a venous disorder. In ischaemia, swelling of the foot can be due to the patient's hanging the leg out of bed in order to relieve rest pain; this is not rare, and if the limb is elevated because it is misdiagnosed as a venous disorder, the severity of the condition is greatly aggravated and may lead to loss of the limb.

An overall view of the venous disorders described in Chapters 4–9 is shown diagrammatically in Fig. 2.5.

Box 2.6   Symptoms of venous disorder

If obvious varicose veins are present patients tend to ascribe any symptoms in limb to them—complaint must be matched by venous changes

Displeasing appearance

Aching discomfort and 'heaviness' on standing

Premenstrual discomfort in vicinity of veins

Swelling

Pruritis: an early indication of venotension and possible eczema

Nocturnal cramps: but these are common in the elderly and in ischaemia (check arterial pulses)

Increased pain and discomfort: usually due to an ulcer, particularly if infected with a pathogen

Venous claudication: only occurs when extensive deep vein obstruction is present (check arterial pulses)

Fig. 2.5   Overall view of the basic patterns of venous disorder. It is possible for more than one pattern to be present in the same limb so that the clinical state does not fall easily into one particular category although usually one pattern will predominate. All illustrations show the patient in the position where venous problems become evident, i.e. upright.

Chapter 1. Normal vein with functioning valves throughout. This fulfills the essential requirement of returning blood against gravity when upright.

Chapter 4. (a) Incompetence in superficial veins due to insufficient number, or poor quality, of valves. Downflow in the incompetent veins after exercise when upright is characteristic. This may be large enough to overwhelm a weak pumping mechanism and cause venous hypertension and ulceration. (b) A typical of pathway of superficial vein incompetence. In this example the long saphenous vein and its arcuate branch have no functioning valves, and form the pathway. The source of downflow is the saphenofemoral junction, with flow reentering the deep veins through perforators in the lower leg and foot to give a retrograde circuit of incompetence.

Chapter 5. (a) Extensive absence of functioning valves in both superficial and deep veins (probably a primary inborn condition). This valveless syndrome has a grossly defective pumping mechanism and causes severe venotension. (b) An ill-defined group in which the vein walls appear weak so that superficial and deep veins become oversized and baggy. Valve cusps, which are no longer supported, become incompetent with inevitable severe venous hypertension. There is likely to an inherited factor here.

Chapter 6. A typical problem of deep vein impairment. The deep veins are obstructed (usually from previous deep vein thrombosis or from injury). To overcome the obstruction, venous blood is forcefully pumped out through perforators in the lower leg and up superficial veins acting as collaterals. In addition, damaged deep vein valves and valves in collateral vessels may be incompetent. The musculovenous pump is severely impaired and this causes venous hypertension, with all its undesirable consequences, particularly ulceration.

Chapter 7. The perforators play a variable role in venous disorders. In superficial vein incompetence, at higher levels they may act as a source of downflow through incompetent superficial veins (this includes the upper leg, for example in gastrocnemius vein incompetence), whereas lower down they act in their normal role of allowing blood from superficial veins to enter the deep veins. In deep vein obstruction, the perforators form part of a collateral mechanism with blood forcefully pumped out through them and up the limb. A combination of deep, perforator, and superficial vein incompetence will cause a heavy surge back and forth through the perforators with each muscle contraction.

Chapter 8. Congential venous anomalies can lead to failure of development in the main deep veins, giving rise to a form of obstructed venous outlet syndrome. A massive unnatural venous channel, the lateral vein, which is valveless, is often seen in these limbs, and this may be accompanied by an inborn general lack of valves in both superficial and deep veins. Venous hypertension becomes manifest as the child grows. Congenital multiple arteriovenous fistulas can vary from a small localized lesion to massive involvement of the limb; in the latter, peripheral ulceration arises from the high venous pressure and a characteristic overgrowth of bone length occurs.

Chapter 9. Ulcers of the leg: most are venous in origin but an important minority are not. A diagnostic scheme is shown here.

NORMAL PATTERN OF
FLOW IN DEEP AND
SUPERFICIAL VEINS OF
LOWER LIMB

When upright and
exercising, venous
return is up the main
deep veins, with
segments of
superficial veins
emptying into slack
deep veins through
nearest perforator

*Example:
This segment
of superficial
vein empties
into deep veins
as soon as they
become slack*

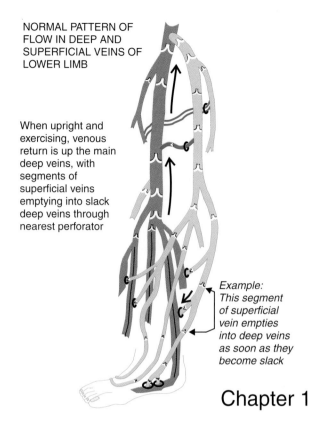

Chapter 1

SUPERFICIAL VEIN
INCOMPETENCE
WITH VARICOSE VEINS

In upright posture,
blood spills from deep
veins at upper level and
down incompetent
superficial veins to
re-enter deep veins via
perforators at a lower
level.
This gravitational
downflow occurs
whenever deep
veins are made
slack by exercise.
It is maximal when
upright but
diminishes to zero
as horizontal position
is assumed.

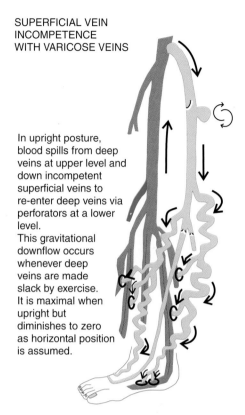

Chapter 4

(a)

A TYPICAL PATHWAY OF
SUPERFICIAL VEIN
INCOMPETENCE

THE RETROGRADE
CIRCUIT OF
INCOMPETENCE

SOURCE

Profunda femoris vein

Long saphenous vein

PATHWAY OF
INCOMPETENCE

RETURN
PATHWAY UP
DEEP VEINS

Short saphenous vein

RE-ENTRY POINTS
VIA
PERFORATORS

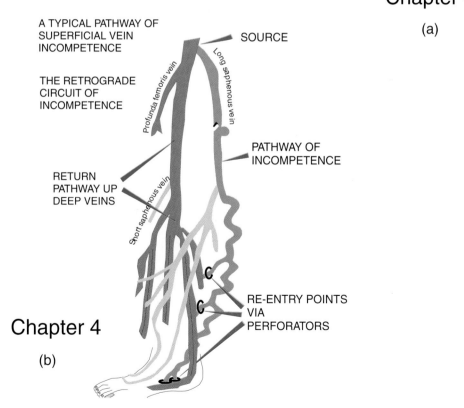

Chapter 4

(b)

Fig. 2.5 (i)

VALVE DEFICIENCY AND WEAK VEIN WALLS

Chapter 5

(a) Inborn (primary) deficiency of valves in both superficial and deep veins leads to surge without effective pumping

(b) Widespread weakness in vein walls (inborn or degenerative) leads to baggy veins with separation of valve cusps and severe impairment of pumping.

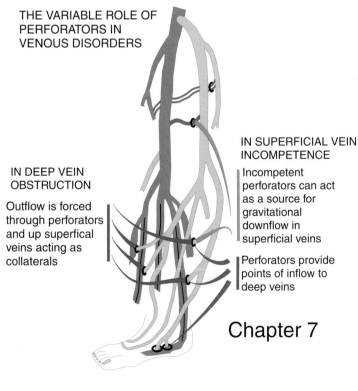

DEEP VEIN OBSTRUCTION WITH ENFORCED UPFLOW IN SUPERFICIAL VEINS

If deep veins are obstructed (for example, by previous deep vein thrombosis) venous return is forced out through perforators and up superficial veins (which are, therefore, important collaterals). Thrombotic damage to valves is also likely to be present increasing difficulties in venous return against gravity.

Chapter 6

THE VARIABLE ROLE OF PERFORATORS IN VENOUS DISORDERS

IN DEEP VEIN OBSTRUCTION

Outflow is forced through perforators and up superficial veins acting as collaterals

IN SUPERFICIAL VEIN INCOMPETENCE

Incompetent perforators can act as a source for gravitational downflow in superficial veins

Perforators provide points of inflow to deep veins

Chapter 7

Fig. 2.5 (ii)

CONGENITAL DEFECTS

Main characteristics of extensive limb involvement are shown.

Anomalous development of veins

Inferior vena cava

External iliac vein

Massive lateral vein running through sciatic notch to join internal iliac vein

Communication with profunda femoris vein

A persistent embryonic vein, massive and valveless, lies in subcutaneous layer and is main venous return for leg. Removing this could be disastrous

Central portion of femoral vein missing

Saphenous vein may be normal and well valved

Extensive angiomatous lesions may be present and limb may overgrow in length.
Much variability in these venous malformations but note how surface vessels may be essential for venous return.

Chapter 8

Multiple arteriovenous fistulas

Features:
Multiple sponge-like communications between a series of large arteries and veins.
Massive hypertrophy of main arteries leading to the fistulas
Overgrowth of bones in region of fistulas
Loud arterial bruits
Pulsatile flow in veins (Doppler)
Strong tendency to venotensive changes in periphery of limb due to high venous pressure

LEG ULCERS

IN ALL ULCERS:
CHECK ARTERIES AND TEST FOR DIABETES
OBTAIN FULL BLOOD PICTURE
CULTURE FOR PATHOGENS
BIOPSY IF ANY SUSPICION OF MALIGNACY.

Chapter 9

4 Out of 5 leg ulcers are venous in origin

BUT 1 in 5 has another cause

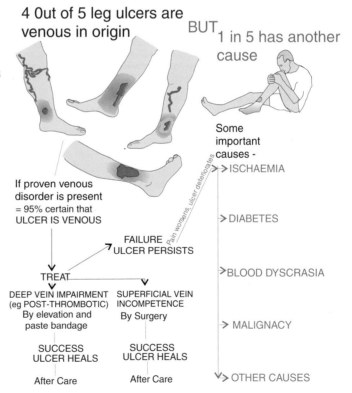

Some important causes -

If proven venous disorder is present = 95% certain that ULCER IS VENOUS

Pain worsens, ulcer deteriorates

FAILURE ULCER PERSISTS

TREAT

DEEP VEIN IMPAIRMENT (eg POST-THROMBOTIC) By elevation and paste bandage

SUPERFICIAL VEIN INCOMPETENCE By Surgery

SUCCESS ULCER HEALS

SUCCESS ULCER HEALS

After Care

After Care

→ISCHAEMIA

→DIABETES

→BLOOD DYSCRASIA

→ MALIGNACY

→ OTHER CAUSES

Fig. 2.5 (iii)

3 Clinical examination and special investigations

Clinical examination

The patient's complaint

It is important that the patient gives a clear statement of his or her complaint and the reason for dissatisfaction with the veins. Visible varicose veins tend to be blamed for any discomfort in the limb, but this may have a very different origin and the symptoms must match the venous abnormality.

History

Certain aspects of medical history are important, particularly the likelihood of a previous deep vein thrombosis, so often long forgotten but still a potent cause of venous disorder. In this respect, any history of 'white leg of pregnancy', major fractures of lower limbs or pelvis, prolonged immobilization in traction or plaster of Paris, or major illness should be enquired about. A family history and the age of first appearance of varicose veins may have a bearing upon the prognosis and policy of management. Knowledge of previous treatment is essential, as this will have fragmented the anatomy of the superficial veins.

Examination

Unless stated otherwise, examination is carried out with the patient upright, i.e. in the position in which venous problems arise and venous defects are most evident. This is best done by asking the patient to stand on a strengthened couch or platform with appropriate handrails on the wall nearby.

Inspection

Careful inspection in good light is fundamental to observe the pattern of prominent veins and detect any skin changes of venous disorder (Fig. 3.1). The feet must be included in this and, if there is any hint of previous deep vein thrombosis, the pubes and lower abdomen must also be inspected. There is much to be learnt from the scars of any previous operations. If tortuous veins are present, these must be traced along their full length; an oblique light throwing the veins into relief is most helpful for this. The following questions should be borne in mind.

- Do the veins fall within long or short saphenous distribution or is this uncertain? Is another and unusual source possible?

- Is visible evidence of venous hypertension present, particularly pigmentation, swelling, and ulceration?

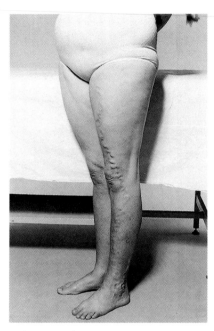

Fig. 3.1 Clinical examination. Careful inspection of all aspects of the limb and foot is essential. If there is any suggestion of previous deep vein thrombosis, the pubic region and lower abdomen must be included.

Touch

Light touch, almost brushing the skin, is very helpful in detecting or locating veins. Consider the following questions.

- If there is apparent swelling, is there any pitting oedema?

- Are varicose veins 'hot' to touch? Do they show a cough impulse?

- If there is an isolated bulge on the inner thigh, is there a thrill on coughing indicating an underlying jet of blood through a leaking valve?

Mapping out

Mapping out is a most important step in which the overall pattern of enlarged veins, including those that are not visible, is defined clearly. The 'tap-wave' test is an essential skill in this respect.

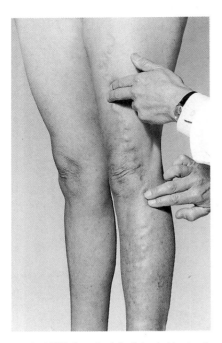

Fig. 3.2 Tap-wave test. With the veins fully distended by standing, the lower hand gives a tap or sharp compression on the vein to be traced. The distinctive percussion wave caused travels along the vein and is detectable by the upper hand even when the vein is not otherwise recognizable.

Tap-wave test (percussion test of Chevrier)

In the standing patient with fully distended veins, a tap or sharp compression of a vein will send a corresponding wave of movement along its length, which is easily detected by light touch. Thus one examining hand 'taps' on the vein in its lower part (so that valves do not dampen the effect), whilst the fingers of the other hand locate the signal in its upper part (Fig. 3.2), moving progressively up the limb. In this way veins that are not detectable by any other clinical means are easily located and traced along their length. This procedure does not reveal much about function and is not reliable in assessing valve competence, but it does swiftly map out the pattern of veins otherwise concealed from touch or sight, and this alone can turn a speculative into a probable diagnosis.

Examination with the patient horizontal and the limb elevated

When the limb is elevated to 45°, the veins will empty so that large subcutaneous veins become a gutter or a hollow. This can prove a valuable addition to mapping out, and in the detection of varicose veins concealed by subcutaneous fat the presence of a hollow helps in the recognition of early venous induration. It has already been pointed out that a hollow is seldom due to a fascial deficiency but is the site of a large varicosity, and does not necessarily signify that an enlarged perforator underlies it.

Clinical tests

The features described so far give the observable changes that may be present in venous disorders. These give indirect evidence of abnormal function in veins, but few are diagnostic of a specific state.

Of the clinical tests, relying solely on the examiner's senses, only two are capable of giving a specific diagnosis. In both the following tests the use of an encircling rubber band to occlude superficial veins is avoided, partly because it may cause artefacts by constricting the deep veins, and also because it does not localize the superficial veins at fault.

The Trendelenburg type of test (selective occlusion test)

This test is based upon demonstration that temporary selective occlusion of one or more superficial veins by localized finger pressure will delay the filling of varicose veins when the patient first stands after the veins have been emptied by elevation of the limb (Figs 3.3 and 3.4). It shows that the varicose veins fill by downflow in the vein selected for occlusion and therefore its valves must be incompetent. This is of great diagnostic value and accurately identifies simple (primary) varicose veins. When positive it is virtual proof of this, but no great reliance can be placed on a negative result in the exclusion of superficial vein incompetence, for example when the likely pathway of incompetence has been misidentified (say, long saphenous) and the real source of incompetence is elsewhere (say, short saphenous) and has been overlooked. Other aspects of this test are considered in Chapter 4 in the section on superficial vein incompetence, the state it is pre-eminent in recognizing.

Perthes' test

This type of test depends upon the change in the distended varicose veins of an upright patient exercising whilst a selected superficial vein is occluded to prevent downflow (Fig. 3.5). In the first stage it is shown that exercise by rising on the toes does not deflate the veins. Then the main pathway of incompetence previously identified by selective Trendelenburg test, often a saphenous vein, is occluded by localized finger pressure and the patient is exercised as before. If the varicose veins become less prominent and softer to touch, it is clear that, when downflow in the superficial vein is prevented, exercise succeeds in emptying the varicose veins. This confirms that the

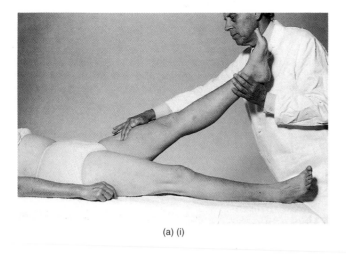

(a) (i)

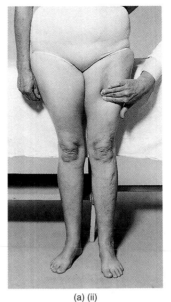

(a) (ii)

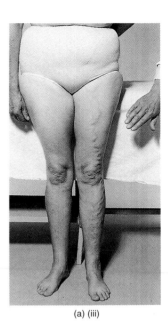

(a) (iii)

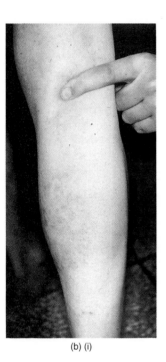

(b) (i)

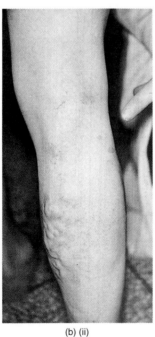

(b) (ii)

Fig. 3.3 Selective occlusion (Trendelenburg) test. (a) Long saphenous vein anterolateral branch: (i) the veins are emptied by high elevation of the limb and the suspected pathway of incompetence is selectively occluded by compression with fingertips; (ii) with compression maintained, the patient stands and the varicose veins are observed (at this stage, the patient may be exercised by rising on toes; absence of vein filling gives additional evidence that there is no significant perforator outflow.) (iii) After a short interval compression is removed. If the veins promptly fill only at this stage, incompetence in the valves of the vein under examination has been demonstrated and the test is considered positive. (b) Short saphenous vein: (i) Fingertip compression controls varicosities; (ii) the veins rapidly fill when compression is removed.

Box 3.2   Trendelenburg test using selective occlusion (Fig. 3.4)

With patient lying elevate the limb to empty the veins.
Occlude suspected pathway of incompetence with the fingertips (not encircling band).
Bring to standing position with finger pressure still applied.
Wait 20 s to see if veins fill.
If not, release finger pressure. Do varicose veins now fill promptly? If so, this gives positive confirmation of simple varicose veins and identifies of the pathway of incompetence.
If the veins filled prematurely, the test is inconclusive—reconsider and repeat.

deep vein pumping mechanism is functioning satisfactorily and the fault lies in the superficial vein being tested which is capable of filling the varicosities as fast as they are emptied by the deep veins. A positive response gives meaningful confirmation of this; an uncertain or failed response raises suspicion of deep vein insufficiency but does not give acceptable proof of this. This test is referred to again in Chapter 4 in the section on superficial vein incompetence.

With superficial vein incompetence the tests described above can give a firm diagnosis, sufficient to act upon clinically. In other venous disorders reliance has to be placed on investigation with instruments measuring the speed and direction of flow, pressure change, or volume change, or outlining the veins and displaying their function by phlebography or ultrasonic imaging (ultrasonography).

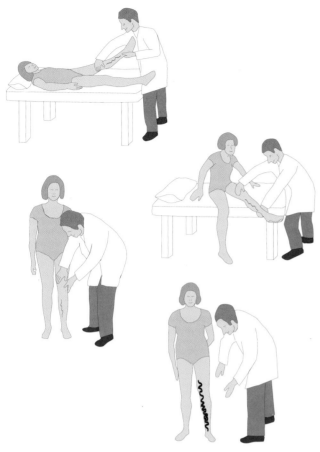

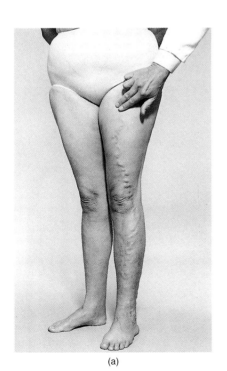

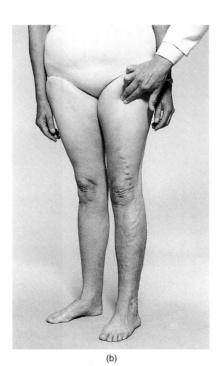

Fig. 3.4 Sequence of moves in the selective Trendelenburg test. A constricting band is not used but the suspected pathway of incompetence is occluded by finger tips. In this way, not only is simple superficial vein incompetence demonstrated but the location of the pathway of incompetence is confirmed.

Box 3.3   Perthes' test with selective occlusion

With patient standing allow varicose veins to fill.

Exercise by rising on toes five times to check that there is no change in prominence of the veins

Occlude the pathway of incompetence with the fingertips and again exercise five times

Maintain finger pressure and assess whether the veins are less prominent and softer to touch.

Release finger pressure. Do veins promptly become prominent and firm to touch?

If undoubtedly so, the test is positive and confirms that chosen pathway of incompetence is correct and that the musculovenous pump to deep veins is effective (i.e. it can deflate the veins of the lower leg provided that downflow in superficial veins is prevented).

Fig. 3.5   (*Below*) Selective Perthes' test. (a) With the patient standing and the veins well filled, the suspected pathway of incompetence is compressed with the fingertips and the patient is asked to rise on the toes three times. (b) With compression maintained, the veins are assessed. A positive response is shown if the veins have become visibly less prominent and have softened to touch. (c) On release of compression full prominence and firmness return promptly.

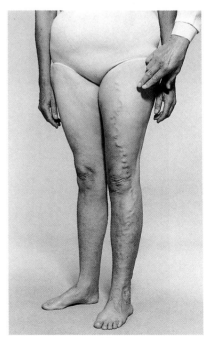

(a)   (b)   (c)

Tests using electronic instruments and radiography

The basic defects that characterize venous disorder become apparent when exercising in an upright position and are readily detected by instruments and imaging techniques.

Demonstration of flow by ultrasound: the continuous-wave directional Doppler flowmeter and pulsed-beam ultrasonic imaging

Abnormal direction of flow

Flow in the direction that should be opposed by valves is abnormal and its presence indicates that the valves are incompetent or absent. A directional Doppler flowmeter (or, more correctly, velocimeter) can detect this with great clarity. In this instrument a piezoelectric crystal in the probe emits a continuous ultrasound signal that is reflected back by red cells to a receiving crystal. According to the speed and direction of movement of the red cells, there is a Doppler shift in the phase of the signal which is recognized by the machine and made apparent audibly, by a needle gauge, by a light-emitting

diode display, or by oscillograph; a permanent record is provided by either a chart recorder or some form of computer printout. In order to facilitate the passage of ultrasound between probe and tissues a coupling gel is used on the skin. If a light-weight flat-headed probe is used, this can be held in the hand against skin without displacement when the patient moves (Fig. 3.6) and allows rapid repositioning of the probe so that several different sites can be examined in quick succession. The signal generated represents the speed of flow but not the volume; thus a high-speed jet of blood leaking through valve cusps may cause a strong signal which can be misleading if more representative flow a short distance away is not sampled. However, such sharply localized high-velocity flow in itself confirms the presence of a leaking valve, although it does not necessarily indicate the overall severity of incompetence. In tortuous veins, confused directional signals may be obtained owing to the close proximity of conflicting flows or uncertainty about the orientation, upwards or downwards, of the segment of tortuous vein under the probe. These difficulties can be resolved by asking the patient to cough in order to create a spurt of downward flow, or by deliberately giving the vein below the probe a sharp press to cause a small peak of upward flow. The Doppler flowmeter is at its best over superficial veins such as a saphenous vein or its varicose branches. Much useful information can also be obtained from the deep veins, but here there may be uncertainty in distinguishing which deep vein

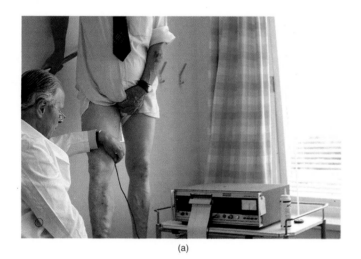

(a)

Fig. 3.6 Directional Doppler flowmetry (or, more correctly, velocimetry because it is measuring velocity of flow) to the superficial veins is a simple but highly informative examination. (a) The probe is placed over the vein to be examined whilst the patient is standing, and the response to coughing, calf compression, and exercise movements is given by audible and visible signals, and also by chart recorder. (b) A chart recording of the responses in Doppler flow in an incompetent long saphenous vein. A diagram of the flow pattern is also shown.

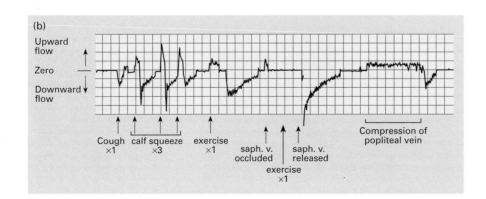

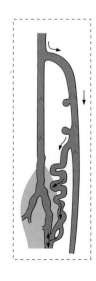

is being picked up or, indeed, whether the signal is coming from an intervening superficial vein, for example a short saphenous vein overlying the popliteal vein. The characteristic superficial vein flow patterns found in the various venous disorders are described in Chapters 4–6. It is sufficient to say here that the directional Doppler flowmeter used in this way can give immediate positive confirmation of incompetence in superficial veins or give warning that deep vein problems may be present.

Pulsed-beam ultrasonography provides a much more sophisticated demonstration by giving an image of veins and their valves on a display screen. It will show movement of these structures and also the direction and speed of blood flow within them. This is particularly valuable for detailed study of short lengths of deep veins and will be described further in the section on imaging techniques. Similarly, phlebography may be used to visualize the pattern of flow within superficial and deep veins.

Box 3.4 Continuous-wave Doppler flowmeter (velocimeter) to superficial veins

Measures velocity and direction of flow. Velocity is not a reliable measure of the volume of flow but gives a broad indication with readings at several levels.

Used to show direction and degree of flow in response to exercise movement in the standing patient.

Downward flow demonstrates the presence of incompetent downflow and gauges the severity of this.

Strong upward flow may be collateral upflow past obstructed deep veins.

Method

It is used after full clinical examination mapping out superficial veins and locating the likely pathway of incompetence in which flow is to be studied. Likely veins to be examined are the long saphenous vein (lower thigh often very suitable and usually representative), the short saphenous vein (but in popliteal fossa the underlying popliteal vein can cause confusion), and any obvious run of varicose veins.

Jelly (KY), a coupling agent, must be used between the probe and the skin

The probe is applied without any pressure as this will impede flow in the underlying vein.

The flow is recorded in the following circumstances:
- with the patient standing still
- on coughing
- when the calf is given three firm squeezes
- during and after exercise by rising on toes once or twice

If there is no response, the patient is asked to raise the foot off the ground with the knee straight (testing flow to the underside of the foot which can be substantial). The vein under examination is now compressed with the fingers well above the probe (to prevent downward flow) and the patient is again exercised; the compression is released after 5 s. Flow occurring now indicates that exercise has effectively lowered venous pressure in the lower leg and incompetent flow runs to this when allowed to.

Enhanced flow in the normal direction

Increased flow in superficial veins in the normal direction can be highly significant and occurs in two circumstances. It may occur when superficial veins, including saphenous veins, are acting as collaterals past occlusion in the underlying deep veins (see Figs 1.13 and Fig. 6.3(b)). It will also be found in the veins above an arteriovenous fistula, but here an added feature will be strongly pulsatile return flow in time with the heartbeats. This must be distinguished from the weak pulsation often noticed in fully distended veins, congested by a short period of standing without movement, which is due to transmission of pulsation from neighbouring arteries. It is most evident in venous disorders where valve incompetence causes rapid congestion within the limb; pulsation may also be found, and is easily seen, in cardiac failure with tricuspid valve incompetence.

Measurement and estimation of venous pressure in leg or foot

Failure in response of venous pressure to exercise

With exercise in the upright position, the venous pressure within the limb normally falls, and when exercise ceases (Fig. 1.15) the original pressure is not regained for at least 20 s (restitution, refilling, or recovery time). In states of superficial or deep vein valvular incompetence the refilling time may be decisively shortened by reflux of venous blood down the limb; this is characteristic of conditions causing venous hypertension (Fig. 3.7). Measurements of venous pressure changes in response to exercise may be obtained by the following means.

- By direct insertion of a needle or plastic cannula into a foot or ankle vein. The pressure is best measured by a calibrated electronic transducer and the changes shown as a tracing on a chart recorder as they occur.

- By indirect methods without the need to puncture a vein, indicating the scale and rate of pressure changes rather than giving accurate measurement. Photoplethysmography, which is described below, is a simple but effective way of doing this and in most circumstances can give a good estimation of valvular competence by gauging the recovery time.

Measurement of change in limb volume: photoplethysmography

Failure in response of limb volume to exercise

The limb volume closely parallels the venous pressure so that when the patient is standing still it is maximal, but after exercise, which has expelled blood from the limb, both venous pressure and limb volume will fall. The reduction in volume will indicate the amount of blood expelled by exercise; the time taken for the volume to return to its original value is a good indication of valve competence. With fully competent valves this will be at least 20 s, but when superficial or deep valve incompetence is present this will be shortened according to the severity of the condition. Various methods can

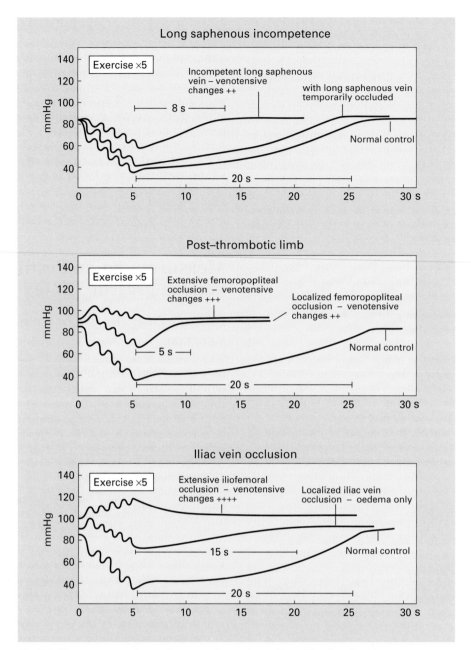

Fig. 3.7   Venous pressure changes in response to exercise and the refilling times in various venous disorders compared with the normal state.

be used for measuring and recording volume changes as they occur (plethysmography).

Fluid plethysmography   The leg or foot is immersed in water within a fixed chamber and the amount of fluid displaced from this is measured. The weight of fluid may cause artefacts, and the range of exercise possible for the patient is rather limited. Nevertheless, it is capable of giving reliable results.

Air plethysmography   The leg is surrounded by an air-filled PVC chamber and the amount of air entering or leaving is measured to give changes in limb volume. This allows the patient more freedom of movement but must be carried out in conditions of

stable temperature to prevent errors due to thermal expansion or contraction of air within the container. In use, this proves to be a practical method, reliably indicating the speed and degree of volume change with exercise.

Electrical impedance plethysmography   This method estimates the volume change within the limb by alteration of its electrical resistance which varies with the volume.

Strain gauge plethysmography   The limb is encircled by a slender elastic tube containing mercury or similar electrically conducting fluid, the resistance of which will vary as the diameter of the elastic tube changes. Thus, when exercise reduces the volume,

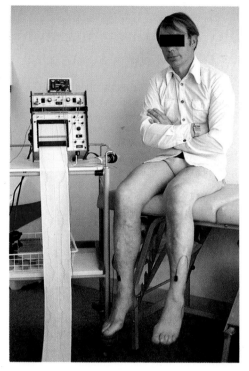

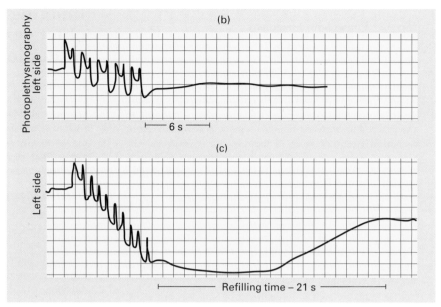

Fig. 3.8 Photoplethysmography. This form of plethysmography offers a simple test which can be carried out within a few minutes and is able to confirm venous insufficiency and, often, to show whether the fault lies in superficial or deep veins. It measures skin capillary filling which is closely related to venous filling and pressure. (a) The examination is carried out with the legs dependent. (b) Recording of response to five exercise movements from a patient with gross incompetence of the long saphenous vein and venotensive changes near the ankle. A small fall is shown but this rises again in under 6 s (the refilling time), indicating rapid refilling by venous reflux. (c) The saphenous vein has been selectively occluded by fingertip pressure and the examination repeated. The recording now shows a much stronger response to exercise and prolongation of the refilling time to near normal at 21 s, confirming that the fault lies in this vein.

the elastic tube will shorten to give a broader diameter and the resistance will fall; as the volume is regained the tube is stretched and the resistance increases again. This method is simple to apply and gives a good indication of the volume changes occurring in the limb. However, it is only sampling the changes at one or two levels and cannot measure the expelled volume; its main value is in gauging the recovery time.

Photoplethysmography   This method (Fig. 3.8) photoelectrically estimates the number of red cells in the skin capillary bed underlying the transducer. A light-emitting diode, which gives off no heat likely to cause artefacts, illuminates the capillary bed with infrared light. This is absorbed by haemoglobin in the red cells, and the amount of light transmitted back to a photoelectric sensor will vary in accordance with the number of red cells underlying it. The signals are recorded as a line tracing on a chart recorder or computerized display (Fig. 3.9). It has been shown that the degree of congestion of red cells in the skin capillaries is closely related to the venous pressure in the limb, and thus the signal from the photoplethysmograph closely parallels the venous pressure changes. It can certainly give a good estimation of the recovery time following exercise, and this is its chief value. If two successive recordings are made, without changing the probe position or the instrument settings, comparison of the rate and extent of venous pressure change in different circumstances can be achieved, for example, in response to exercise with and without saphenous occlusion (see Fig. 4.5(c)). The method has certain vagaries but, with experience, can give a good portrayal of venous changes in the limb,

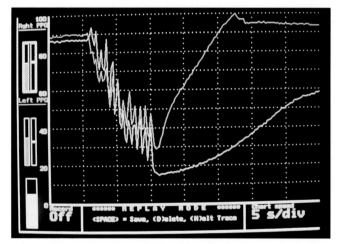

Fig. 3.9   Simultaneous photoplethysmography recordings from both limbs by a machine programmed to present these superimposed for easy comparison. It is immediately apparent that the left side shows a diminished response to exercise and a shortened recovery period typical of an impaired musculovenous pumping mechanism.

taking only a few minutes and with no discomfort to the patient. It is a very practical method for assessing the effectiveness of musculovenous pumping, the overall competence of valves, and the likelihood of the presence of venous hypertension.

Box 3.5   Photoplethysmography

Is non-invasive, easy, and rapid.

It estimates the degree of congestion in skin capillaries; this runs parallel to venous pressure and will rise and fall with it. Its main value is to detect when venous pumping is proving inadequate in which case it will show a reduced response to exercise and a shortened time for 'venous pressure' to return to normal (recovery time). If the response is small and the recovery time is abnormally shortened, venous pumping is inadequate. If this is due to overwhelming by superficial valve incompetence, it should be possible to restore temporary normality by occlusion of the appropriate superficial vein; in deep vein insufficiency this is not possible by any manipulation. In oedema of uncertain origin it can demonstrate normal venous function and exclude this as a cause.

Method

Patient sits upright with feet clear of floor.

Sensor heads are applied to the fronts of both legs just above the ankles, using transparent double-sided adhesive tape.

The patient is asked to give both feet five full movements and the response is charted. If the response is shallow and the recovery time is under 15 s, repeat the procedure whilst suspected superficial vein occluded by finger pressure. If this causes a larger response, with a recovery time of 25 s or more (i.e. normal), the fault lies with the superficial vein and its removal is indicated. If there is no improvement, either the wrong superficial vein has been chosen or it is a deep vein problem. Reconsider and repeat.

Note: The method is only applicable to superficial vein incompetence when this is severe enough to overwhelm the pumping mechanism. It is particularly useful in distinguishing between venotension (pigmentation or ulcer present) caused by deep vein problems and superficial incompetence.

A similar routine is suitable for all forms of plethysmography.

Maximum venous outflow (MVO)   Plethysmography, usually by strain gauge, can be used to measure the maximal speed at which venous blood can leave a limb and, from this, estimate any restriction in venous outflow. With the patient horizontal and the lower limbs elevated, a pneumatic cuff is used to cause venous congestion. The cuff is then abruptly released and, from the tracing on a chart recorder, the reduction in volume (limb circumference if a strain gauge is used) over the first few seconds is expressed as a percentage of the total fall in volume. For example, in a normal limb 90 per cent of the total fall in volume will occur in the first 3 s (Fig. 3.10, left side), but in ileofemoral obstruction with poor collaterals a fall of perhaps only 45 per cent would occur in the same time (Fig. 3.10, right side). Although useful, estimation of maximal venous outflow does not give specific information and adds little to that gained from the other tests with the instruments described above. However, it can help in excluding a venous cause in an oedematous limb, so that unnecessary phlebography is avoided. However, overall, the information gained is greatly inferior to that obtained from techniques visualizing veins.

Imaging techniques: functional phlebography and ultrasonography by duplex or colour flow scanning

If the special tests with instruments have not satisfactorily explained the nature of the venous disorder, a technique visualizing the veins can be used. This will not only display abnormal outline to the veins, such as occlusion or deformity, but will show if valves are defective or absent. In addition, abnormal patterns of superficial or deep venous flow in response to exercise can be demonstrated. The two main techniques are functional phlebography and ultrasonography.

Functional phlebography

Phlebography has been transformed over recent years by several factors, particularly the use of a non-irritating osmolar opaque medium, such as Iohexol, which causes no discomfort and does not precipitate phlebitis, the introduction of the image intensifier which allows prolonged viewing without exposing the patient to excessive radiation, and the realization that the patient must be examined in the position that causes venous problems, i.e. upright (Fig. 3.11(a) (i)). With the exception of acute thrombosis in the deep veins, it is only when the patient is near upright and exercising intermittently that many features of venous disorder become apparent. The essence of functional phlebography is to study the functioning of the veins whilst they are working to return blood against gravity. This will allow valve function to be assessed and the causes of inadequate musculovenous pumping to be identified; occlusion or severe deformity in deep veins can be recognized, unnatural enlargement or tortuosity can be seen, and unusual flow patterns (e.g. collateral flow in superficial veins) are recognized. It is essential that the pattern of venous return should not be distorted by using such artefacts as constricting bands (Fig. 3.11(a) (ii)). The opportunity to witness events is very brief and is limited by the fact that only part of the limb can be viewed at one moment, the need to keep the amount of opaque medium within safe limits, and the rapidity with which the changes come and go with exercise.

It is not really possible for a radiologist to perform a comprehensive functional examination of a limb without knowing the likely nature of the problem that should be concentrated upon. It is essential that the radiologist should be well briefed by the surgeon or, even better, that the surgeon should be present, to give guidance on the features to be looked for. For these reasons, functional phlebography is a skilled and rather specialized examination. It is important to record the rapidly changing events in some fashion for subsequent study and much can be learnt from this. Depending on the sophistication of the apparatus, either multiple static films can be taken or the whole procedure can be recorded videographically. One problem is knowing the relationship in depth between veins, and misinterpretation is all too easy without some method of clarification. The simplest way is to take two views of the limb in different rotations so that the relative shift in the veins gives an immediate understanding of their relationship. Before starting, various manoeuvres are rehearsed with the patient, such as exercise by rising up on the toes or rotating the limb inwards and outwards. Any movement by the patient causes immediate changes within the veins, dispersing the opacified blood and quickly creating a confused picture. For this reason requests to exercise or rotate the limb must be carefully timed. Throughout the examination it must be remembered that only streams of opacified blood are seen and it is quite possible for a large vein to remain invisible because the opacified

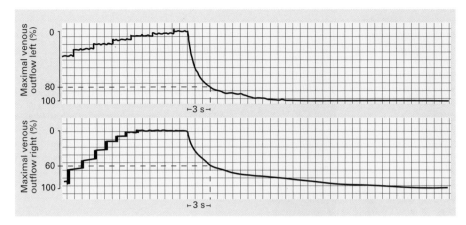

Fig. 3.10 Maximal venous outflow tracings from a patient with a history of a right deep vein thrombosis during pregnancy 20 years previously. The level of the recording is related to the volume of the calf, and changes in this are due to variation in the amount of blood in veins. The initial rise shown is due to venous congestion caused by a pneumatic cuff on the thigh; the sharp fall is on release of the cuff and gives a measure of the rapidity with which venous blood can leave the limb. Left side: 80 per cent of the total fall occurs within the first 3 s, which is within the normal range. Right side: only 60 per cent of total fall occurs in the first 3 s, indicating restriction in venous outlet from the limb. Phlebography confirmed right iliac vein occlusion, but well compensated by pubic varicosities crossing to the opposite side.

stream has chosen other channels; failure of a known vein to appear does not necessarily mean that it is occluded, and different ways may have to be found to persuade opacified blood to enter it. Functional phlebography is not an easy method, but it is immensely rewarding to those who familiarize themselves with it. It is not possible to describe functional phlebography in detail here, but some of the main manoeuvres will be outlined and examples of the results that can be obtained are given in the sections describing the various disorders. The method preferred by the Oxford Vascular Service is described here (Fig. 3.11(a) (iii)), but other centres have evolved their particular techniques for dynamic phlebography and obtain similar results.

Functional phlebography in the normal subject

If the patient is tilted foot down to 50° or more and contrast medium is introduced by needle into a superficial vein on the calf, it will be seen to drift down the superficial veins until checked by a valve and will soon appear in the deep veins of the leg. This downward movement takes place because the specific gravity of the opaque medium is higher than that of blood. If injection is continued up to, say, 100 ml, the deep veins will fill steadily so that they are clearly outlined up to the iliac veins and beyond (Fig. 3.11(b) (i)). Even a small exercise movement will cause rapid movement upwards in the deep veins with partial emptying of the superficial veins and segmentation of opacified blood between their valves. If movement continues, the picture will quickly become confused and all opaque medium will soon leave the limb. During the phase of static filling, opacified blood enters the tibial and peroneal veins by multiple perforators, but often it will similarly enter large venous sinuses (the pumping chambers) lying within muscles. This is a normal phenomenon but if, for instance, a single large gastrocnemius vein fills in this way it may be mistaken for a short saphenous vein. Static filling of the deep veins, as just described, is the first stage in functional phlebography and will test the ability of the deep veins to fill normally. Judicious exercise movements may be given during this stage and subsequently to study the patterns of flow. The valves of the deep veins can be shown by lowering the head of the table to near horizontal, so that the veins deflate slightly;

the table is then rapidly returned to near vertical again (the swill test), which causes the valve cusps to fill and gives a clear impression of their number and, to some extent, their competence (see Fig. 1.1, Fig. 3.11(b) (ii), and Fig. 4.19(e)).

Functional phlebography in venous disorders

The procedure is carried out as described above, with the needle introduced through any convenient enlarged vein on the calf; this has the advantage that the direction of movement of the blood from these veins with slight exercise gives an important indication of function. When about 5 ml of medium has been injected the patient is asked to make a small exercise movement and the effect of this is watched on the screen. In simple incompetence of superficial veins the medium will sweep downwards and appear in deep veins (Fig. 3.11(b) (iii)); in occlusion or severe deformity of deep veins the medium will be swept up the superficial vein as collateral flow (see Fig. 1.13). In other cases, where both superficial and deep valves may be incompetent, heavy surge back and forth may be seen with exercise (Fig. 7.2(b)).

Other sites for injection may be used, including varicosities on the thigh. If the deep veins fail to fill and the opacified blood streams up superficial veins, as may happen in post-thrombotic syndrome, it may be necessary to reposition the needle to a foot vein to give maximum opportunity for outlining deep veins in the leg.

Varicography

Contrast medium injected moderately quickly, with the patient in only slightly head-up tilt, will tend to outline the vein in an 'upward' direction and, in effect, trace it to its 'origin'. In superficial incompetence this method is of value in showing the source of incompetence, for example a short saphenous termination (Fig. 3.11(c) (i)) or a recurrent set of varicose veins of uncertain origin (see Figs 4.29(a) (iii), 4.29(b), 4.29(c), and 4.29(d)). This method gives little information on function but it can be combined with information gained from functional phlebography to give comprehensive views of the veins at fault (Fig. 3.11(c) (ii)). However, the filling of veins by varicography is capricious and results can be misleading until experience is gained.

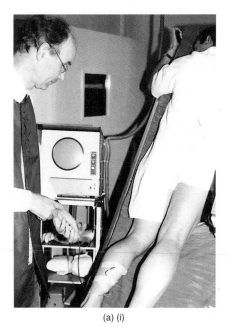

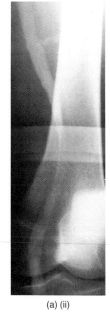

(a) (i)   (a) (ii)

Fig. 3.11 Functional phlebography.

(a) General features. (i) The patient is on a tilting table in the near-upright position for most of the procedure. Outlining of the veins is observed by the image intensifier and static films are exposed as required. (See Fig. 4.19 (c) for the phlebograms obtained from this patient.) (ii) Constricting bands are not used because they distort the pattern of venous flow. (iii) Diagrams summarizing the main features of functional phlebology.

(iii)

	Superficial vein incompetence	**Post-thrombotic syndrome**	**Valveless syndrome** Inborn deficiency of valves deep and superficial
Needle into any convenient enlarged calf vein, small amount of contrast injected. Patient exercised (on toes) × 2 4 ml ex × 2	Flow down and into deep veins	Preferential flow up lower saphenous vein — accentuated by exercise ? move needle to foot vein	Contrast surges back and forth but appears in deep veins or leg via often large perforator(s)
Patient remains still whilst up to 150 ml injected 100-150 ml Passive filling	Outlines deep veins up to iliac veins (valves not shown)	Contrast travels upwards preferentially in lower saphenous vein and superficial veins Deep veins deformed or not outlined	Fills both deep and saphenous vein in parallel fashion
Patient exercised two or three times Ex × 3	Spills over from upper deep vein to fall down saphenous vein	Blood pushed up superficial veins and collaterals Deep veins deformed or fail to fill	Blood in deep veins surges back and forth with each movement
Patient still. Table lowered to near horizontal until femoral vein shows distinct 'deflation' — but not emptied. Table then rapidly put to near vertical Swill test	Valves shown as blood 'swills' back	Opacified blood rapidly cleared by fall-back. No valves seen in deformed veins	When returned to upright blood in deep vein falls down rapidly and contrast in upper thigh 'disappears' Valves absent or defective
Patient still. Posture and table tilt varied to find optimal position to assist contrast 'up' superficial veins (varicography) Upward trace	Further details of origin may be shown but unpredictable	Variably shows superficial and collateral veins	

(a) (iii)

Fig. 3.11 (continued)

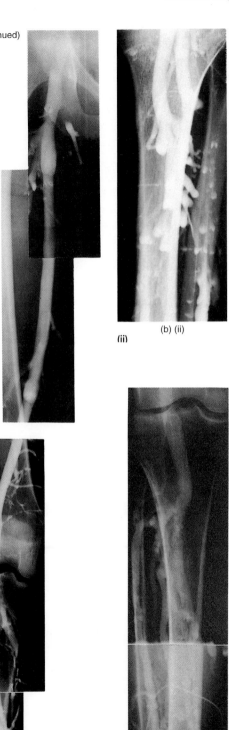

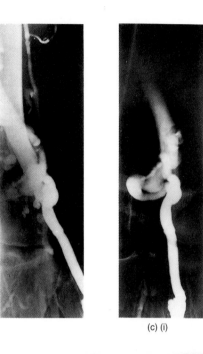

(ii)

(b) (ii)

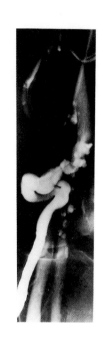

(b) Some basic manoeuvres (see also Fig. 4.19). (i) Opaque medium, injected into calf veins while the patient remains still, fills the principal deep veins passively but the valves are not well shown. (ii) The swill test is used to display the valves. The patient is tilted to near-horizontal and up again to empty partially and then refill the veins. This procedure may require repeating to show different levels, and in this illustration well-valved tibial veins are shown. Since it disperses opacified blood, it is best performed as the last stage in functional phlebography. (iii) In superficial incompetence opaque medium injected into calf varicosities will be swept down and into deep veins after an exercise movement (rising on toes), as shown here. If deep vein deformity or occlusion is present, the medium is likely to be swept upwards, outlining superficial veins acting as collaterals (see Fig. 1.13).

(c) (i)

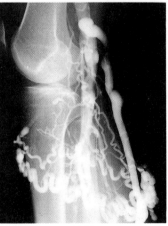

(c) (ii)

(b) (i)

(b) (iii)

(c) Varicography. (i) When functional phlebography has been completed, varicography can be carried out to clarify anatomical details of superficial incompetence. In this illustration, a short saphenous termination is shown in three different rotations. Varicography usually requires a near-horizontal position to give an upward trace and this has the drawback of collapsing veins so that their size is misleading. It only gives the outline and not the function of the veins but this has already been ascertained by the preceding examination.
(ii) Combination of functional and varicography techniques can give an excellent demonstration of the venous disorder. In this example an enlarged incompetent short saphenous vein gives rise to varicose veins that encircle the leg and join the long saphenous vein.

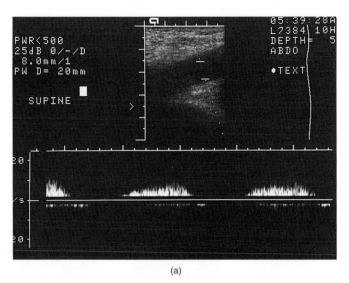

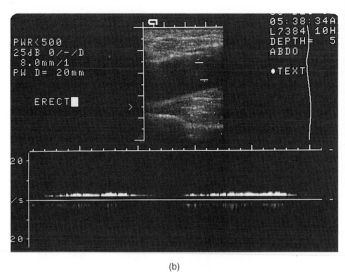

(a)   (b)

Fig. 3.12 Imaging of vein and measurement of flow velocity by duplex ultrasonography. The sonograms were taken during examination for suspected deep vein thrombosis. Phasic flow was recorded wherever sampled and this, together with the easy distension and compressibility of the vein, clearly indicated that thrombus was not present. In fact, this is a good example of normality. Two frames are shown from a pulsed ultrasound scanner using a phased array of transducers (Acuson 128) with a pulsed-beam Doppler velocimetry facility. This has no moving parts and gives a rectangular image, unlike the rotating beam or sector scanner which gives a wdge shaped image. Structures lying beneath the probe are shown on the screen alongside the vertical scale giving the depth from the skin surface in 0.5-cm divisions. Where flow in blood vesssels is to be studied, a gate of variable width, indicated by two parallel cursors, may be positioned within the vessels and set to define the width to be sampled; the angle of the Doppler ultrasonic beam is shown by an interrupted line. The direction and speed of flow are shown in the lower part of the frame; vertical graticules represent velocity in centimetres per second; a time-scale runs horizontally in seconds; signals above the baseline indicate flow away from the probe and, below the baseline, towards the probe; when both are present simultaneously this indicates turbulence or poor positoning of the probe.
(a) Right common femoral vein with the patient supine without movement. The vein outline is clear and the Doppler signal shows intermittent flow away from the probe (towards the heart) in phase with respiration. A maximum velocity of flow of 8 cm/s is reached and there is no significant downflow. The gate measuring flow has been adjusted across the vein lumen at 8.0 mm width with its centre 20 mm deep, and the mean velocity of flow is taken from within this gate.
(b) The same vein with the patient in the erect posture without movement and the instrument settings unchanged. As might be expected, the vein width has increased by over 25 per cent, and this increased capacity has reduced the velocity of flow to 4 cm/s (the cross-sectional area has been doubled and therefore the same volume is conveyed at half the speed). (Courtesy of Dr D.R. Lindsell, John Radcliffe Hospital, Oxford.)

Ultrasonography (ultrasonic imaging)

Pulsed-beam ultrasound scanning creates an image of tissue interfaces and moving blood on a video display unit. This can be used to portray a section through arteries and veins in any plane, from horizontal to vertical. The plane is chosen to show the structure under study to best advantage. In this way a portion of vein over some inches can be shown with its walls and valves clearly outlined and any movements by them demonstrated. The direction and speed of blood flow within the vessel at any point can be individually picked out by a Doppler flow facility and recorded separately (duplex) (Fig. 3.12). Colour flow scanning (triplex) has the additional feature of displaying flow in a colour representing its direction of movement and showing the velocity by the intensity of the colour (Figs 3.13–3.16). Thus the vein walls and lumen can be outlined and the flow studied, clot can be recognized by the absence of flow and immobile vein walls, and the structure of valves and their competence can be scrutinized in detail. The anatomy of veins can be visualized preoperatively, for example, to demonstrate the level and manner of short saphenous termination; individual deep veins and their branches can be distinguished and flow patterns displayed, so that, for instance, incompetence in a gastrocnemius vein can be recognized (immediately apparent by colour flow) and the reflux within it estimated to assess its significance. This is possible because the diameter and speed of flow within any designated vessel can be measured, and the volume of flow, either expelled upwards or refluxed downwards, can be calculated from this. In the popliteal vein this will indicate the effectiveness of the musculovenous pump below the knee or, conversely, the severity of reflux in the deep veins at that level.

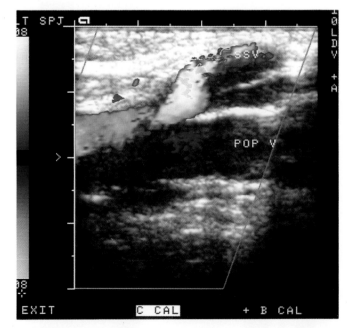

Fig. 3.13 Ultrasonographic colour flow imaging can give a rapid display of veins, their valves, and the direction and velocity of flow. In this illustration, the red colour outlines downward flow (away from heart) in the popliteal vein and into an incompetent short saphenous vein, the origin of varicose veins; upward flow (towards the heart) is represented in blue, but this is minimal here because this phase has ceased with relaxation of calf muscle. This is an ideal method for the non-invasive examination of limited areas of special interest, such as the popliteal fossa.

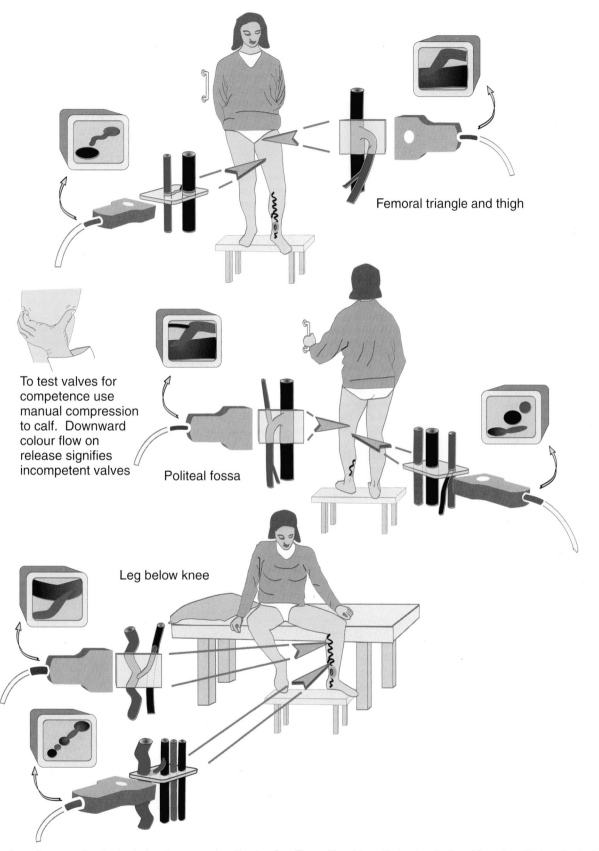

Femoral triangle and thigh

To test valves for competence use manual compression to calf. Downward colour flow on release signifies incompetent valves

Politeal fossa

Leg below knee

Fig. 3.14 Assessing venous function by duplex ultrasonography with colour flow. The position of the patient and application of the probe at the key sites is shown. At each site the probe is moved around freely, and at appropriate points valve competence is checked by manually compressing and releasing the limb beneath the valves to see if reflux occurs. The probe projects ultrasound and scans in a rectangular slice, and the probe can be turned to give vertical, transverse, or oblique cuts.

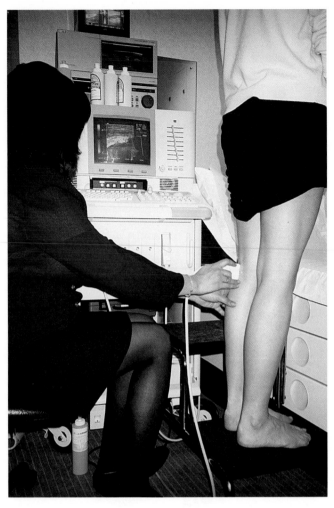

The advantages of ultrasonography are that it is non-invasive and can be used for prolonged viewing with repeated cycles of exercise in a way that is not possible with phlebography. Moreover, the running costs are decidedly less. It is an excellent method for special study of localized areas of vein, both for research and in the practical management of some venous problems. It is already a practical alternative to phlebology for detecting acute thrombosis or in the display of specific structures, such as a short saphenous termination or a valve suspected of leaking. Its potential for future development is considerable and it will continue to displace phlebology for many purposes in the lower limb; moreover, it is increasingly finding a role in practical pocedures by its ability, for example, to guide the entry of a needle into an inaccessible vein during sclerotherapy.

Keeping a record of the duplex ultrasonography findings is greatly helped by direct use of a computer, keying in results as they are obtained. An example of a diagrammatic representation suitable for vascular work is shown in Fig. 3.17. A template of this sort uses very little computer memory and encourages a systematic approach.

Fig. 3.15 Ultrasonography in use. The transducer head can be moved quickly from one site to another and used to exert pressure to test for deformability of veins. The operator's left hand is ready to squeeze and release the calf to test for reflux if the valves are incompetent. This will be immediately recognizable as a brief downward coloured flow.

Fig. 3.16 (*Right*) Illustration of the capabilities of colour flow ultrasonography. The video screen gives a continuous moving display of the tissues under its probe, but at any given moment this is only a ultra-thin slice. A static picture, such as those shown here, captures this only at the instant of being taken. It cannot do justice to the mass of information passing before the operator as the probe is shifted, angled, rotated, and pressed, and is only a reminder of one moment. The operator's skill and interpretation abilities are of key importance in acquiring information far beyond that conveyed by the static pictures. The patient is examined in the upright position, where abnormal states become apparent, but note that the picture has a horizontal lie because the 'slice' illuminated by the probe is always displayed that way, no matter how the probe lies.

Scans (a) and (b) illustrate testing competence of valves, in this example at the saphenofemoral junction. (a) Compression at calf level causes a surge upwards to give a blue colour. (b) On release of compression, blood refluxes downwards by gravity and this is shown by red colour whilst the flow lasts; duration of more than 0.5 s demonstrates incompetence of valves, here in the long saphenous vein. (c) Competence of valves can be similarly checked at any level in the superficial veins. Here the long saphenous vein in mid-thigh shows the typical (red) downflow of incompetence.

The following show deep veins with normal upward (proximal) flow in blue and the artery alongside with normal downward (distal) flow in red: (d) superficial femoral (deep) vein; (e) upper popliteal vein; (f) saphenopopliteal junction (artery not visible); (g) paired posterior tibial veins with artery in between.

Thrombosis in deep veins (see also Fig. 10.5): (h) the outline of the popliteal vein is clearly discernible but it cannot be compressed (narrowed) by pressure with the probe nor can any flow can be elicited, confirming that it is filled with thrombus; (i) a thrombosed popliteal vein after 3 months, with patchy areas of flow indicating that recanalization is taking place.

The following are examples of other features that can be shown by ultrasonography: (j) Baker's cyst in popliteal fossa (this may rupture and simulate deep vein thrombosis); (k) perforating vein near the ankle (marked by +), with the echogenic deep fascia shown as a line of increased density indicated by arrows; (l) oedema at the ankle shown by increased density and interstitial spaces.

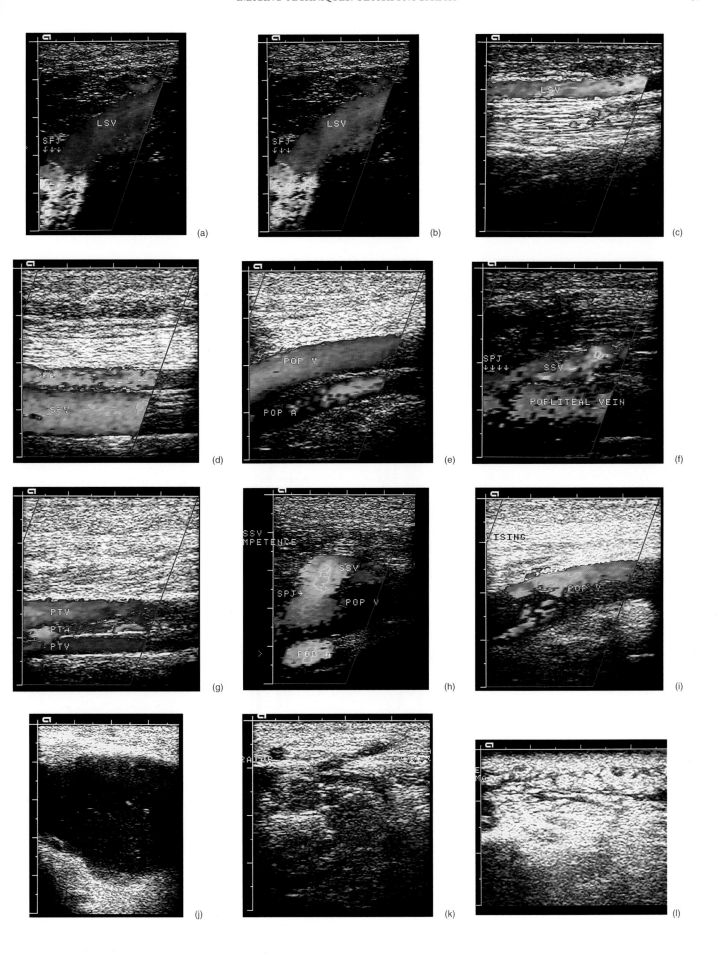

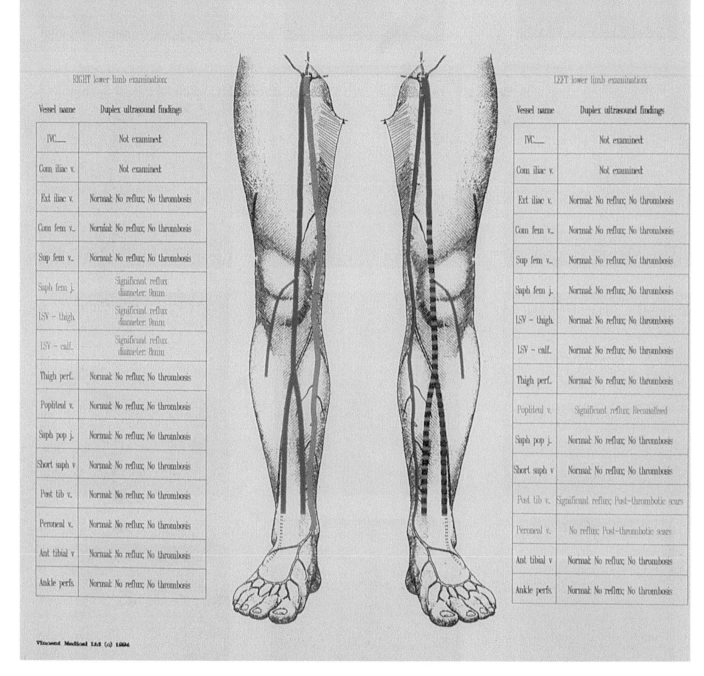

The Middlesex Hospital
Vascular Laboratory
Venous Duplex Examination

Patient:
Mr A Patient Number: pp Exam date: 28 Sep 1994.

RIGHT lower limb examination:

Vessel name	Duplex ultrasound findings
IVC___	Not examined
Com iliac v.	Not examined
Ext iliac v.	Normal: No reflux; No thrombosis
Com fem v_	Normal: No reflux; No thrombosis
Sup fem v_	Normal: No reflux; No thrombosis
Saph fem j.	Significant reflux diameter: 9mm
LSV – thigh.	Significant reflux diameter: 9mm
LSV – calf.	Significant reflux diameter: 8mm
Thigh perf.	Normal: No reflux; No thrombosis
Popliteal v.	Normal: No reflux; No thrombosis
Saph pop j.	Normal: No reflux; No thrombosis
Short saph v	Normal: No reflux; No thrombosis
Post tib v.	Normal: No reflux; No thrombosis
Peroneal v.	Normal: No reflux; No thrombosis
Ant tibial v	Normal: No reflux; No thrombosis
Ankle perfs.	Normal: No reflux; No thrombosis

LEFT lower limb examination:

Vessel name	Duplex ultrasound findings
IVC___	Not examined
Com iliac v.	Not examined
Ext iliac v.	Normal: No reflux; No thrombosis
Com fem v_	Normal: No reflux; No thrombosis
Sup fem v_	Normal: No reflux; No thrombosis
Saph fem j.	Normal: No reflux; No thrombosis
LSV – thigh.	Normal: No reflux; No thrombosis
LSV – calf.	Normal: No reflux; No thrombosis
Thigh perf.	Normal: No reflux; No thrombosis
Popliteal v.	Significant reflux; Recanalised
Saph pop j.	Normal: No reflux; No thrombosis
Short saph v	Normal: No reflux; No thrombosis
Post tib v.	Significant reflux; Post-thrombotic scars
Peroneal v.	No reflux; Post-thrombotic scars
Ant tibial v	Normal: No reflux; No thrombosis
Ankle perfs.	Normal: No reflux; No thrombosis

Vincent Medical Ltd (c) 1994

Fig. 3.17 With a suitable computer program results can be keyed in and added to the appropriate part of a template diagram, such as that illustrated here. It requires little computer memory but gives a comprehensive visual representation of the findings.

Box 3.6   Imaging techniques

Functional (dynamic) phlebography
Essential capabilities and drawbacks
Purpose is to display function and outline, not merely anatomical shape. Window of examination is large and the full limb is covered by three or four windows. Response to muscle contraction (pumping) and resulting flow can be seen and recorded.
Demonstrates valves and their competence.
Allows varicography to be included and this can give extra details.
BUT
It is invasive requiring injection of medium; nevertheless should seldom cause trouble.
Gives only a brief opportunity to see events and is not easily repeatable.
Requires a special interest and skill to obtain good results.
Key requirements
Use of modern non-irritant opaque medium for injection to allow maximal dose with safety.
Use of image intensifier so that more prolonged viewing is possible within permitted radiation dosage.
It must be carried out in an upright position, in which venous problems become apparent, with judicious exercise to create typical flow patterns
Method
Summarized by the diagram in Fig. 3.11(a)(iii)

Ultrasonic imaging
Non-invasive and can be repeated as often as required.
Gives the outline of veins, with direction of flow in response to exercise or compression indicated on the display by colouring the flow so that incompetence is immediately recognizable.
Can display vein outline, valve status, and presence of clot in the area examined.
It is the easiest and quickest way to outline the saphenopopliteal junction before surgery.
Low running costs.
BUT
It has a small window of viewing and is most suitable for a selected area rather than overall coverage, for example to look for short saphenous or gastrocnemius vein incompetence. However, it is easy to move quickly between a number of key areas and in this way carry out a more general assessment.

Box 3.7   Understanding the basics of diagnostic ultrasound: technical details and terms

Ultrasound is central to diagnosis in venous disorders and it is an advantage to have some understanding of its basic principles and the terms used.

Ultrasound: Piezoelectric crystals and materials
The human ear hears sound up to a frequency of 20 KHz; sound above this frequency, beyond the range of human hearing, is termed ultrasound. In medicine, frequencies between 1 and 15 MHz are used for a variety of diagnostic purposes. These frequencies are generated by piezoelectric crystals or materials which have unique characteristics.

   A piezoelectric crystal or material changes its shape when an electric voltage is applied to it, and this property is used to generate high frequency sound. Conversely, any stress put upon a piezoelectric material (including sound waves) generates an electric voltage. Thus the material can be used both to emit and detect ultrasound. When applied to a limb the emitted ultrasound is reflected back (an echo) by tissue interfaces and at each point of reflection generates a signal which can be displayed on the video screen. This signal will be located on the screen according to the fractional time interval taken for ultrasound to travel the distance, back and forth, between the transducer and that point of the tissue, and in this way a pattern is built up corresponding to the tissues it is targeting. The frequency of the emission can be varied by using piezoelectric discs of different sizes.

Continued

Box 3.7 *Continued*

Penetration of tissues by ultrasound

A coupling agent (a gel) is used to join the face of the probe to the skin since the ultrasound will not cross even a thin layer of air satisfactorily. The depth of penetration of ultrasound varies with its frequency. A high frequency has little penetration, but the lower the frequency the greater the penetration. Thus, at 15 MHz it can barely pass beyond the surface, at 5 MHz it will penetrate a depth of 5 cm, and at 2.5 MHz it will penetrate to a depth of 15 cm. However, there is a trade-off, because at lower frequencies there is a severe loss of resolution (the detail that will be shown) which limits its use at depth. Fluid transmits ultrasound well, but although gas reflects well, it transmits very poorly and this is a handicap in the abdomen. Bone is also a barrier to ultrasound. Muscle, blood vessels, and other soft tissues transmit satisfactorily and reflect well from their surfaces to give a good image.

Echogenicity

This is the strength of reflected ultrasound and varies according to relative change in density of tissue at interfaces. The strength of the representation of tissue on the video image depends on this. Red blood cells have a high echogenicity because of their much greater density compared with the fluid plasma around them, and it is this strong reflection that makes possible the measurement of velocity and direction of flow by Doppler shift. The echogenicity of a thrombus varies with its age. Thus it is poorly imaged in the early stage but after a week or two may visualize well.

Grey scale

The brightness of the image components on the screen indicates the density of the tissue interface being shown and is depicted in a range of grey colour, the grey scale. This portrayal by varying shades of grey is known as *B mode*.

Continuous- and pulsed-wave ultrasound: angle of probe

For simple measurement of velocity in moving blood, as in *Doppler flowmetry*, ultrasound is used as in a *continuous-wave form* and this detects the amount of Doppler shift by the change in frequency as it is reflected back from moving red blood cells. This can only be elicited if the beam is in line with the flow and angled to it at about 45°. This is achieved by suitable manual alignment of the probe. Most modern units are bidirectional, i.e. the direction of flow, towards or away from the probe, will be indicated as well as the velocity.

Pulsed-wave ultrasound is used when an image is to be produced. This can also be used to measure Doppler shift by aligning the probe's sonic field parallel to the flow and also by adjusting the angle of projected ultrasound with marker lines shown on the screen. To obtain a satisfactory reading the operator has to ensure that these settings are favourable, but there is reasonable latitude here. Ultrasonography that is capable of creating an image and also measuring the velocity of moving blood by the Doppler shift is referred to as *duplex*.

Colour scanning

This is an extra facility that depicts flow of blood in a colour code to indicate the direction of movement; for example flow towards the probe may be red and flow away from the probe, blue. In this case, if the probe is pointed up the limb, arterial blood will be red and normal venous return will be blue.

Real-time imaging

This is the term describing the ability to depict movement as it occurs. Since the image is scanned many times each second, this creates a rapid sequences of images giving, in effect, a moving picture.

The probe: sector and linear array scanning

The piezoelectric material is usually arranged as a disc to form a transducer capable of transforming electrical energy into physical change and vice versa. The term 'transducer' is often loosely used to denote the probe itself.

For *Doppler velocimetry* only a single fixed piezoelectric transducer is required and a variety of probe frequencies are available to be used according to the depth at which it is to operate.

For *imaging* there are two basic types. For *rotating-beam or sector scanning* a piezoelectric transducer that sweeps back and forth inside the probe through an arc of about 90° is used to give a wedge shaped image. In the *linear array* of piezoelectric transducers the probe contains a battery of fixed transducers that fire in sequence to give a rectangular image in the same proportion as the tissues being scanned. This is the form most often used for vascular work in the lower limbs.

Many styles of ultrasonographic equipment are available and the description above can only give a general outline. Whatever the instrument, the user must be aware of the direction, shape, and depth of the field of ultrasound projected by the probe. The orientation of the image is always related to the position of the probe, not the patient.

Box 3.8 Duplex ultrasonography and colour scanning

Duplex ultrasonography combines the ability to provide a real-time video image (i.e. a rapid sequence of images giving a moving picture) of the tissue interfaces underlying the transducer probe, with a facility for measuring velocity of flow by Doppler shift within blood vessels. Colour scanning shows the direction of flow coded in colour so that movement towards the probe is, say, red, and away from it, blue, with the intensity of colour increasing with its velocity. This gives immediate distinction between normal arterial and venous flow, or of abnormal direction of flow as occurs in venous reflux. A pair of adjustable cursors on the video screen can be placed over the vein being studied and used as a gate to select the width of Doppler sample required; this can also be used to measure the vein lumen. The depth beneath the surface and the width of the adjustable gate are indicated on the screen. The velocity and direction of flow are displayed as a series of signals above or below a base line according to the flow direction. The size of these signals can be measured against scales of velocity and time. The display can be frozen at any time and print-outs can be obtained whenever required.

Advantages over functional phlebography
No injection of medium is required, there is no discomfort, and the procedure can be repeated as often as is required. Permanent record is provided by colour image print-outs or video tape, and these will include the Doppler velocimetry display. The window of viewing is less than in phlebography, but the ease of moving from one area to another largely outweighs this. Another advantage is that it allows local examination of valve function in a way that is not possible with phlebology, for example to demonstrate incompetence in the popliteal vein when the valves above this level are competent and would hinder distribution of opaque medium to that level. Functional phlebography, limited by dosage of radiation and medium, offers only one, possibly two, opportunities for displaying the features required and considerable skill is needed to achieve this; with ultrasonography, the procedure can be repeated without any reserve to obtain an optimal demonstration. Nevertheless, functional phlebography can give details not obtainable by ultrasonography and still has a role, but as a matter of practical expediency ultrasound is the first choice for imaging the veins of the lower limb.

Protocol for examining the patient
Preliminary clinical examination and Doppler flowmetry is important so that attention is focused on the likely areas of abnormality. During assessment of venous function the patient must be examined in the position in which venous abnormality becomes evident, i.e. standing. The patient's weight should be on the opposite limb held straight, and on the side being examined the hip and knee should hang slightly flexed in order to relax the muscles. In this way the veins will fall slack on release of manual compression (or relaxation of muscle after contraction), ready to receive any downflow that may occur; taut muscles will prevent this from happening. Coupling gel should be used between the scanner probe and the skin.

The movement of venous blood is essential for the full display of a vein and only its outline is visible without it. Venous flow is created by either muscle contraction during an exercise movement or a firm squeeze by the examiner's hand to an area below the veins being observed. This will empty the veins compressed and cause an upward movement of blood which in normal veins will be held by valves and not fall back again on release of compression (or relaxation of muscles). However, if valves are defective, there will be a downward movement of venous blood, made obvious by colour scanning. If this occurs over more than 0.5 s (timed on the video display), it signifies reflux in that vein. The severity of this is judged by the velocity and the volume (width of gate) of flow; clearly, a thin slow trickle may have little significance but a massive leak of gravitational downflow is of major importance.

This is the basic manoeuvre used to assess functional competence and it is repeated at various points in the limb. The following sites are particularly important.

Deep veins
Common femoral, superficial femoral, popliteal, tibial and peroneal veins, and branches arising from them, including mid-thigh perforators and gastrocnemius veins, should be examined. Study of these veins will show whether they have an adequate set of functioning valves or whether there is deep vein insufficiency. An occluded vein shows as a dark incompressible outline not illuminated by any blood flow.

Superficial veins
The saphenofemoral and saphenopopliteal junctions are common sources of downflow in incompetent superficial veins, and this is evident immediately *after* calf muscle contraction or manual compression. Incompetent saphenous veins and their varicose branches can be identified and reflux in them can be demonstrated. If the patient has had previous surgery to veins, then likely areas for the source of recurrent incompetence must be examined, particularly at the site of previous ligation, and a search made for perforators acting as a new source of incompetence, for instance in the mid-thigh. Alternatively, the source of incompetence may be in the other saphenous system which must be checked. In most cases of superficial vein incompetence, the source can be demonstrated by ultrasongraphy and the gravitational downflow from here traced through the superficial veins to give convincing proof.

Continued

Box 3.8 *Continued*

Perforators

When deep and superficial veins have been assessed without satisfactorily defining a venous disorder, a special effort must be made to see whether the perforators can offer an explanation. The perforators have varying roles and significance in the various disorders (see Chapter 7). Some major distinctions that must be made are as follows.

In *superficial vein incompetence* a perforator in the lower part of the limb will allow inward flow of blood immediately after relaxation of calf muscle contraction or release of manual compression; of course, this flow is in the normal direction and does not in itself indicate that the perforator should be removed at surgery. However, if there is impairment of neighbouring deep veins there may be a strong surge back and forth with each muscle contraction or manual compression, and the surgeon will wish to know about this because this perforator is probably best removed. With recurrent veins, a perforator may take over as the source of incompetence and this must be looked for, particularly in the mid-thigh.

In the *post-thrombotic limb*, with extensive deep vein obstruction, the perforators and superficial veins may be forced to act as collaterals so that there is strong outflow through perforators and up the superficial veins, accentuated by each exercise movement. This may be a valuable compensatory mechanism which should be preserved, and the deep veins must be assessed to know the extent of occlusion or reflux in them.

Finding outflow from a perforator should not lead to an automatic diagnosis of 'incompetent perforator' but a careful search should be made to demonstrate its significance. If it is due to deep vein occlusion, a very different policy of treatment will be required.

Locating perforators, whatever their significance, is carried out by moving the transducer in stages down the limb in the line of likely perforators and at each stage setting up venous movement by manual compression. The transducer must be aligned to project its sonic field along the probable lie of the perforators and this will usually mean turning it to give a transverse cut horizontally across the limb parallel with the perforators. At the same time the deep and superficial veins between which the perforator may run should be keep in view.

This is an area where misinterpretation is all too easy! Just locating a perforator is not sufficient. The direction and pattern of flow through it during a cycle of manual compression and release, or a muscle contraction and relaxation, must be ascertained, and the significance of this considered in conjunction with the state of the deep and superficial veins.

Outlining anatomical arrangement of veins as guidance for the surgeon

There is considerable variation in the anatomy of veins about which the surgeon should be forewarned. In this respect the popliteal fossa is particularly important because of the differing level and arrangement of the saphenopopliteal junction lying surrounded by major vessels and nerves. Ultrasonography can define this, much to the advantage of the surgeon who can then avoid a futile and damaging search in the popliteal fossa. The identification of the saphenopopliteal junction by ultrasonography is an essential preliminary to operation upon it.

Special features

It has already been mentioned that a gate between cursors can be set to measure the width of any vein on the video screen. This can be used by the computer software to calculate the volume of blood within that portion of vein. Since the velocity of flow is also measured, the volume per second can be estimated. In this way, the amount of blood expelled up the popliteal vein at each calf muscle contraction can be calculated together with the volume of blood that refluxes back. The computer program can be set to give this and to provide a valuable indication of deep vein insufficiency.

In suspected acute deep vein thrombosis the patient will usually be examined in the supine position and ultrasonography can reliably assess thrombosis in the calf region as well as in the major veins above this level. The outline of an occluded vein will be seen, usually alongside an artery, but will not narrow with external pressure in the way in which a normal vein does. This is an indication of clot within it and is confirmed by the absence of any blood flow within it (see Part II for discussion of diagnosis of acute deep vein thrombus)

The soft tissue imaging capabilities of ultrasonography are valuable in revealing conditions, previously unsuspected, that are of importance in their own right and may have a direct bearing on the condition being investigated. A good example is the presence of a Morrant Baker cyst which is causing oedema or simulating deep vein thrombosis because it has ruptured. Similarly, tumours and haematomas can be displayed.

Box 3.9 Duplex ultrasound examination with colour flow

The assessment of patients with venous disorder in practice

The medical history must include any previous varicose vein surgery or episodes suggestive of deep vein thrombosis in the past. The patient sits on an examination couch with the feet on a low platform. Since patients may forget about old operations, and the limb should be inspected carefully for any surgical scars. Even if there is no history of deep vein thrombosis, the deep vein system should always be scanned for evidence of this.

Technical details

The ultrasound machine used to obtain the various illustrations of ultrasound colour flow in Part I of this book was an Acuson computed sonography duplex machine 128 XP10 with ART technology, which is easy to use and gives good-quality images. It uses a multi-Hertz 5–7 MHz frequency probe longitudinally, supported by a curve linear 3.5 MHz probe, used for specific indications, particularly when looking at oedematous legs where veins can be difficult to reach unless the better penetration of this low-frequency probe is used. It is also useful in obese patients or when looking deeply at the iliac veins. However, the majority of assessments are carried out using the 5–7 MHz probe. Coupling gel is used as required throughout (disposable paper underpants are helpful).

The duplex ultrasound machine initially provides a B-mode image which is displayed in a range of grey shades (grey-scale). This is used to locate superficial and deep veins at the start of the examination. Once they are found, colour flow can be switched on. This will require the angle of the projected ultrasonic field to be adjusted electronically so that it is slanted at approximately 45° to the axis of flow. It is usually best to arrange this pointing up the limb so that upward flow, retreating from the ultrasonic field, and downward flow, advancing into the field, are distinguished decisively one from the other in a consistent fashion. In this way any blood flowing away from the probe, up the limb (depending on settings chosen), is shown as blue, and downward flowing blood (including venous gravitational reflux) as red, so that arterial flow is picked out in red, venous return in blue, and venous reflux is in red. If there is significant reflux, this will be recognized by a long duration of flow and is usually obvious from the colour flow. If this is uncertain or shows a slight red blip, it is wise to measure the reflux by spectral Doppler flow analysis to decide its significance. This samples blood flow within an adjustable gate on the video screen at any selected point, usually just below a valve. The calf is compressed to create upward flow (blue) and, on release, this will be followed by reverse flow (red) if the valves are incompetent. The criterion for reflux is reverse flow lasting for more than 0.5 s or a velocity of reverse flow greater than 10 cm/s.

Investigation procedure (see Fig. 3.14)

The femoral triangle. The investigation is started with the patient standing on the platform facing the examiner and with the weight on the opposite limb so that the muscles of the limb to be examined are relaxed. The groin is examined first, locating the saphenofemoral junction and checking its competency. At the same time the common femoral vein is looked at to make sure that there is no scarring (increased density and deformity in the vein wall) or incompetence from past thrombosis. Examination of patients with primary varicose veins is usually straightforward. The long saphenous vein is checked for incompetence and the presence of competent perforating veins is noted. However, with recurrent varicose veins following surgery, it is necessary to determine whether there has been a satisfactory ligation of the saphenofemoral junction or whether surviving branches, a second saphenous vein, or even neovascularization have re-established a source of incompetence. Remnants of the long saphenous vein should be looked for. If it has not been stripped, it will probably be filling from an incompetent mid-thigh (Hunterian) perforating vein and this can be accurately located; a search for other feeding veins is also made. In patients with recurrence who have had ligation of the saphenofemoral junction, the external branches of the pudendal vein should always be examined because they can be the source of continuing incompetence. These veins often become prominent in pregnancy, and may persist as incompetent communications with an unstripped long saphenous vein after an otherwise satisfactory ligation at the saphenofemoral junction.

The thigh. Next, the thigh is examined with the patient's leg turned outwards so that its medial aspect is exposed. In the first instance the long saphenous vein is followed throughout the thigh, noting the size and reflux, and it is also scanned for incompetent perforating veins. In those patients with recurrent varicose veins it is important to see whether the long saphenous vein is still present and, if so, to look for any incompetent veins joining it. The lateral thigh veins are then scanned and the state of the anterolateral vein is checked. Lateral thigh perforating veins are noted and their position measured from the lateral condyle. The deep veins are then scanned, looking for scarring or incompetence from previous deep vein thrombosis. In a swollen leg, the presence of recent acute venous thrombosis must be excluded.

The popliteal fossa. When examination of the thigh is complete, the patient is turned so that the popliteal fossa can examined with the patient still standing. The popliteal vein is of major importance, and incompetence or active thrombosis in it must not be missed. The patient faces away from the examiner with the knee slightly bent and muscles relaxed to prevent possible compression of the vein by artery or muscle. The anatomy of the fossa is looked at in transverse section by turning the probe to a horizontal lie.

The position and arrangement of the junction of the short saphenous vein with the deep vein and the position of gastrocnemius veins are noted. It is important to see whether the short saphenous vein is joined by gastrocnemius veins before entering the popliteal vein, or whether they join it separately. Alternatively, the short saphenous vein may extend through the fossa without joining the popliteal vein (but there may be an interconnecting branch) and continue up the posterior thigh superficially to end in the long saphenous vein in upper thigh.

Continued

Box 3.9   *Continued*

After establishing the venous anatomy, the short saphenous vein is examined, looking for incompetence at several levels. The presence of a Giacomini vein extending from it up the back of the thigh is noted, and any reflux in it is recorded. If the patient has recurrence of varicose veins after saphenopopliteal ligation, the popliteal vein must be inspected for a saphenous stump with surviving branches that have reconnected with remnants of the short saphenous system lower down. Varicose veins over the back of the calf may not arise directly from the short saphenous vein, and connections with the long saphenous system or with perforating veins should be looked for. The deep veins are then examined. The popliteal vein above and below the gastrocnemius branches is inspected and the presence of segmental reflux is noted. The presence of scarring from old thrombosis is noted. If a thrombus is present, the vein becomes incompressible, and either no flow is seen or the clot is outlined by irregular flow.

Below the knee. Once the popliteal fossa has been examined, the patient sits facing the examiner with both feet on the platform. The leg to be examined is swung outwards so that the medial aspect of the calf is accessible. The long saphenous vein below the knee is examined first for segmental incompetence. If incompetence has been found in the thigh, it is important to determine whether this extends into the saphenous vein below the knee. Varicosities over the lower calf usually fill from an incompetent long saphenous vein or its posterior arcuate branch, but any additional varicose veins should be scanned for possible origin from incompetent perforating veins, and here the upper and lower aspects of the calf must be searched specifically for Cockett's perforating veins (near the ankle) and Boyd's perforating vein (just below the knee). The location of any incompetent perforators is marked, their diameter is measured at the fascial outlet, and the distance from a bony anatomical landmark, such as a medial malleolus or condyle, is measured. The lateral aspect of the calf is then checked for incompetent perforating veins and their position is noted. Once the superficial system below the knee has been examined, the posterior tibial veins and the peroneal veins should be inspected for scarring and incompetence. The absence of these changes implies that there has been no previous deep vein thrombosis.

Diagnosis of acute deep vein thrombosis

Duplex ultrasound imaging now plays a major role in the diagnosis of acute deep vein thrombosis. This depends on the following.

- Finding that the outline of a vein cannot be compressed by external pressure in the way possible in a normal vein, and that it will not change width with pressure alterations within it, such as those caused by posture or by transmission of abdominal pressure (Coughing and Valsalva's manoeuvre).
- Direct imaging of thrombus is often possible, particularly in the older thrombus which has acquired greater density and echogenicity.
- Blood flow, shown most strikingly by colour flow, will either be absent or will be seen flowing around a thrombus.

With these criteria it is possible to detect thrombus reliably in the major veins from common iliac down to the tibial and peroneal veins (see Figs 3.16(h)(i), 6.2, and 10.5).

4 Clinical patterns of venous disorder I
Incompetence in superficial veins: simple or primary varicose veins

Incompetence in superficial veins

The retrograde circuit of incompetence

In the upright position, each contraction of the muscles in a normal limb pumps blood upwards and it is prevented from returning by effective valves. The immediate reduction in the venous pressure and slackening of the deep veins in lower leg and foot caused by this provides an opportunity for superficial veins to empty into the deep veins, ready to be pumped up with the next movement. Normally the valves in the superficial veins limit this inward flow, so that only a short segment between each valve can empty through the corresponding perforating veins and disorderly widespread transfer of blood from superficial to deep veins is prevented. However, if there is extensive incompetence in the superficial valves, it is possible for blood to spill over from deep veins at high level, flow down the superficial veins, and finally enter the deep veins at low level every time these veins fall slack after muscle contraction (Fig. 4.1). This is the mechanism underlying simple or primary varicose veins and is, by far, the most common venous disorder.

Such abnormal downflow is gravitationally determined. It only occurs when the patient is upright, or nearly so. In addition to muscular activity, it occurs as a single episode, when the patient rises from the horizontal to the vertical position, or when external pressure to calf or foot partially empties the deep veins. It will not occur with exercise unless there is a reasonably effective deep vein pumping mechanism. In this way, a retrograde circuit of flow is set up, spilling over from a deep vein somewhere above a musculo-venous pumping mechanism, down incompetent superficial veins, and through perforators to enter deep veins below the pumping mechanism. This may be any group of muscles in the leg or the foot itself, as described earlier. Endless repetition of this cycle of reversed flow causes the superficial veins to become enlarged and tortuous, i.e. to become varicose veins. However, the main stem of the saphenous veins appears too robust to develop this change and it is the branch veins that do so. Varicose veins are the response to a dynamic process of strong reversed flow and not just static distension.

A typical retrograde circuit (Fig. 4.2) is based on a superficial vein, often a long or short saphenous vein with defective or absent valves. The circuit has four components:

(1) a source of outflow from deep to superficial veins at high level;

(2) a pathway of incompetence running down the limb;

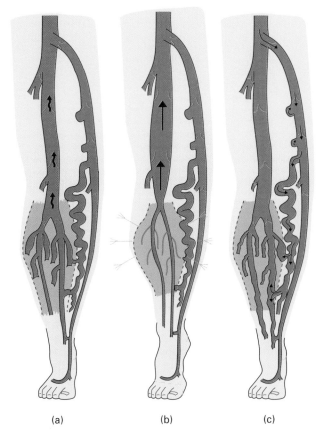

(a)   (b)   (c)

Fig. 4.1   The retrograde circuit of superficial vein incompetence in a standing patient. (a) Standing still. The veins are well filled with a slow upward drift in the main conduit veins. (b) On contraction of muscle. The leg veins are compressed and the blood is driven upwards, emptying the deep veins. (c) On relaxation of muscle. The deep veins, protected from reflux by valves, are now slack. This allows a rush of blood down the pathway of incompetence (here the long saphenous vein and its varicosities) and, via perforators, into the deep veins so that they are filled prematurely from this unwanted source. This process is endlessly repeated in movements such as walking.

(3) re-entry points where superficial downflow joins the deep veins;

(4) a return pathway provided by the deep veins and the musculovenous pumping mechanisms.

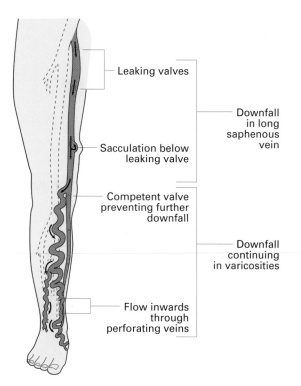

Leaking valves

Downfall
in long
saphenous
vein

Sacculation below
leaking valve

Competent valve
preventing further
downfall

Downfall
continuing
in varicosities

Flow inwards
through
perforating veins

Fig. 4.2 The components of a typical retrograde circuit of superficial incompetence: a source (in this example, the saphenofemoral junction), a pathway of incompetence (the long saphenous vein and varicosities), re-entry points to the deep veins (perforating veins), and a return pathway up the deep veins (activated by the musculovenous pump). The other essential factor is gravity; the circuit's activity is maximal in the upright position but diminishes to extinction as the horizontal is approached.

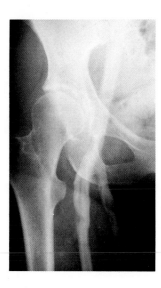

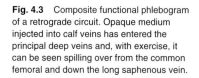

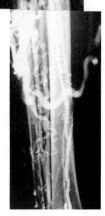

Fig. 4.3 Composite functional phlebogram of a retrograde circuit. Opaque medium injected into calf veins has entered the principal deep veins and, with exercise, it can be seen spilling over from the common femoral and down the long saphenous vein.

In a retrograde circuit based on an incompetent long or short saphenous vein, its upper end provides the source, its main stem and incompetent branches form the pathway of incompetence, and one or more perforating veins are the re-entry points (Figs 4.3 and 4.4). The deep veins receiving this downflow may be principal conduits, such as the tibial veins, or the venous sinuses (pumping chambers) within any muscle group in the leg, or the veins of the foot (Fig. 4.4(b)). Although the source is usually the upper end of a saphenous vein, any communication between deep and superficial veins at high level may take on this role; not infrequently pelvic veins provide a source, particularly during pregnancy, giving varicosities in the vulva and upper thigh, and these may persist after childbirth (see Fig. 4.10). Less usual sources are particularly likely to occur when the superficial vein anatomy has been fragmented by previous surgery; for example, after high saphenous ligation, a mid-thigh perforator may become the source of recurrence (Fig. 4.29(d) (iii)). There are numerous variations on this theme, but each has the same components: a higher-level source, a pathway of incompetence, and re-entry point(s) provided by perforating veins at lower levels including the foot. This state is usually curable by removal of the source and the pathway of incompetence, but enlarged re-entry points (one or more perforators) that allow backflow may also require closing off. An understanding of the retrograde circuit in superficial vein incompetence is essential in the good management of varicose veins, and treatment will not be successful unless these components to the circuit are accurately recognized and effectively obliterated by sclerotherapy or removed by surgery. The more completely that this is done, the more effective and permanent treatment will be. Several typical retrograde circuits of superficial vein incompetence are illustrated in Figs 4.5–4.16.

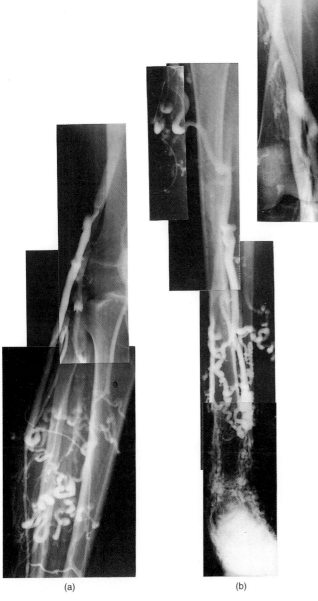

Fig. 4.4 Short saphenous incompetence. (a) Composite pictures of short saphenous incompetence obtained by functional phlebography. (b) A retrograde circuit runs from a high level down to a low pressure area created by a venous pumping unit, and this includes the foot. Varicose veins, as part of the pathway of incompetence, often run to the underside of the foot, as shown in this composite phlebogram of short saphenous incompetence.

Box 4.1 The retrograde circuit of superficial incompetence

This is an essential concept in understanding superficial incompetence and varicose veins (see Fig. 4.1). It is maximal when upright and virtually ceases when lying—**gravity is the prime mover**. The components are as follows:

- a **source** of outflow from deep veins at the apex of the circuit
- the **pathway of incompetence**—the incompetent superficial veins including the varicose veins allowing downflow
- one or more **re-entry points** of flow back into the deep veins—provided by perforating veins to pumping chambers (venous intramuscular sinuses) or to main conduit veins emptied by recent muscle contraction
- a **return pathway** provided by the deep veins, usually normal, mostly taking blood back to heart but some spilling over at the source to join the retrograde circuit once more

Thus, when walking, there is a continuous dynamic turbulent flow down the pathway of incompetence.

Mixed patterns of superficial incompetence

These arise when there are two or more sources of incompetence causing the varicose veins (e.g. long and short saphenous vein incompetence both contributing to varicosities on the calf) or a pathway of incompetence that starts in long saphenous vein and then crosses over to join the short saphenous vein from which the varicose veins arise, or vice versa (Fig. 4.8).

Unusual or unexpected sources of superficial vein incompetence

It has already been mentioned that there are many possible unexpected sources of incompetent downflow in superficial veins, such as the internal pudendal vein from the pelvic deep veins or when previous surgery has fragmented normal anatomy; moreover it is also possible for retrograde circuits of incompetence to arise in conjunction with other forms of venous disorder. Some examples of these less usual states are given below.

Unexpected sources

Varicosities from a long saphenous source may be visible in short saphenous territory or vice versa; one variant of this is a vein running upwards for a short distance before linking on to a branch of the other saphenous system and so giving rise to the apparent paradox of upward flow in a simple varicose vein (Fig. 4.9). During pregnancy, vulval varicosities arising via pudendal veins from the pelvic veins may appear and persist to provide an obscure source of superficial vein incompetence down the thigh and leg (Fig. 4.10). In its most extreme form, this will be even more extensive, taking its source from massive incompetence in the ovarian veins and through the pelvic veins (Fig. 4.11); it will be accompanied by severe premenstrual discomfort in the pelvis and in limb varicosities (pelvic congestion syndrome). This is closely comparable with the equivalent state, in the male, of incompetence in a testicular vein leading to varicose veins at its lower end, but here outside the pelvis and showing as a varicocele in the scrotum; the venous return from this is to pelvic veins, but it also has easy communication with veins in the upper thigh.

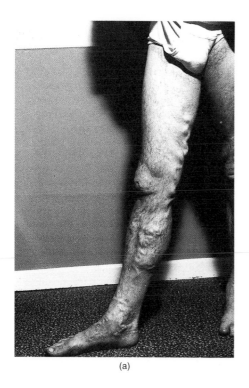

(a)

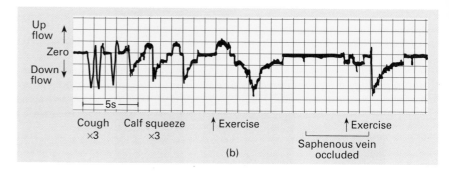

(b)

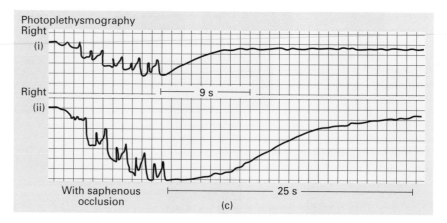

(c)

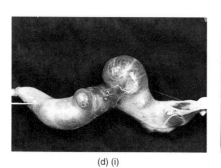

(d) (i)

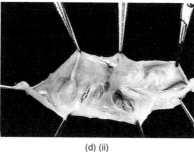

(d) (ii)

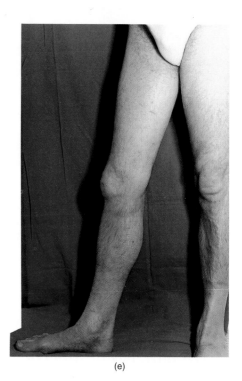

(e)

Fig. 4.5 Long saphenous incompetence: clinical features and investigations.

(a) A massive varicose vein arises from the long saphenous vein in the upper thigh (posteromedial branch in continuity with the arcuate vein) and runs down the length of the limb with branches continuing on to the foot. The presence of skin pigmentation indicates that downflow in the superficial veins is overwhelming the musculovenous pump sufficiently to cause venous hypertension. Selective (Trendelenburg) occlusion and Perthes' test were strongly positive.

(b) Doppler flowmetry to the long saphenous vein shows downflow after squeezing the calf and after exercise, but it is delayed when the saphenous vein is occluded by finger pressure.

(c) (i) Photoplethysmogram showing a refilling time of 9 s after five exercise movements.

(ii) Photoplethysmogram repeated whilst the saphenous vein is occluded by finger pressure. The response is much stronger and the refilling time is now 25 s. These tests strongly indicate that surgery to remove the long saphenous vein and varicosities should give a good result.

(d) Portion of the thigh varicosity after surgery: (i) Distended with saline to show sacculation in thinned and weakened walls; (ii) The vein opened to show its interior. Deep saccules are evident but no valves can be recognized. It is not known whether the weakened and expanded walls are a primary phenomenon or are secondary to the stress of turbulent downflow.

(e) Appearance 3 months after surgery. Discomfort has been relieved, there are no visible varicose veins, and pigmentation is much less. Photoplethysmography showed refilling in the normal range at 25 s.

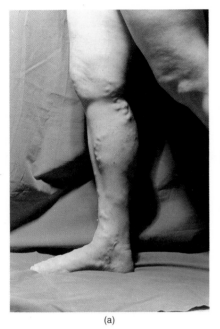

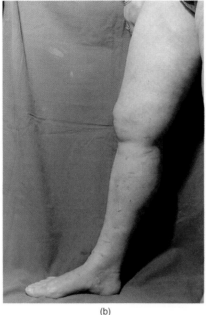

(a)　　　　　　　　　　(b)

Fig. 4.6 Long saphenous incompetence: relief of symptoms with improved appearance and minimal scars. (a) Varicose veins, following two pregnancies, causing much discomfort, particularly around time of menstruation; large varicose veins can be seen running across the front of the ankle on to the foot. All tests and investigations were similar to those of the patient illustrated in Fig. 4.5. (b) Three months after surgery. Discomfort has gone and the patient is pleased with the appearance. Only small incisions closed with subcuticular stitches were used, or stab incisions and adhesive tape, in order to minimize scars.

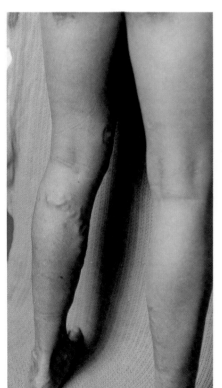

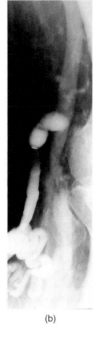

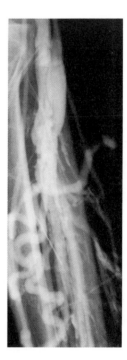

(b)

(a)

Fig. 4.7 Short saphenous incompetence and varicose veins in a young woman with a strong family history of vein problems. (a) Appearance of left limb. All clinical tests and special investigations confirmed short saphenous incompetence. (b) A phlebogram was obtained to show the level and manner of saphenous termination to guide the surgeon. It shows an enlarged saphenous vein terminating at the most common level and the varicose vein arising from it in upper calf.

Fig. 4.8 Interconnection between the long and short saphenous systems. This is commonplace, and the phlebogram here shows a varicose vein running obliquely from the short saphenous vein in the upper calf to join the long saphenous vein down which incompetent flow continued.

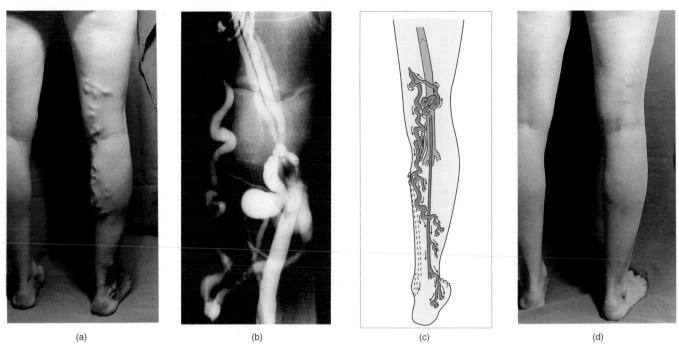

(a)   (b)   (c)   (d)

Fig. 4.9 Deceptive varicose veins. This varicose vein, in the mother of three children, had recently enlarged and caused discomfort. (a) On inspection, the vein shown here might be assumed to have an origin in the long saphenous vein, but a selective occlusion test showed this was not so; however, pressure behind the knee controlled the entire varicose vein and its branches at the ankle. Doppler flowmetry confirmed that, after exercise, flow came up from the popliteal fossa and across to the uppermost visible point of the vein, and then down its length; this flow could be intercepted by finger pressure over the midpopliteal fossa. (b) Phlebography confirmed the origin of the varicosity as a tortuous vein arising from the short saphenous termination and winding upwards before descending posteromedially. (c) Diagram of the distribution of the vein shown by functional phlebography. In the lower leg it connects with both long and short saphenous veins as well as the deep veins by perforators. (d) With a good understanding of the unusual arrangement of this vein it was possible to remove it completely, with relief of symptoms and the improved appearance shown here.

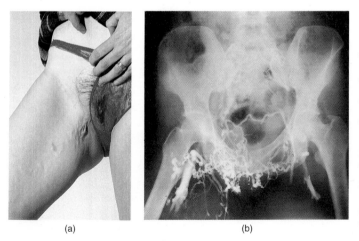

(a)   (b)

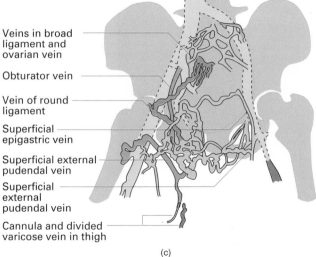

Veins in broad ligament and ovarian vein

Obturator vein

Vein of round ligament

Superficial epigastric vein

Superficial external pudendal vein

Superficial external pudendal vein

Cannula and divided varicose vein in thigh

(c)

Fig. 4.10 Pelvic source of superficial incompetence. (a) A pudendal varicose vein taking its source from pelvic veins. The patient had developed large vulval varices during pregnancy, but these subsided after childbirth leaving the vein shown here. (b) Phlebogram obtained through the pudendal varicosity during surgery. (c) Explanatory diagram of connections with pelvic veins. The internal pudendal vein, not identified here, is commonly implicated.

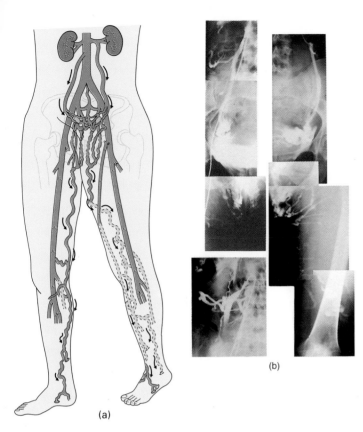

(a)

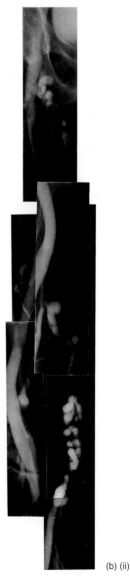

(b)

Fig. 4.11 Ovarian vein incompetence. (a) Diagram of ovarian vein incompetence. One or both ovarian veins becomes the source of a pathway of incompetence, leading down to the pelvic veins and through internal pudendal, round ligament, and obturator veins to emerge as pudendal varicosities in the upper thigh; from here an extensive pattern of varicose veins runs down the limb. (b) Clinical example (pelvic congestion syndrome) in a patient aged 39, the mother of three children. Bilateral descending ovarian phlebograms obtained by transfemoral vein catheterization are shown; the lower left frame gives further detail of ovarian vein catheterization. On both sides medium flows down the ovarian veins and via a plexus of pelvic veins to perivulval and thigh varicosities; on the left side it reaches knee level. At operation both ovarian veins and the pelvic plexuses arising from them were largely removed, together with extensive removal of varicose veins in both lower limbs. This brought the patient complete relief from long-standing disabling premenstrual pain and frequency of micturition. (By courtesy of Mr J. Hobbs.)

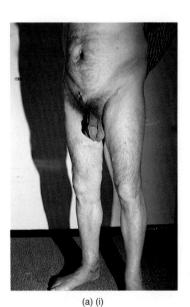

(a) (i)

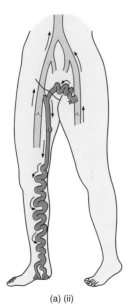

(a) (ii)

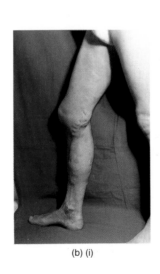

(b) (i)

(b) (ii)

Fig. 4.12 Other patterns of incompetence.
(a) Intricate patterns of incompetence. (i) Crossover incompetence. Clinical appearance showing pubic varicosities, originating from the stump of a ligated long saphenous vein on the left side and providing the origin for substantial long saphenous incompetence, with venotensive changes, on the right side. (ii) Explanatory diagram.
(b) Paradoxical upflow. (i) These recurrent varicosities followed long saphenous surgery and appeared to have their source in midthigh. However, the varicose veins and the Doppler downflow in them were controlled by pressure in the upper popliteal fossa, and from here Doppler upflow to the midthigh was detected after exercise and in unison with the pattern of downflow in the varicose veins. (ii) Composite phlebogram explaining this paradoxical flow. The varicosity originates from an upward extension of the short saphenous vein; there is also a lesser contribution from a long saphenous stump in the groin.

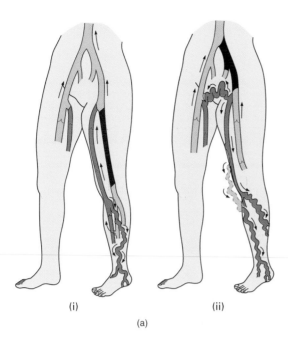

(i)　　　　　(ii)

(a)

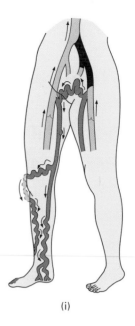

(i)

Fig. 4.13 Complex patterns of incompetence.
(a) Diagrams of complex patterns, combining deep vein impairment with superficial vein incompetence. (i) Varicosities running down to the foot and originating from a long saphenous vein acting as collateral to an occluded femoropopliteal deep vein. (ii) Typical long saphenous incompetence and varicosities below left iliac vein occlusion. This is not uncommon and surgery may endanger pubic collateral veins originating from the saphenous termination.
(b) Crossover incompetence in iliac vein occlusion. (i) Long saphenous incompetence on right side arising from pubic varicosities acting as collaterals to left iliac occlusion. Surgery to the right side could damage this collateral mechanism. (ii) An example of complex crossover incompetence shown by functional phlebography in left iliac occlusion. After three exercise movements, opaque medium injected into calf veins on the left side has travelled preferentially up the left long saphenous vein, across to the opposite side via public collateral varices, and down an incompetent right long saphenous vein, and is seen entering varices in the right thigh. Injection of medium was made at one site on the left leg only.

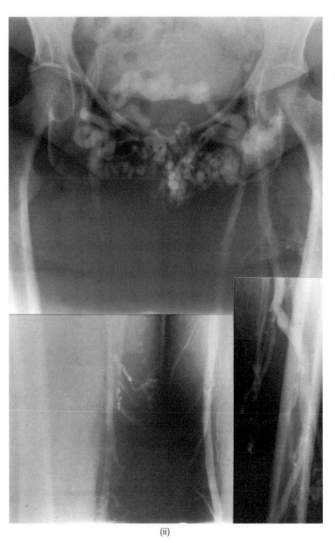

(ii)

(b)

Intricate patterns

These patterns of incompetence follow an unexpected course, either by crossing over from one limb to the other or because flow passes from the source in an upward direction for an appreciable distance before cascading down the limb. An example of the former is long saphenous incompetence taking its origin via pubic varicosities crossing over from a surviving branches in a saphenous stump of the opposite side following inadequate surgery there (Fig. 4.12(a)). An example of paradoxical upward flow can be seen in an extension from the short saphenous vein running upwards to emerge on the inner aspect of mid-thigh and acting as the source of downflow in a long saphenous vein incompetent below this level (Fig. 4.12(b)); high ligation of the long saphenous vein will not cure this condition as the fault does not lie here.

Complex patterns

These occur when deep vein impairment and superficial vein incompetence coexist. Certainly, a saphenous vein acting as a collateral past deep vein occlusion is often oversized and incompetent but, as the predominant flow is continuous collateral upflow, confusion in diagnosis seldom arises. However, when the lower part of the limb has been spared thrombotic damage and is capable of effective pumping to produce an area of low venous pressure, it is possible for incompetent saphenous branches to spill down to the low pressure area and show the features of typical simple varicose veins. For example, if the femoral vein is occluded in mid-thigh, but there is no thrombotic damage to the deep veins below the knee, a saphenous vein acting as collateral may develop varicose side branches running down to the foot (Fig. 4.13(a) (i)). These veins may have no collateral function but become varicose by allowing flow down to the low pressure areas created in foot or lower leg by exercise. Similarly, in iliac vein occlusion, a typical long saphenous vein incompetence, with varicose veins, may develop in the limb beneath this, taking its source from the collateral flow passing from the common femoral vein to the uppermost saphenous branches and across the pubic region (Fig. 4.13(a) (ii)). A crossover variety of this type occurs when an incompetent long saphenous vein of the opposite limb takes its source from pubic collaterals that have crossed over to join its superficial epigastric and pudendal branches (Figs 4.13(b) (i) and 4.13(b) (ii)). It is important to recognize this, since otherwise surgery to treat apparently simple saphenous incompetence may damage valuable collateral vessels.

Box 4.2   Sources of retrograde circuit

Most common sources:

- saphenofemoral (long saphenous) junction
- saphenopopliteal (short saphenous) junction
- upper level (relative to pathway of incompetence) perforating veins, for example mid-thigh or mid-leg to varicose veins running to foot

Less common sources:

- ovarian vein via pelvic veins to up thigh
- pelvic veins to upper thigh
- crossover incompetence via pubic veins from saphenous stump of opposite side
- from pubic or inguinal veins that are collaterals for obstructed iliac veins on the same or opposite side
- from superficial veins (such as long or short saphenous veins) acting as collaterals to obstruction in main deep veins in the limb

Deceptive sources:

- From veins running upwards for an appreciable distance from the uppermost short saphenous vein or its Giacomini branch.
- From one or more gastrocnemius veins via a mid-leg perforator.

Causation of incompetence in valves of superficial veins

The central feature of superficial vein incompetence is lack of effective valves in these veins. This may arise because there is an inborn weakness in the valve cusps or the vein wall, or there is a deficiency in the number of valves. Many patients give a family history suggesting an inherited defect, and the fact that simple varicose veins not infrequently first appear at the age of 14 or 15 supports the belief that some form of inborn weakness is responsible in at least some patients. Some authorities believe that the fault is in the vein walls which allow valve cusps to separate and leak. This may certainly be true, but examples are seen where virtually no valves are present, or only vestigial ones, in the superficial veins concerned. It is likely that there are several different causes for valve failure, each leading to the same final result of incompetence and varicose veins. (See also the section on the spectrum of valve deficiency in Chapter 5, p. ??).

Aggravating factors

Many varicose veins first appear in pregnancy, and although most will recede again others will persist (Fig. 4.14). A probable mechanism is the dilating effect of oestrogen upon the vein walls, affecting their role in retaining valve cusps in good apposition and uncovering any imperfections. Apart from this, women are more prone to superficial vein incompetence than men in a ratio of about 2:1, again probably due to hormonal influence; this is supported by the fact that women's varicose veins are always more troublesome and prominent just before menstruation. Jobs involving prolonged standing have been shown to increase the likelihood of varicose veins and the incidence increases with age.

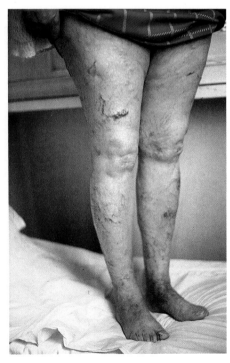

Fig. 4.14 Pregnancy can produce a widespread profusion of varicosities, including intradermal venules. These usually disappear when pregnancy is over but persisted in this patient.

Box 4.3 What causes veins to become varicose?

Three theories

1. Valves, perhaps deficient in quality or number, become incompetent with time so that turbulent downflow occurs, expanding veins in width and length to become tortuous.

2. Vein walls which have an inborn weakness give way to form varicosities, but in this process the valve cusps separate and become incompetent. Thus the leaking valves and retrograde flow are secondary to changes in the walls and are incidental.

3. Forceful outflow from low level perforators expands superficial veins to cause varicosities and leaking valves; this process extends sequentially up the limb. However, most varicose veins do not show outflow in low-level perforators although the veins from high level downwards have obvious incompetence. Moreover, in deep vein obstruction, where heavy outward collateral pumping through perforators is occurring in mid-leg the superficial veins may enlarge but do not become varicose.

Conclusion

It is possible that several varieties of varicose veins and valvular incompetence occur, each developing in differing ways. Certainly weak vein walls giving way seems the most likely explanation of a large group, but in others a deficiency in number and quality of valves is evident from examination of saphenous veins removed at operation. Weak vein walls and turbulent flow from leaking valves will combine to enhance the changes caused by the other.

Manifestations

Unsightly varicose veins are the most common expression of superficial vein incompetence and women are more likely to complain of this than men. Varying degrees of discomfort are attributed to the clearly visible defect and, although this is usually correct, the possibility of another cause should not be overlooked. However, it is possible for the reverse to be true, and for the patient to have heavy uncomfortable legs caused by substantial superficial vein incompetence but without any visible varicosities. This 'concealed' incompetence is not uncommon and is caused by a 'straight through' variety of saphenous incompetence which connects with perforators without any intervening varicosities (Fig. 4.15); it is essential to confirm this by Doppler flowmetry before making and acting on this diagnosis. Conversely, obvious varicose veins may seem unrelated to symptoms elsewhere in the limb; an example is the misleading pattern of varicosities found in the thigh when a large clearly visible varicosity arises from the saphenous termination and 'bypasses' a competent valve in the uppermost long saphenous vein but then joins this vein in its incompetent lower part (Fig. 4.16).

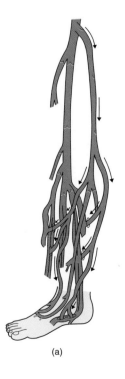

(a)

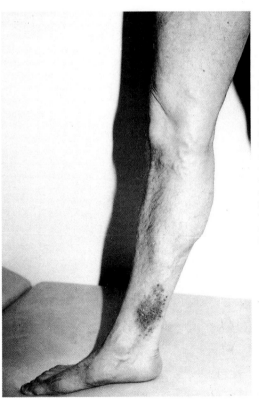

(b)

Fig. 4.15 Concealed superficial vein incompetence. Severe venotensive changes arising from superficial incompetence but not accompanied by obvious varicose veins. (a) Usually a pathway of incompetence includes visible varicose veins arising from a saphenous vein. However, it is possible for retrograde flow from a saphenous vein or posterior arch vein to enter perforating veins directly, without intervening varicose veins, and cause venotension in a relatively concealed fashion as shown in this diagram. (b) Clinical example. This patient's only complaint was of an uncomfortable, itching, and discoloured patch above the ankle. Only one small varicose vein at knee level could be seen but, in fact, a massive incompetence in the long saphenous vein was present, which was detectable by tap-wave and proved by Doppler flowmetry and photoplethysmography. Surgery to this vein relieved the symptoms and the skin changes subsided.

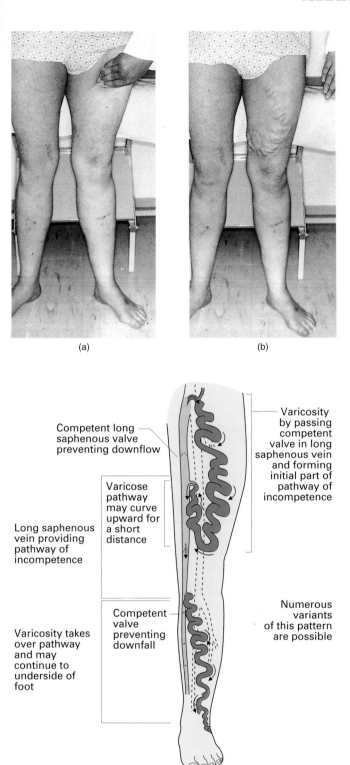

(a)   (b)

Competent long — saphenous valve preventing downflow

Varicosity by passing competent valve in long saphenous vein and forming initial part of pathway of incompetence

Varicose pathway may curve upward for a short distance

Long saphenous vein providing pathway of incompetence

Competent valve preventing downfall

Numerous variants of this pattern are possible

Varicosity takes over pathway and may continue to underside of foot

(c)

Fig. 4.16 Bypassing a valve in superficial incompetence. A functioning valve in a superficial vein is bypassed by a varicose vein which re-enters the incompetent portion of the vein below the valve. (a) Fingertip compression to the upper part of a thigh varicosity (anterolateral branch of saphenous vein) gives complete control, including varicose veins below the knee. (b) Release of compression causes immediate filling to varicose veins in the thigh and leg. At surgery, syringe testing confirmed the presence of a functioning valve in the upper third of the saphenous vein but with gross incompetence below this level. (c) Explanatory diagram. This bypassing phenomenon occurs in many variants and is a common cause of confusion.

The more severe forms of superficial vein incompetence, with or without varicosities, may overwhelm the pumping mechanism and give rise to venous hypertension. In mild cases this may cause an area of pigmentation, swelling, and slight induration near the ankle, perhaps with a tendency for eczema as shown in Fig. 4.17(a); in more severe cases venotensive changes will be more extensive and often include ulceration (Figs 4.17(b) and 4.18, see also Figs 4.28 and 9.2(b)) which is considered later in this chapter and in Chapter 9; the severe states may be aggravated by lymphatic impairment (see 'venous' oedema in Part III) These changes are not specific to superficial vein incompetence (primary varicose veins) and it is important to remember that other venous conditions which create venous hypertension, such as deep vein impairment, can be an even more potent cause but require rather different management.

Box 4.4   Causes of venous hypertension (venotension)

Superficial vein incompetence overwhelming the deep vein pumping mechanism, either because downflow is so heavy or because pumping is relatively weak.

Deep vein impairment
- Post-thrombotic.
- Following injury
- Inborn (primary) deficiency of deep vein valves.
- Congenital failure in normal development of deep veins.

Arteriovenous fistula
- Traumatic
- Congenital

Consequences
Venous hypertension, however caused, results in:
- excess capillary exudate, oedema and pericapillary cuffs of fibrin
- trapping of leucocytes in capillaries with further damage to endothelium and walls, and slowing of microvascular circulation
- reduced nutritional exchange to skin and subcutaneous tissue (fibrosis).
- extravasation of red cells and accumulation of haemosiderin

Clinical changes in affected area:
- oedema
- induration (fibrosis)
- skin pigmentation (haemosiderin)
- increasing damage to skin, eventually with necrosis and ulceration
- vulnerability to infection

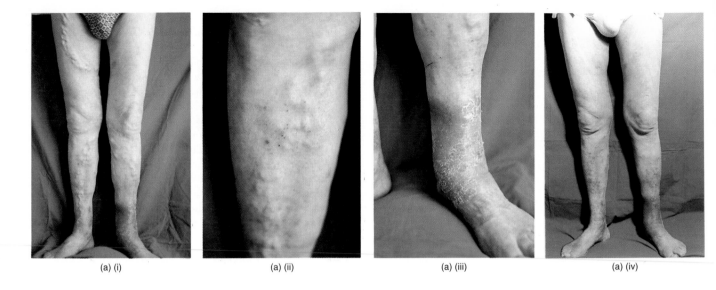

(a) (i) (a) (ii) (a) (iii) (a) (iv)

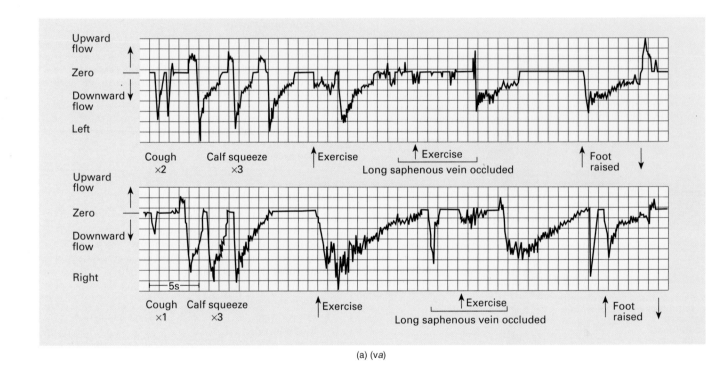

(a) (v*a*)

Fig. 4.17 Consequences of venous hypertension (venotension) in superficial vein incompetence.

(a) Skin changes. (i) A patient with long-standing bilateral long saphenous incompetence. His main complaint was of discomfort and pruritus. (ii) Scratch marks over a varicose vein on the right shin confirm severe pruritus. (iii) Pronounced pigmentation and eczema at the left ankle are accompanied by induration and oedema. An area of eczema on the left inner thigh indicates a general skin sensitization. (iv) All tests confirmed simple incompetence in the superficial veins. Appropriate surgery completely relieved his symptoms and the improved state of the limbs 3 months later is shown here. (v) Preoperative recordings: *a* Doppler flowmetry (long saphenous veins); *b* and *c* Photoplethysmography on both sides. (vi) Postoperative photoplethysmography.

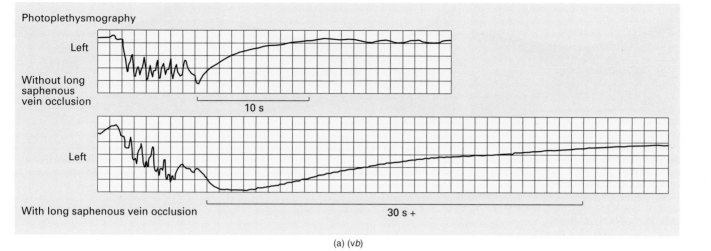

Photoplethysmography

Left

Without long
saphenous
vein occlusion

10 s

Left

With long saphenous vein occlusion   30 s +

(a) (v*b*)

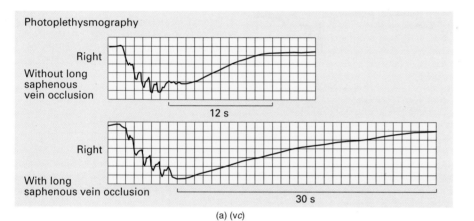

Photoplethysmography

Right

Without long
saphenous
vein occlusion

12 s

Right

With long
saphenous vein occlusion   30 s

(a) (v*c*)

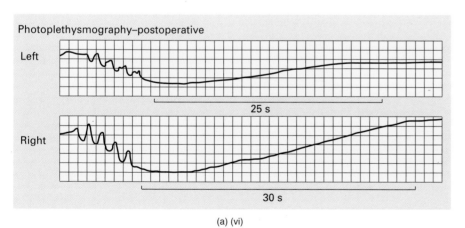

Photoplethysmography–postoperative

Left

25 s

Right

30 s

(a) (vi)

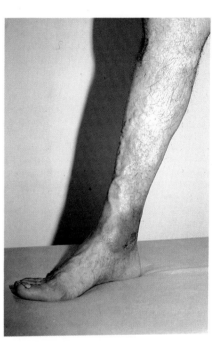

(b) Venotensive changes with a large varicose
vein to the foot. This patient presented with
venotensive pigmentation and a small painful
ulcer near the ankle. A massive anterolateral tibial
varicose vein originated from an incompetent long
saphenous vein and ran on to the foot; Doppler
flowmetry and photoplethysmography fully
confirmed the diagnosis of venous hypertension
from this cause. Surgery was advised but the
patient would only accept sclerotherapy. This
successfully obliterated the tibial varicosity with
complete relief of symptoms and healing of the
ulcer. The ulcer remained healed 1 year later.

Fig. 4.17 (continued).

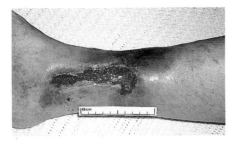

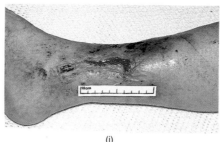

(i)

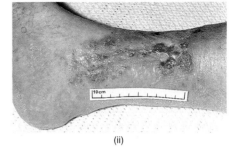

(ii)

(a) The ulcer is surrounded by pigmentation and induration. Its edges show areas of epithelial ingrowth indicating that it is in a healing phase following 10 days of elevation and active movements. Surgery to the long saphenous system was carried out at this stage and the patient was mobilized immediately afterwards.

(b) (i) The ulcer, shown in (a), 1 month after surgery. It is healing well with active epithelial ingrowth. (ii) Two months after surgery the ulcer has healed except for a crusted area in the upper part. At 3 months healing was complete.

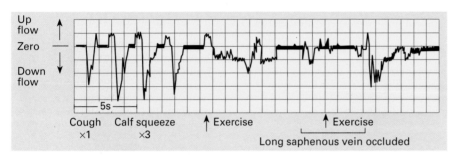

(c) Preoperative investigations. Doppler flow in the long saphenous vein whilst standing, showing downflow on coughing, after calf squeezing, or after exercise, but prevented during saphenous occlusion by finger pressure.

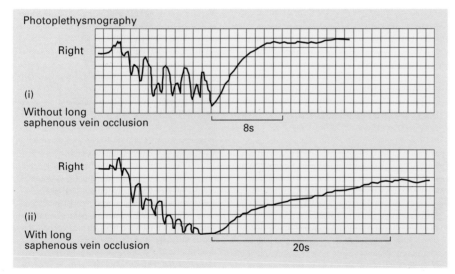

(d) Preoperative investigations.
(i) Photoplethysmography with refilling time of 8 s.
(ii) Refilling time improved to over 20 s when the saphenous vein is occluded by finger pressure.

Fig. 4.18   Severe ulceration caused by long saphenous incompetence. It should be noted that severe ulceration such as this often develops because the musculovenous pumping mechanism is relatively weak and easily overwhelmed by superficial vein incompetence. Removing the factor of superficial incompetence makes it much easier to prevent ulceration but is not a complete cure because the weak musculovenous pump remains barely adequate. This was so in the patient illustrated who returned a year later, threatened with renewed ulceration because she had ceased taking any protective measure. With a policy of elevation whenever possible, and elastic support to the knee, the limb returned to good condition; the patient was urged to maintain these simple protective measures.

Clinical examination and special investigations

The general aspects of this have already been considered in some detail in Chapter 3 and will only be summarized here in relation to superficial vein incompetence. The history must always include enquiry for possible previous deep vein thrombosis with pregnancy, serious illness, or limb fractures. This will give warning that deep vein impairment is possible; it is then essential to examine the lower abdomen and pubic region for varicosities acting as collaterals past occluded iliac veins. The following procedure is appropriate and is carried out with the patient standing, the position in which venous problems become evident.

1. Inspection The general pattern of prominent veins and varicosities on all aspects of the limbs and on the lower abdomen is noted, together with any suggestion of saccules on the saphenous veins (see Fig. 3.1). The lower leg and foot are scrutinized for signs of venotension. If there is any possibility of diabetes the underside of the foot should be inspected to exclude neuropathic ulceration. General medical considerations should not be overlooked at this stage; because varicose veins are an obvious defect, symptoms are often wrongly attributed to them.

2. Mapping out The importance of commencing examination with a careful mapping out of the abnormal veins and other veins connecting with them cannot be overstated. This is done by inspection, palpation, and use of the tap-wave technique (see Fig. 3.2); the foot must be included and, if there is any suspicion of previous deep vein thrombosis, the lower abdomen and pubes. It may be combined with other observations on the varicosities, such as cough impulse and increased warmth; if there is a palpable saccule on a saphenous vein, check for a thrill (by touch, auscultation, or finding a high Doppler velocity) on coughing in keeping with a leaking valve here.

3. Pathway of incompetence The likely pathway of incompetence from which the varicosities arise should be selected, based on the findings at mapping out.

4. Trendelenburg test A selective Trendelenburg test, using compression by finger tips and not any form of tourniquet, should be applied to the suspected pathway of incompetence (see Fig. 3.3). This is the key test upon which diagnosis and decision for treatment depends. Perthes' test, exercising by rising on the toes with the pathway of incompetence occluded, is carried out as useful confirmation of the diagnosis (see Fig. 3.5).

In many cases the examination so far will have given clear evidence of the diagnosis and will have accurately identified the pathway of incompetence. However, sometimes the tests are inconclusive and, in any case, it is always useful to have further confirmation. This is easily and quickly provided by use of the directional Doppler flowmeter.

5. Directional Doppler flowmetry The probe is usually placed over the saphenous vein in the lower thigh or upper calf, and the response to coughing, squeezing the calf, and rising on the toes us noted (see Fig. 3.6). If the pathway of incompetence has been correctly identified, a burst of downflow should follow each exercise movement (Fig. 4.5(b)). If this does not occur, it is possible that the

muscles so far exercised are not involved in the retrograde circuit and the effect of raising the foot clear of the ground, with the knee straight, should be tried. If varicosities run to the foot, this may produce a surprisingly vigorous response.

When downflow has been demonstrated, the test is repeated with the suspected pathway of incompetence occluded by finger pressure well above the probe to confirm that this eliminates the downflow (Fig. 4.5(b)). The Doppler flowmeter is also a valuable tool in mapping out and demonstrating interconnection between veins, for example, between varicose vein and saphenous vein, or long and short saphenous systems. This is done by placing the probe over one vein and giving sharp compression with the fingers to the other vein; if there is any connection the brief movement of blood this causes is easily transmitted to the vein under the probe.

6. Photoplethysmography If obvious venotensive skin changes are present, and particularly if there is ulceration, further evidence will be needed to give positive confirmation of the cause as superficial vein incompetence. This may be elegantly provided by some form of plethysmography, and a simple practical way of carrying this out is by photoplethysmography (see Fig. 3.8). It can be used to demonstrate that an abnormally brief recovery time after exercise is restored to near normal when the suspected pathway of incompetence is selectively occluded by finger pressure (not a constricting band) (Fig. 4.5(c)). An unequivocal response can be accepted as sufficient evidence, but if there are any remaining doubts, functional phlebography or ultrasonography may be advisable to exclude deep vein impairment.

7. Functional phlebography This should not be carried out routinely in varicose vein cases but only when there are special features that require clarification. This method has already been discussed (Fig. 3.11), but the indications and findings in superficial vein incompetence are summarized here.

- It gives positive identification of simple incompetence and demonstrates its source if other means have failed to do this.

- It gives reassurance that the deep veins are normal and well valved or, conversely, that some form of deep vein impairment is present.

- It assists the surgeon by displaying variable anatomy such as the termination of the short saphenous vein.

- It identifies an unusual source of incompetence, such as the pelvic veins.

The features of superficial vein incompetence typical of varicose veins are as follows.

- Demonstration of enlarged and tortuous veins arising from a pathway of incompetence such as a saphenous vein.

- Downward flow in varicosities immediately following an exercise movement and entering the deep veins by perforators lower in the limb (Fig. 4.19).

- When the deep veins have been passively filled, this will confirm their normal outline and also give opportunity to demonstrate the source of incompetence. The patient is asked to exercise by rising on his toes several times and the area of the suspected source is closely watched on the image intensifier. It is often possible to see spillover from deep to superficial veins, with flow down the pathway of incompetence (Figs 4.19(b), 4.19(c), and

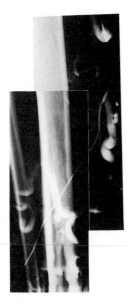

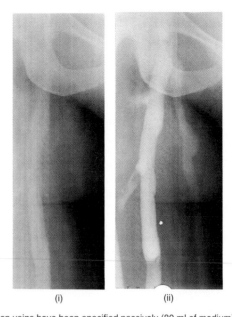

(i)   (ii)

(a) Opaque medium (3 ml) has been injected into a varicose vein in mid-calf and is shown here after one exercise movement. The opacified blood was seen to sweep down the varicose vein and enter the tibial deep veins. This is characteristic of the retrograde circuit in superficial vein incompetence.

(b) (i) The deep veins have been opacified passively (80 ml of medium), with the patient standing still. The common femoral vein is weakly outlined.
(ii) The patient is asked to make two exercise movements, rising on the toes and down again. The view shown here was taken immediately afterwards. Opacified blood has been pumped upwards and some has outlined an incompetent long saphenous vein as blood spills down it and to the deep veins of the leg made slack by the muscle contractions.

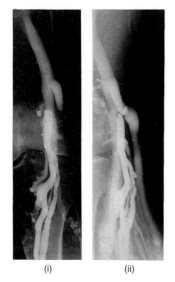

(i)   (ii)

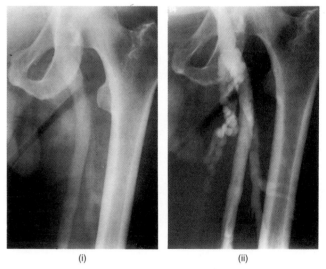

(i)   (ii)

(c) Similar spillover and down an incompetent short saphenous vein.
(i) Before exercise. (ii) After exercise.

(d) Spillover outlining a recurrence after ligation of the long saphenous vein.
(i) Before exercise. (ii) After exercise. There is increased density of medium in the femoral vein and a varicosed reconnection has been outlined by downflow to join an unstripped long saphenous vein.

Fig. 4.19 Functional phlebography (also Fig. 3.11). Patient in the near-vertical position.

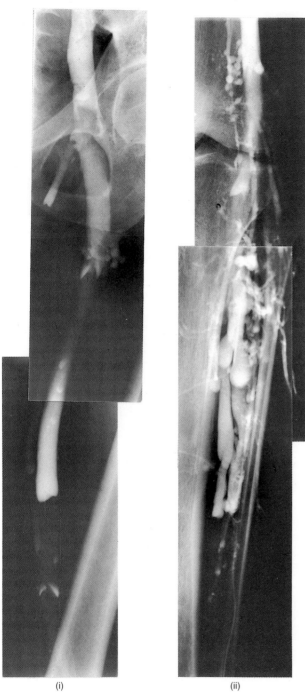

(i)   (ii)

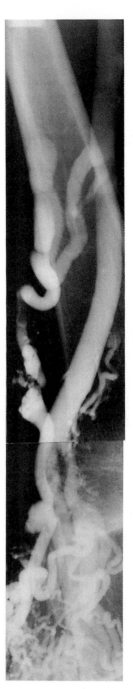

Fig.. 4.19 (continued).

(e) Assessment of valves in deep veins by the swill test. (i) Good valves shown in superficial femoral vein. A valve at the commencement of the profunda femoris is faintly shown and the upper long saphenous vein shows two competent valves. (ii) A series of valves displayed in the tibial veins.

(f) Phlebogram displaying the short saphenous termination prior to surgery. This vein shows unexpected tortuosity and terminates at an unusually high level.

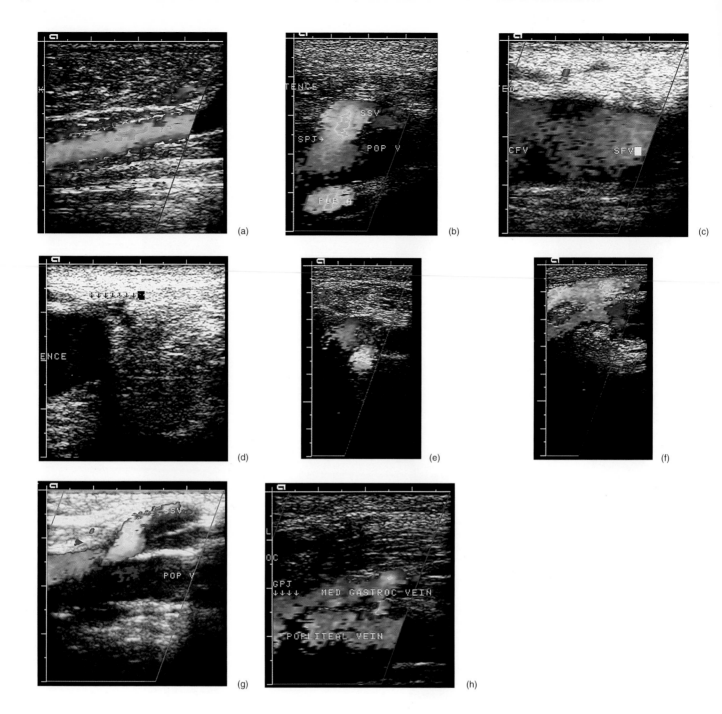

Fig. 4.20   Ultrasonography allows rapid assessment of superficial veins at any level (a) a long saphenous vein in mid-thigh shows incompetent downward (red) flow after release of manual calf compression. It is joined by a perforator. (b) Incompetence in short saphenous system shown by reflux at saphenopopliteal junction (see also Fig. 3.13).

Looking for recurrence at sites of previous ligations of saphenofemoral junction. (c) On the right side there is no recurrence. (d) On the left a definite surviving tributary is seen (marked by a series of arrows). This may account for recurrent varicosities but other possibilities, such as a mid-thigh perforator, should also be looked for. Looking for the source of recurrence. (e) There is no sign of recurrence at previous ligation in groin; (f) The saphenopopliteal junction shows heavy reflux into the short saphenous system. The double channel in its upper part denotes a Giacomini vein which shares in the incompetence and should be removed at surgery.

Preoperative viewing of the popliteal fossa may show anatomical features important to the surgeon. (g) An incompetent saphenopopliteal juction at normal level is shown by strong downward flow but the dark outline of a gastrocnemius vein joins the short saphenous vein close to the junction; this showed no evidence of incompetence and could be preserved at surgery. (h) A gastrocnemius vein is seen to join the popliteal vein and showed only upward flow without any incompetence. This is a normal vein and should be left undisturbed.

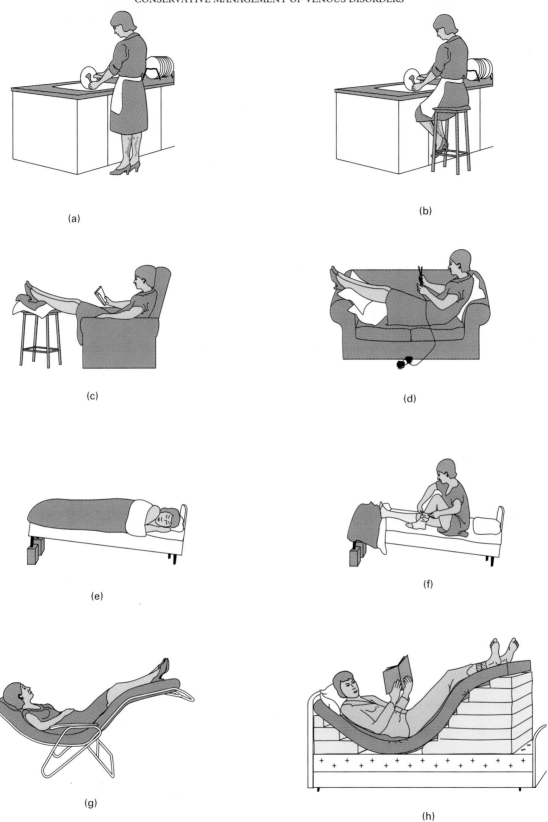

Fig. 4.21 Conservative management of venous disorders. General instructions for the patient, designed to minimize venous hypertension. (a) Avoid standing like this. (b) Sit whenever you can. (c), (d) Make several opportunities during the day, and particularly in the evening, to sit with legs raised high, above the level of your heart. (e) Many hours of valuable elevation can be achieved at night by raising the foot of the bed. (f) Put on elastic stockings before getting up. (g) Investment in a specially designed chair may be better than improvisation, and will encourage maximal use. It should be remembered that every moment that the legs are fully elevated they are improving, but when down, even with stockings, they are deteriorating, particularly when standing still. The patient should be active, but take every opportunity to elevate, particularly if ulceration threatens. (h) Sustained high elevation will be required for active venous ulceration. Blocks of 10 cm (4 in) polyurethane foam can be used to form a shaped overlay on a bed. The limbs and feet should be moved frequently.

4.19(d)), but the radiologist must be given clear guidance by the surgeon upon the probable source.

- The swill test will give an overall impression of valves in the deep veins and will often give additional information about the source and pathway of incompetence (Fig. 4.19(e)).

- In short saphenous and recurrent varicosities it may be easiest to locate the source by varicography, using the upward trace technique as described in Chapter 3. The flow of medium will often follow the pathway of incompetence upwards and, via the source, into the deep veins (Fig. 4.19(f)). This upward flow is capricious and may be diverted before it reaches the objective, but usually succeeds. The fact that the patient is now near horizontal means that the veins are semicollapsed and this makes it more difficult to evaluate the importance of veins displayed.

8. **Ultrasonography** Ultrasonography by B-mode duplex scanning or colour flow imaging, as described in Chapter 3 (see Figs 3.13–3.16) is particularly useful in short saphenous incompetence where it can give positive confirmation of downflow in an incompetent vein and display the level of short saphenous termination. Similarly, it can be used to display details of incompetence in a gastrocnemius vein causing perforator outflow in the calf, or in a groin recurrence (Fig. 4.20).

Treatment of superficial vein incompetence and its manifestations

Varicose veins without accompanying venotensive changes

Three levels of treatment can be recognized: cosmetic, alleviation of symptoms, and elimination of the underlying incompetent veins to give a lasting cure.

Cosmetic treatment

Lesser varicose veins can be disguised by appropriate make-up or the use of elastic support hose. Some patients will settle for these options, but most will want the unsightly varicosities banished so that in summer the uncovered limb is blemish free. Sclerotherapy can accomplish this, often with lasting benefit, but in more gross varicose veins the best cosmetic result, and the most lasting, will be given by appropriate surgery, eliminating the source of incompetence without obvious scars, a skill the surgeon should be able to offer.

Dermal flares of fine intradermal venules and telangectasia can be treated successfully by microslerotherapy, using a very fine needle and diluted sclerosant and probably requiring several sessions (see Figs 4.24(c), 4.25, and 4.26). These disfiguring small veins can also be treated by laser or high-intensity light therapy, which is increasingly being used.

Relief of symptoms

Symptoms of heaviness and tiredness accompanying varicose veins can certainly be relieved by use of elastic support hose or elastic stockings (see Fig. 6.5(c)), combined with a policy of elevating the limb whenever possible (Fig. 4.21). However, this is not a cure and elastic support is often tedious to wear, particularly in hot weather. The most effective method will be the elimination of superficial vein incompetence by sclerotherapy or by surgery.

Elimination of the underlying cause

Treatment here will aim at a cure, i.e. complete elimination of the superficial incompetence which causes the unsightly varicosities and symptoms from venous stress. The essentials are correct identification of the source and pathway of incompetence, and their obliteration by sclerotherapy or by surgery (Fig. 4.22). Most failures in these aims are the result of inaccurate identification of the source or inadequate elimination of the pathway.

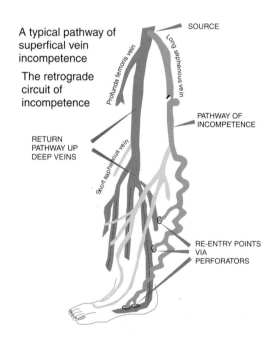

Fig. 4.22 The pathway of incompetence to be obliterated by sclerotherapy or surgery. This should include the source whenever possible. Sclerotherapy or multiple varicectomy through stab incisions, obliterating a major part of the pathway but leaving the saphenous vein intact, may give a satisfactory result in selected cases in order to preserve the saphenous vein for possible arterial reconstruction or coronary artery bypass. However, an incompetent saphenous vein is not always suitable for this purpose.

Box 4.5 The key principle in treating superficial incompetence and varicose veins

Accurate identification and obliteration of the pathway of incompetence and its source (Fig. 4.22)
The more completely this is done, the better the immediate and long-term result. The varicose veins are the peripheral part of the pathway of incompetence and must be eliminated as far as possible.
Obliteration can be achieved by:

- **sclerotherapy** — using the empty vein–compression technique to obliterate the pathway, including the varicosities
- **surgery** — removing the source, the main pathway, and the peripheral pathway (the varicosities)

Pros and cons
Sclerotherapy is very successful in eliminating the varicose peripheral pathway but less satisfactory in closing the proximal or truncal pathway, typically a saphenous vein, and may be unable to eliminate the actual source (but many Continental specialists dispute this and regularly inject the saphenous vein at high level). It is easily done in an outpatient clinic and full mobility is encouraged immediately afterwards; there is usually little discomfort but the patient may find the bandages tedious. It requires several weeks of compression bandaging, may leave brown staining for several months, and has an appreciable recurrence rate.

   Surgery aims to remove the source and main pathway of incompetence directly; the peripheral pathway of varicosities is removed by multiple stab incisions. Scars should be insignificant with a good cosmetic result. It can be done as a day patient under general or local anaesthesia, but a brief admission may be preferred. Early active mobility is encouraged with only light elastic support. Usually, there is little discomfort and a good long-term result, but residual veins and recurrences are again possible. Is considered more likely to be successful than sclerotherapy when a large set of veins have to be treated.

Indications
Sclerotherapy:

- suitable for lesser or localized varicosities, as a first form of treatment, or when the source is not clear
- for residual or small recurrent varicose veins after surgery
- for intra- and subdermal venules and telangectasia
- may be used in selected cases of ulcer or to eliminate a vein prone to haemorrhage when surgery is contraindicated.

Surgery:
Where there is a well-defined source and pathway with substantial varicose veins

- when sclerotherapy has not been successful or is contraindicated
- when superficial vein incompetence is causing venotensive changes, such as pigmentation or actual ulceration
- in the long-term treatment of haemorrhage or superficial thrombophlebitis

Contraindications

- the patient who is unable to walk is *not* suitable for sclerotherapy and surgery should seldom be advised; conservative treatment should be employed.
   General infirmity or ill health.
   The contraceptive pill: this offers a very small risk depending on its content but there may be greater risks in withdrawal. The patient should discuss this with her physician (see also Box 4.8).
   Pregnancy: active treatment is best postponed until several months after childbirth when the varicose veins will have subsided spontaneously in many cases. Suitable elastic support is a much wiser alternative to active treatment in pregnancy.

Note: Certain specific contraindications to sclerotherapy are given in the next section

Comment
Assuming that treatment is of a high standard, both methods can give good result. The authors believe that in well-established varicose veins surgery is most likely to give a good long-term result with least disturbance to the patient. There is a considerable variation in patient response and the skill of application of the method employed. **In general it seems reasonable to use sclerotherapy for the lesser problems and surgery for the more extensive ones.**

   Whichever method is used, a saphenous vein should never be sacrificed without good reason; it may be required sooner or later for reconstructive arterial surgery. However, an incompetent long saphenous vein often has areas of weak wall and is not satisfactory for use as an arterial conduit so that undue efforts to preserve it may not be justified.

Compression sclerotherapy

In this method a suitable chemical, such as 3 per cent sodium tetradecylsulphate, is injected into the varicose veins or the pathway of incompetence leading to them; this will destroy the endothelium and create a reaction within the veins that eventually seals them into a fibrous cord. An 'empty vein–compression bandage' technique is used to achieve this goal. The veins to be treated are identified whilst the patient is standing (Figs 4.23 and 4.24(a)) and likely sites of injection are marked with a felt-tipped pen. Injection into an artery is a grave hazard likely to cause extensive gangrene; this is most likely to happen in the vicinity of the ankle and this area should be avoided as far as possible. Although anaphylaxis is rare, measures to combat it must be at hand (adrenaline, hydrocortisone, antihistamine, intubation).

Box 4.6   Basic principles in compression sclerotherapy (see Fig. 4.24)

A small quantity of sclerosant is injected into a vein emptied by elevation of limb to ensure maximal effect on endothelium.

After a short interval, with the limb still in elevation, compression bandage is applied to press vein walls together. This is to prevent entry of blood which would clot and allow eventual recanalization; equally importantly, it will hold vein walls together whilst a fibrous bonding forms between them over the next few weeks to permanently seal the vein.

Immediately after injection and bandaging the patient is asked to exercise vigorously and to follow a daily programme of exercise. This is to combat clotting extending into the deep veins.

Compression bandaging is maintained for at least 3 weeks.

The patient is then repositioned sitting up on a couch with the lower limbs horizontal (Fig. 4.23(c)), or with the legs over the edge in moderate dependency to give slight distension of the veins (Fig. 4.24(a)). Needles, with syringes containing sclerosant attached, are inserted into selected veins and taped to the skin (Figs 4.23(d) and 4.24(a)). The patient then lies flat, the limb is elevated to empty the veins, and the sclerosant is injected (Figs 4.23(j)–4.23(n) and 4.24(b)). In this way, a small quantity of sclerosant produces maximum effect without causing blood clot. While the limb is still in elevation, pressure pads are placed over the sites of injection and a firm bandage is applied (Figs 4.23(o)–4.23(v) and 4.24(b)). This prevents blood from re-entering the veins when the patient stands and minimizes clot formation; it also presses the inner walls together to ensure that they will bond firmly with fibrous tissue. Provided that the veins are kept empty in this fashion, little discomfort follows the procedure and obliteration of the vein is likely to be permanent (Figs 4.23(w) and 4.23(x)). Compression is maintained for at least 3 weeks and the patient is asked to exercise freely to discourage clotting spreading to the deep veins (Fig. 4.24(b)). Failure to apply effective compression will cause the injected veins to distend with clot (Fig. 4.24(b)) so that they are painful (in fact, an induced superficial thrombophlebitis) and eventual recanalization of

---

Box 4.7   Materials required for compression sclerotherapy (medium to large veins)

Skin sterilizing swabs and marking pen
Needles (25 G × 5/8 in)
Syringes (2 ml disposable)
Ampoules of sclerosant: 3 per cent sodium tetradecyl sulphate (STD or Fibro-vein), or 3 per cent hydroxypolyethoxydocan (polidocanol) (Aethoxyskerol) (see note below)
Pads for compressing vein locally
Cotton crepe bandage (3 in) for applying next to skin
Elastic adhesive bandage (3 in) for putting as crossply over the crepe bandage
Elastic support as stocking or tubular bandage
Plastic foam block 18 in high upon which is elevate the limb
Rayon (Micropore) adhesive tape (1/2 in)

To have nearby as safety measures:

- Adrenalin for intramuscular injection (1 ml of 1:1000)
- Hydrocortisone for intravenous use (100 mg ampoule)
- Antihistamine for intravenous use (10 mg chlorpheniramine maleate)
- Heparin (and normal saline) (1000 units in 1 ml ampoule)
- Means of laryngeal intubation

Additional information
The sclerosants listed above are supplied in a range of concentrations used according to the size of veins being treated.
Sodium tetradecyl sulphate (formerly marketed as STD but now as Fibro-vein):
3 per cent — suitable for medium to large size veins and varicostities.
1 per cent — suitable for small veins and larger venules. Use 27 G needle.
0.5 per cent — suitable for medium-size venules. Use 27 G needle.
0.2 per cent — suitable for fine telagectasia and fine venous flares. Use 30 G needle. Best used with a microsclerotherapy set where the needle is mounted on flexible tubing with an attachment for the syringe at the near end. This arrangement gives maximum sensitivity, without the weight of the syringe, for insertion of the needle into very fine vessels. (See Figs 4.24(c), 4.25 and 4.26.).

Similarly, polidocanol (Aethoxyskerol) is sold in a range of concentrations appropriate for their intended use.

---

the vein is likely to occur; in a substantial vein, such as a saphenous vein, this will destroy any remaining valve function so that if the vein reopens it is a large conduit devoid of any restraint by valves and the recurrent state may be more severe than the original one. Although the method is very effective in small to medium calibre veins it does tend to give only temporary occlusion of the larger veins, particularly the saphenous vein itself, so that not infrequently recurrence occurs here after a year or two and further treatment is needed.

Fig. 4.23 (a-x) Compression sclerotherapy: empty vein technique.

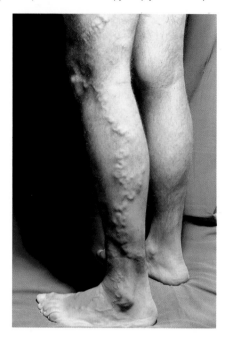

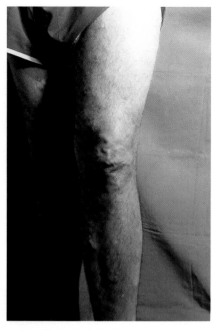

(a) Tortuous outlying varicose veins like this are ideal for compression sclerotherapy.

(b) All veins are identified and suitable sites for injection marked whilst the patient is standing.

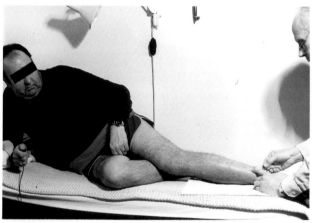

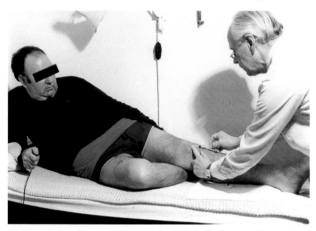

(c) The patient is repositioned on a couch; sitting up helps to keep veins slightly distended.

(d) The needle, with a syringe containing 0.5 ml of sclerosant attached, is inserted into a selected vein.

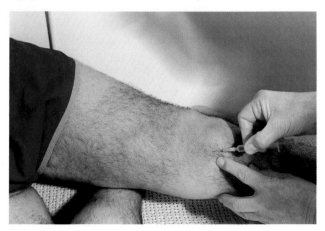

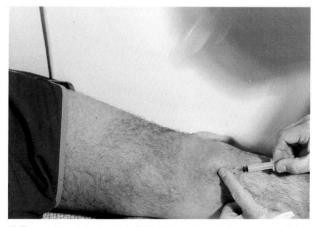

(e) Details of needle insertion. Skin is drawn down and the needle inserted with a lifting action of point to open a vein lumen.

(f) The needle hub is steadied whilst slight suction withdraws a spot of blood to check correct entry into the vein lumen. If there is any hint of arterial backflow reposition needle to vein nearby.

Fig. 4.23   (continued).

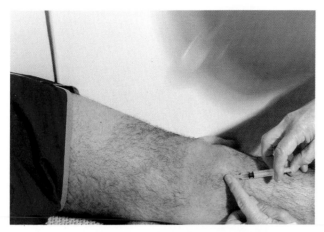

(g) The needle is cleared of blood by a small injection of sclerosant.

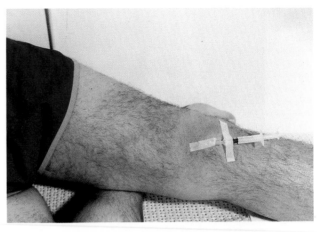

(h) The needle and syringe are taped to the skin.

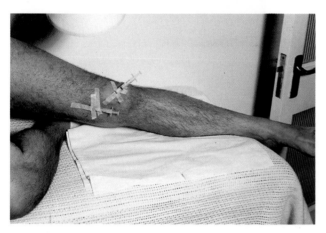

(i) This is repeated at selected sites.

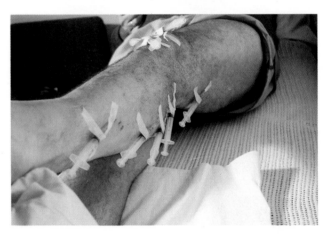

(j) Multiple syringes up the length of the varicose vein, all taped to skin; the foot is elevated to empty the veins.

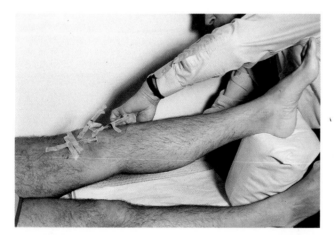

(k) Each syringe delivers the chosen dose (0.5 ml or less, total dose in limb not exceeding 3 ml).

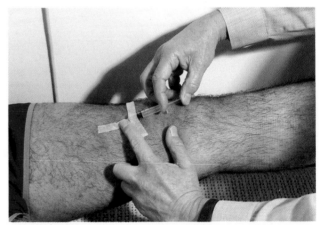

(l) Details of sclerosant delivery. The hub is steadied before the plunger is depressed.

Fig. 4.23 (continued).

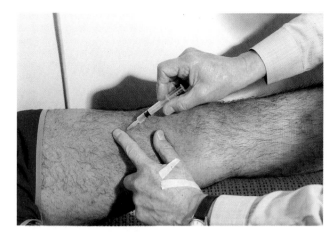

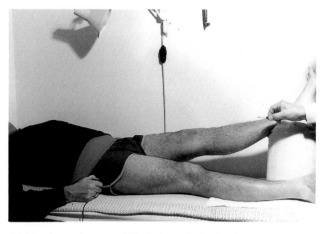

(m) Removing syringes: tapes are removed and the needle is withdrawn with finger pressure over the injection site.

(n) All syringes are removed. The limb remains in elevation.

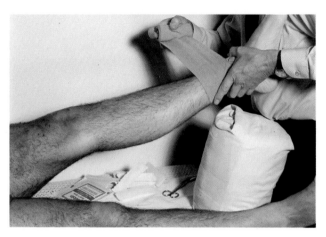

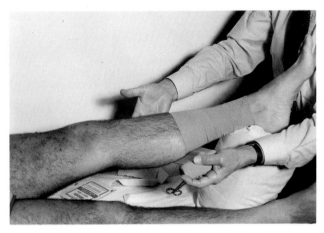

(o) Crepe bandage is applied over cotton pads at each injection site.

(p) Crepe bandage is applied over cotton pads at each injection site.

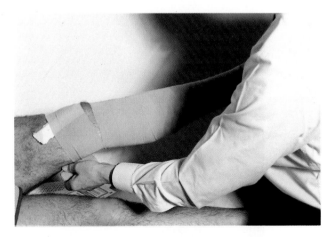

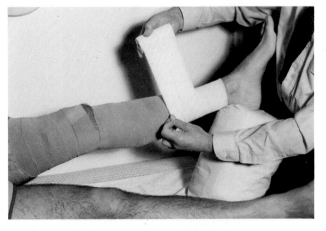

(q) Crepe bandage is applied over cotton pads at each injection site.

(r), (s), (t) The crepe bandage is now locked together by elastic adhesive bandage. A gap is left to permit knee flexion.

Fig. 4.23 (continued).

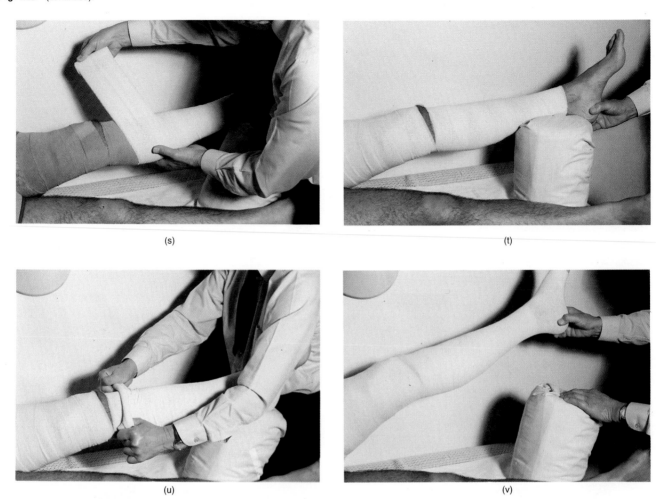

(s)   (t)

(u)   (v)

(u), (v) A tubular bandage or elastic stocking is applied to ensure that the injected veins are kept as empty as possible. This remains in place for 3 weeks, followed by elastic support alone for 2 months.

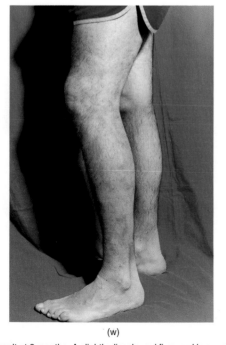

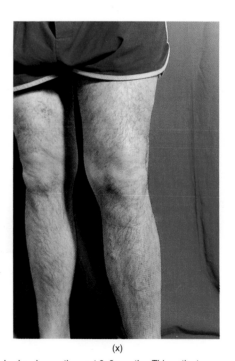

(w)   (x)

(w), (x) Result at 3 months. A slightly discoloured firm cord has replaced the vein: this will slowly absorb over the next 6–9 months. This patient was seen 3 years later and the good result was confirmed.

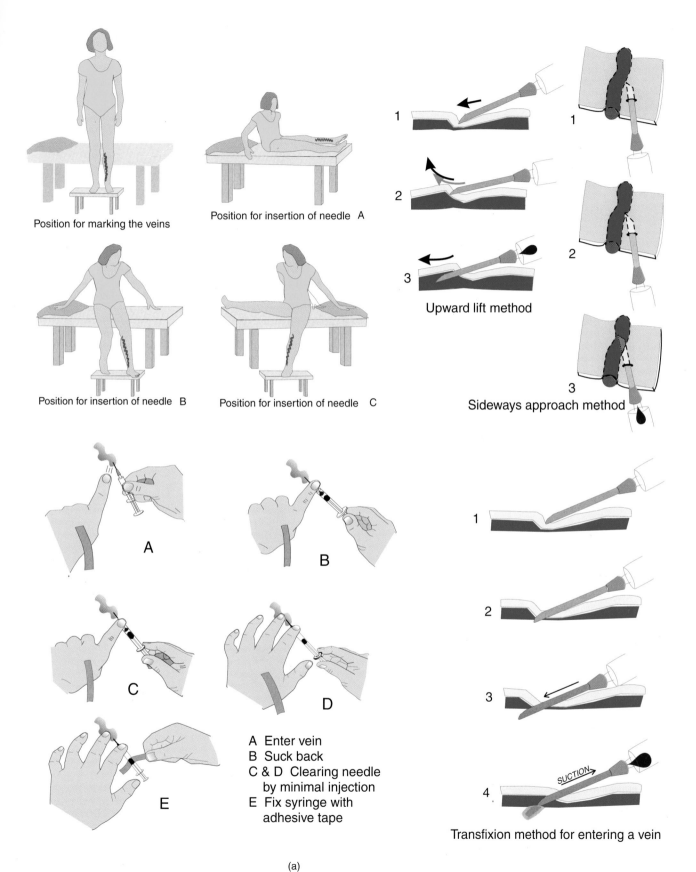

Position for marking the veins

Position for insertion of needle   A

Position for insertion of needle   B

Position for insertion of needle   C

1

2

3

Upward lift method

1

2

3

Sideways approach method

A

B

C

D

E

A Enter vein
B Suck back
C & D Clearing needle
   by minimal injection
E Fix syringe with
   adhesive tape

1

2

3

4 SUCTION

Transfixion method for entering a vein

(a)

Fig. 4.24   Procedure in empty vein–compression sclerotherapy.

(a) *In standing position.* Identify pathway of incompetence, and select and mark sites for injection. *Sitting up on couch with limbs horizontal (or sitting on edge of couch with some dependency of limb).* Insert needle (with attached syringe containing 0.5 ml of sclerosant) into selected vein(s), test aspirate, and then clear needle of blood by a minimal injection. Tape syringe to skin. This can be repeated at up to six sites.

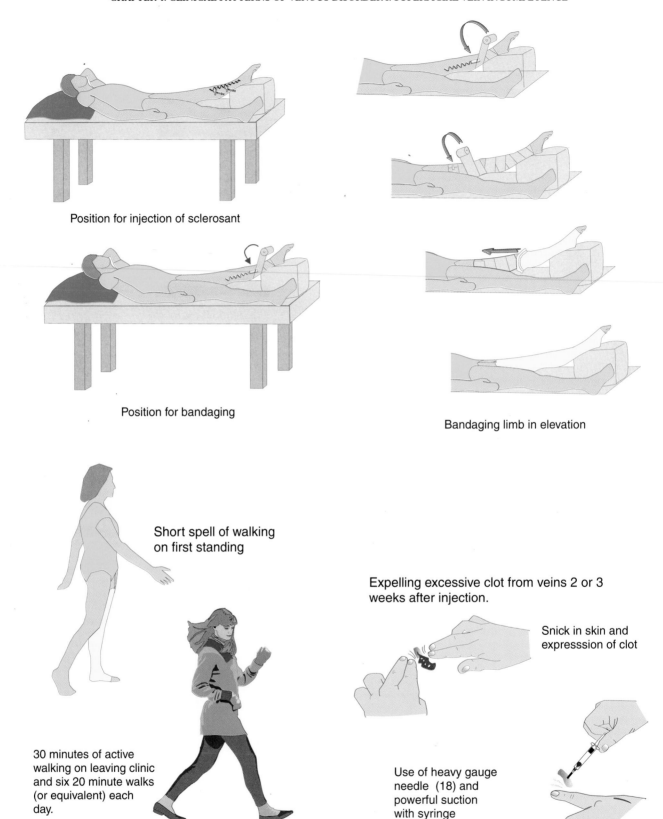

Position for injection of sclerosant

Position for bandaging

Bandaging limb in elevation

Short spell of walking
on first standing

30 minutes of active
walking on leaving clinic
and six 20 minute walks
(or equivalent) each
day.

Expelling excessive clot from veins 2 or 3
weeks after injection.

Snick in skin and
expresssion of clot

Use of heavy gauge
needle (18) and
powerful suction
with syringe

Fig. 4.24

(b) *Patient lying with limb elevated.* Sclerosant now injected at each site. All syringes and needles are removed with brief pressure over injected veins. Cotton or rubber compression pads are placed on each site and a cotton crepe limited-stretch bandage is applied moderately firmly. Elastic adhesive bandage is applied obliquely over the crepe bandage to lock it in position. Elastic support is applied over this, using either an elastic stocking or a tubular elastic bandage (shaped Tubigrip). *The patient is asked to stand and walk about for a minute or so, to turn over vein circulation and disperse any remaining sclerosant.* The patient dresses and sets out immediately on a 20-min walk. An appointment is made for 3 weeks and an instruction sheet is given which includes advice to take 15-min walks at least six times each day, to elevate the feet whenever possible and certainly in the evenings, and to move the feet frequently by ankle movements, perhaps every 5 min. These measures are used to minimize unwanted clotting in stagnant veins. When seen 2 or 3 weeks later some of the injected veins may be uncomfortably distended with dark clot. This should be aspirated through a large-gauge needle or, if necessary, expressed through a 2-mm incision. This immediately relieves the discomfort and avoids a brown staining that can persist for many months.

Microsclerotherapy for telangiectasia (intradermal venules and dermal flares)
Only very dilute (0.25%) sclerosant to be used
For prominent venules a syringe with 30 G needle attached may be used

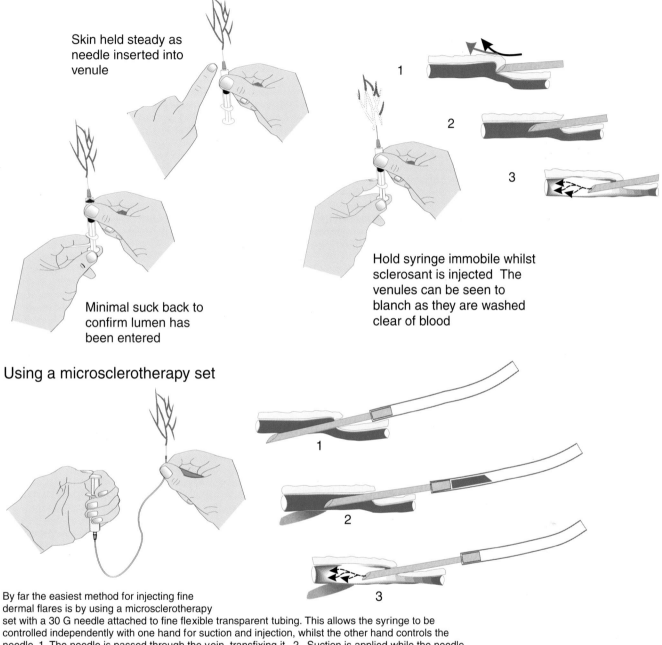

Skin held steady as
needle inserted into
venule

Minimal suck back to
confirm lumen has
been entered

1

2

3

Hold syringe immobile whilst
sclerosant is injected The
venules can be seen to
blanch as they are washed
clear of blood

Using a microsclerotherapy set

1

2

3

By far the easiest method for injecting fine
dermal flares is by using a microsclerotherapy
set with a 30 G needle attached to fine flexible transparent tubing. This allows the syringe to be
controlled independently with one hand for suction and injection, whilst the other hand controls the
needle. 1. The needle is passed through the vein, transfixing it. 2. Suction is applied while the needle
is slowly withdrawn until a fleck of blood appears in the tubing. 3. Sclerosant is then injected - (about
0.25 - 0.5 ml) - which should be seen to wash through the neighbouring area of vessels. This can be
repeated with the same set at a dozen or more sites. Cotton pads and a crepe bandage are used for
24 h afterwards.

(c)

Fig. 4.24

(c) *Microsclerotherapy*. Banishing disfiguring dermal flares by sclerotherapy is an important skill requiring a delicate touch. Once the needle has entered a venule it must be held immobile whilst the other hand depresses the syringe plunger. The same needle and syringe can be used at several sites, and at each the venules should be seen to clear as the sclerosant flushes through them. An easier method using a microsclerotherapy set is also shown. This separates the syringe from the needle (see also Figs. 4.25 and 4.26).

Box 4.8   Difficulties and dangers – how to overcome them

Fainting

Quite common if the patient is standing when needles are inserted — it often occurs before any material is injected (vasovagal attack). Never attempt to inject with the patient standing (particularly on a couch) because the fall accompanying faint may injure patient!

Attack is preceded by restlessness, sighing, perhaps sweating. Lie the patient down immediately and check the pulse — it is probably slow. When the pulse returns to normal strength and rate complete injections with the patient in the lying position.

This is a harmless episode if properly managed but minimize its occurrence by always having the patient in the sitting or lying position during the insertion of needles.

Injection into an artery — a major catastrophe

This will cause rapid onset of severe pain, soon followed by pallor in the affected area, which turns to irreversible gangrene within hours and, if extensive, can lead to loss of limb.
Essential precautions
- Avoid injections near the ankle where arteries are close to the surface and easily entered.
- Always keep the needle tip in sight; never go deeply.
- Always suck back before injecting any sclerosant — if bright red or pulsatile abandon that site and withdraw the needle immediately.
- If pain occurs whilst injecting, cease immediately
- If there is severe pain and pallor develops in the area below the needle, detach the syringe and allow bleed back; inject dilute heparin before removing the needle; admit to hospital and consult with an arterial surgeon urgently.
- Always be conscious of this possibility. *It does happen — do not let it be you!!*

Dosage

Do not exceed the permissible maximum dosage of the sclerosant being used. With 3 per cent sodium tetradecyl sulphate this is 3 ml spread over six sites; the maximum dosage at one site should be 0.5 ml. An excessive dose can enter skin capillaries and cause a scattered skin necrosis.

Subcutaneous injection of the recommended sclerosants is relatively harmless at low dosage, but other older materials not so forgiving and sloughing of skin can follow.

Intradermal injection of sclerosant will cause a small area of skin necrosis. When this is happening the resistance to the syringe plunger is obvious and gives warning that the needle is misplaced — *never force in an injection.*

Allergy

Always enquire about allergies and do not inject a patient known to be allergic to a previous sclerosant.

Anaphylactic shock

Fortunately, this is rare but it is potentially dangerous. It occurs within a few minutes of injection — the patient shows obvious distress, with pallor and breathlessness, rapid weak pulse, and fall in blood pressure. Unlike a fainting attack it does not improve quickly when lying flat but may show progressive severity. *Immediate action must be taken.*

- Give 1 ml of 1:1000 adrenalin intramuscularly
- Follow with 100 mg of hydrocortisone by slow intravenous injection
- Follow with an antihistamine (such as chlorpheniramine maleate 10 mg in 1 ml) by slow intravenous injection (intravenous drip advisable).

(Ampoules of these materials should always be at hand when injecting varicose veins)
Admit to hospital and alert anaesthetist in case intubation is needed

Problems following sclerotherapy

Deep vein thrombosis and pulmonary embolism are known to occur occasionally after sclerotherapy but are rare if the patient follows a programme of active exercise immediately after and in the following few weeks. If the leg is uncomfortable, exercise it! A policy of 'resting the leg' is not permissible after sclerotherapy.

Another important factor is the *contraceptive pill*. The older version with a high oestrogen content is known to cause thrombosis and should certainly be withdrawn before sclerotherapy. Later versions based on progestogen are considered safer, but the patient should discuss this with her physician and, if necessary, use alternative contraception. Patients on other forms of hormone therapy, such as in carcinoma of the prostate, should not be treated without full agreement of appropriate doctor.

Continued

Box 4.8 *Continued*

Sclerotherapy should not cause pain, and complaints of pain that is not relieved by exercise should be investigated. The bandage should be removed and the limb inspected. One of the following may be the cause.

- The bandage is too tight or has slipped. If nothing else appears wrong, reapplication of the bandage or substitution of elastic support should bring relief.
- The injected veins are tense, tender, and distended with clot, and are dark brown in appearance. This is the most common cause of discomfort and is due to unwanted seepage of blood into the veins to form clot — in effect an active induced thrombophlebitis. If left untreated, it will continue causing pain for some weeks and will give rise to pronounced brown staining that will persist for months. Treatment is not difficult; the clot should be aspirated by strong suction through a large-bore needle (Fig. 4.24(b)) and this may be required at several sites up the vein. This manoeuvre causes little discomfort and brings immediate relief. Do not be reluctant to do this — its benefit is obvious! In some cases it may be necessary to make a small stab incision through which the clot can be expelled by moderate pressure. The compression bandage is reapplied or elastic support is substituted according to the stage at which seen, and the patient is encouraged in continued activity.
- In the elderly, the possibility of ischaemic pain must be excluded. Is the foot of good colour and at least one ankle pulse present? Do not reapply compression bandage if there is any doubt and, if necessary, consult an arterial specialist. (Note: pre-existing ischaemia is a strong contraindication to sclerotherapy.)

Summary of post injection programme
The patient is instructed to walk vigorously for 20 min immediately after injections and bandaging are completed (no taxi home!). Thereafter the patient should take at least three walks of a mile each during the day, with any other walking activity that can be fitted in, and in the evening should elevate the feet above the horizontal and move them frequently. Arrange to see the patient again after 3 weeks, but express every willingness to see him or her earlier if problems or undue discomfort occur. At 3 weeks remove the compression bandage and substitute elastic support. Injected veins should be firm, non-tender, and slightly dark in colour. If there is an obvious excess of clot distending the veins, this should be aspirated through a large-bore needle (see above). See the patient again in 6 weeks for final assessment and/or for injections to the opposite limb.

Contraindications to sclerotherapy
- **Ischaemia** is an absolute contraindication. If there are any doubts about a good arterial supply sclerotherapy should *not* be employed. It is a serious error to apply a compression bandage to an ischaemic limb!
- Inability to walk actively. This may be due to arthritis, general infirmity, or ischaemia. Sclerotherapy must be followed by active walking to minimize the possibility of unwanted thrombosis in deep veins.
- Ill health and general infirmity, known malignant disease.
- History of allergy, deep vein thrombosis in the past.
- The contraceptive pill–see above.
- Pregnancy–see Box 4.5, p. 67.

Do not attempt extensive bilateral sclerotherapy at one session. Only when the areas involved are small is it permissible to treat both sides simultaneously.

Microsclerotherapy is essentially the same technique, but on a miniature scale, used to eliminate disfiguring intradermal flares of fine venules (Figs 4.24(c), 4.25, and 4.26). Laser or high-intensity light therapy can also be very successful here.

Sclerotherapy is seldom as complete as surgery in the obliteration of the incompetent veins, and for this reason the patient will often be asked to attend at regular intervals so that further injections may be carried out to any returning varicosities. In this way, for a large set of veins, sclerotherapy tends to be a long-term policy of maintenance rather than the one-time cure intended with surgery. The use of compression bandaging, necessary with sclerotherapy, is undoubtedly tiresome, and patients who have had treatment by both injection and surgery often say that they preferred the surgical treatment. Sclerotherapy has its drawbacks (e.g. a discoloration that may persist for many months afterwards) and, although its exponents appear to overcome these problems effortlessly, it must not be regarded as an easy alternative to surgery with a requirement for little skill; quite the reverse is true. Injection into an artery, referred to above, is a potential disaster which must never be forgotten; if, on sucking back, the needle produces any hint of arterial blood, by colour or pulsatile reflux, it should not be used but immediately repositioned elsewhere. Nevertheless, sclerotherapy is a most valuable method of treatment and in the case of lesser veins can often accomplish treatment that is scarcely possible for surgery. Perhaps the most reasonable view is to use surgery for the well-defined patterns of saphenous incompetence, and to use sclerotherapy to back this up when necessary or in the treatment of lesser varicosities. The combination of sclerotherapy with surgical treatment is discussed in the section on the treatment of recurrent varicose veins.

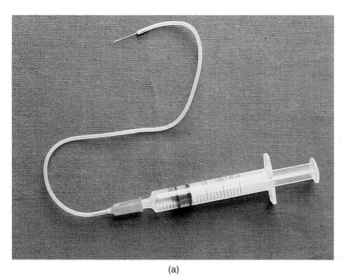

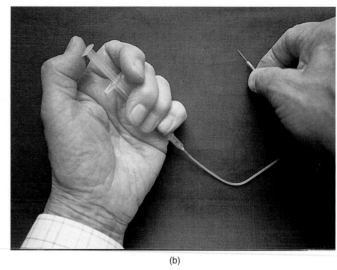

(a)   (b)

Fig. 4.25   (a) Microslerotherapy set. This frees one hand to manipulate the syringe whilst the other steers the needle. (b) If the syringe is held as shown here, the thumb is able to push the plunger in or out, to suck or to inject, without danger of displacing the needle.

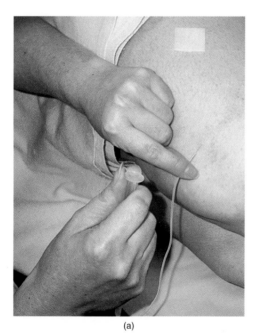

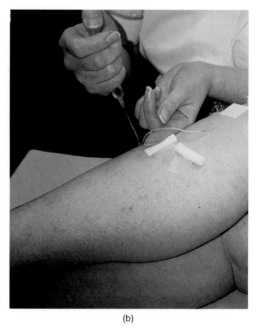

(a)   (b)

Fig. 4.26   Microsclerotherapy in practice: (a) the needle is passed through the vein and then slowly withdrawn whilst suction is applied by the thumb pushing the syringe plunger up; (b) as soon as a fleck of blood appears the needle is held still while the thumb now presses the plunger down to inject sclerosant. This may be repeated at a number of sites. Only a very weak solution should be used (0.2 per cent).

Surgical treatment

The essential principle with surgery is that the source and the main pathway of incompetence are actually removed; in the case of a saphenous vein, this requires high ligation at its termination, flush with the deep vein, stripping a substantial part of its length, and extensive removal of the varicose veins. Some typical procedures are illustrated in Fig. 4.27. If an incompetent saphenous vein is left in place, unstripped, it remains open as a valveless conduit running directly down to the low-pressure areas beneath the musculovenous pumps and is likely to form the basis of a new retrograde circuit of incompetence with renewed varicose veins (see the section on recurrent varicose veins).

Surgical treatment should also remove the main varicosities through a series of minimal incisions (Figs 4.27(o) and 4.27(p)); otherwise these veins are liable to persist, much to the patient's disappointment, and will require final elimination by sclerotherapy. Moreover, these varicosities are the distal part of a pathway of incompetence and directly communicate with the low-pressure areas so that they are constantly available to re-establish flow from higher levels; not only will they remain visible but they may progressively enlarge. Cosmesis is particularly important here, but fortunately the be regarded as the main offender and its varying role in venous disorders is considered in Chapter 7.

The best opportunity for surgical cure is at the first operation because recurrent veins based on a superficial vein anatomy fragmented by previous surgery are much more difficult to treat effectively. The first opportunity must not be wasted by inaccurate identification of the veins at fault or inadequate surgery. Conscientious surgery for varicose veins is time consuming but very rewarding in terms of immediate comfort and lasting benefit to the patient.

majority of varicosities can be removed through stab (1–3 mm) incisions by the hook–avulsion technique shown in Fig. 4.27(o). However, occasionally a massive 'bunch of grapes' varicose vein, long neglected and densely adherent, may be encountered and tunnelling between several larger incisions (Fig. 4.27(q)) placed along Cox's lines of skin cleavage (Fig. 4.27(t)) will be required.

A further aspect that may require special attention is the site of inflow from incompetent superficial veins to the deep veins at low level, i.e. the perforating veins. Usually, these are multiple points and it is neither practical nor necessary to identify and remove them surgically. However, in some cases one or two individual perforators become enlarged and give heavy surge back and forth as the muscles contract and relax. When recognized, it is best to remove these veins, since otherwise they may form the source of a new pattern of varicosities running to the foot. However, the perforator must not

Box 4.10 *Continued*   **Day case surgery for varicose veins**

Day case (ambulatory) surgery under local anaesthesia is widely practised. With good organization it proves entirely practicable with the advantage of low cost and convenience to patient.

Factors to consider   *Selection and safety*   Clearly defined, routine cases only; patient otherwise fit and mobile. Do only one limb at a time, otherwise overdose of local anaesthetic, or adrenalin it contains, may occur. Full mobility must be regained at end of procedure. Do *not* allow patient to drive home if nerve block or diazepam is used. *Anaesthetic agent to use* (and see previous page) 1% lignocaine hydrochloride (Xylocaine) which may be diluted with saline to 0.5% if a large area ia involved. 'With adrenalin' may be helpful but do not use this in a nerve block (muscle paresis may prove too prolonged) or in a 'topping-up' infiltration (for fear of overdose). An alternative is bupivacaine (Marcain) 0.25%, but this is long acting and with a nerve block may prevent early mobility by paralysing muscles.

Outline of procedure. Diazepam (5 mg) may be given orally to an anxious patient, but this can be withheld and later given intravenously if needed. *In standing position*, mark out veins and decide whether local infiltration without exceeding dossge limits will be sufficient or, if groin to knee stripping is planned, a femoral nerve block should be used to anaesthetise anteromedial aspect of limb. If anterolateral aspect of thigh is involved, lateral cutaneous nerve of thigh should be blocked. *With patient supine*, carry out nerve block(s) and allow, say, half an hour for full effect. The saphenofemoral junction will require separate local infiltration.

Femoral nerve block. A 22 gauge needle, directed headwards at 30 degrees, is inserted through the groin skin crease just lateral to the femoral artery (palpated with the finger of the opposite hand) and passed through the deep fascia; suck back to confirm that a blood vessel has not been entered, and inject 20 ml of 1% Xylocaine slowly. Inject the lateral cutaneous nerve as it emerges from under inguinal ligament just medial to the anterior superior iliac supine. For ligation of saphenopopliteal junction use local infiltration down to and just beneath deep fascia, along the line of the short saphenous vein and around varicose veins to be removed. Proceed with surgery, for example saphenofemoral ligation, strip to below knee and removing all varicose veins by multiple stab-avulsions. Subcuticular stitch is used for groin or popliteal incisions but no stitches elsewhere, just simple adhesive strip (Micropore) to stab incisions. Light elastic support up to knee or mid-thigh is applied. If nerve block has not been used patient may walk immediately and return home with suitable instruction sheet.

Box 4.11   Safety in surgery

There are some real dangers for the inexperienced surgeon. Complete division of the common femoral vein in error is not all that rare and requires skilled repair if permanent disability is to be prevented. Even more serious is the introduction of a stripper into an artery and its delivery through the common femoral artery with disastrous results when forceful stripping is carried out! A small number of such cases have been recorded with loss of limb or life.

The popliteal fossa is surrounded by important anatomy and surgery in this area requires an experienced surgeon. The venous anatomy is very variable, and surgery should always be preceded by ultrasonic imaging or phlebography to display the venous pattern so that the plan of operation can be based on this. Similarly, surgery on a recurrence from a common femoral source must be clearly visualized beforehand.

Nerve injury is a relatively common complication. The sural nerve in the lower leg lies close to the short saphenous vein and is easily damaged if special care is not taken by use of an adequate incision and visual identification of the nerve. Near the ankle the saphenous nerve is similarly close to the long saphenous vein and liable to be stripped with it. For this reason stripping to this level is avoided as far as possible. In the vicinity of the ankle there are numerous substantial nerve filaments just beneath the skin which are vulnerable to injury when veins are removed through stab incisions. Nerve-hooking techniques are particularly prone to this error, and it is wisest to use a short incision to give full vision in this area; transverse incisions here leave practically no scar.

Lymphatics and lymph glands seldom cause problems but nevertheless should be treated with respect, particularly in the groin where a route minimizing disturbance to them should be chosen. The incision recommended in Fig. 4.27(e) usually allows them to be displaced harmlessly. There are two circumstance where interference with the lymphatics may lead to a collection of lymph or a lymphatic fistula: (i) an inborn lymphatic deficiency may be present, so be cautious if the limb is oedematous and take care to preserve the lymphatics; (ii) after previous surgery to the saphenofemoral junction, further surgery through the scar tissue may inadvertently damage lymphatics already impaired, and a route should be chosen to avoid this.

In the groin and popliteal fossa keep good **haemostasis** and ligate all branches securely, otherwise substantial haematoma may collect postoperatively; this may be a factor in recurrence. In other areas the surgeon relies on rapid natural haemostasis by the contraction of the vein ends that occurs when veins are evulsed, as in stripping a saphenous vein or removing peripheral varicose veins; this is greatly assisted by pressure to the area for 30 s, particularly if haemorrhage persists. When stripping a saphenous vein, it is best to do this slowly, pausing as each branch dimples the skin, so that the branch veins are given time to contract down. In this way there should be little blood loss or haematoma. Elevation of the limb can also be employed in troublesome cases. In the authors' opinion a tourniquet should *never* be used; it is not necessary and introduces an unwanted hazard. See 4.27(s) for points in dealing with haemorrhage from injured deep veins. Always remember that moderate pressure easily controls venous bleeding and gives time for new tactics to be thought out; a sucker used to see the origin of venous bleeding can swiftly and deceptively exsanguinate the patient.

Tight bandages or strong elastic stocking must be avoided so that the deep veins are allowed unrestricted free flow. A crepe bandage moderately firmly applied up to the knee is all that is required. It soon loosens and when the patient is mobile can be changed to a light elastic support up to the knee. There is no need to support the thigh, which is difficult to do without discomfort to the patient and possible constriction to the deep veins.

Box 4.12 Good cosmetic results with surgery

Perhaps the strongest reason for patients seeking treatment for their varicose veins is because they want a blemish-free leg. Appearance is paramount and the surgeon must ensure that unsightly veins are not replaced by ugly scars.

Factors in minimizing scars

- Use of minimal incisions, as far as is consistent with good surgery. Stab–avulsion phlebectomy is ideal for this (see Figs 4.27(i) and 4.27(o)).
- Alignment of incision with cleavage lines of skin; those described by Cox (see Fig. 4.27(t) are widely accepted.
- Use of continuous subcuticular sutures: these are virtually pain free and heal better and without the ugly cross-hatching of conventional transverse through-and-through sutures. The latter encircle living tissue and create a ring of devitalized tissue with attendant inflammation and scarring. They should never be used.
- Even with subcuticular stitches there are good and bad methods. The subcuticular stitch should not be knotted or fixed at any point but should be free to slide a little when the tissues swell. This is achieved by stretching out the two ends of the stitch on the skin surface and applying a rayon adhesive strip (Micropore or Steri-Strip) to cover the length of the incision and the exposed stitch (see Figs 4.27(k) and 4.27(q)(ii)). The wound is thus supported by both a stitch that can yield slightly and the adhesive strip.
- Choice of adhesive is critical—it must be non-reactive and allow free ventilation so that the skin beneath it does not become sodden.
- The subcuticular stitch can be either self-absorbent or an inert monofilament (Prolene is the authors' choice) which is removed 3–7 days later; continued support is given by reapplying a strip of rayon adhesive. The stitch slides out easily and seldom causes pain.
- Other ways of closing incisions using adhesive strips or film may be equally effective provided that the adhesive is not easily lifted by exudate and the skin edges are held accurately opposed.
- Stab incisions, now widely used for rapid removal of varicose veins from multiple sites, are cosmetically good and require at most only an adhesive strip. However, do not forget the drawback of blindly seeking a vein through a minute opening, for example at the ankle where substantial nerve filaments may be damaged.
- Take care not to remove any subcutaneous fat because this may leave an ugly hollow that is clearly visible is certain lights.
- Staining of the skin, as may occur with sclerotherapy, is not a potential problem after surgery.

Box 4.13 Removal of varicose veins by avulsion through a stab incision

This method of phlebectomy is illustrated in Fig. 4.27(o) but additional points are given below.

It is only suitable for varicose branch veins and must be accompanied by elimination of the source and, usually, the main pathway of incompetence, such as a saphenous vein.

Avoid the dorsum of the foot and the region of the ankle where nerves such as the musculocutaneous nerve, the sural nerve, and important branches lie near the surface and are easily caught by a vein hook (see Fig. 4.27(o). Here visual dissection through a 0.5-cm incision should be used to ensure that it is a vein that is picked up.

Do not go deeply with the hook for fear of damage to structures that are more deeply placed, particularly subcutaneous nerves (most at risk near ankle) and lymphatics; the stab incision is only suitable for veins immediately beneath the skin. *Never* attempt to hook a short saphenous vein, because the sural nerve is closely applied to it and will be damaged, or the long saphenous vein which runs closely with the saphenous nerve.

Fibrosis and adhesion caused by failed injections or phlebitis may prevent use of this method and an appropriate incision for open dissection will be required.

A varicose vein may not be easy to see in the horizontal limb but is recognized by preoperative marking, a palpable groove, or feeling the vein against the curved arm of a hook passed under it.

The procedure illustrated in Fig. 4.27(o) is carried out at intervals adjusted to the length of vein previously removed, usually about 5–8 cm. Such small incisions can be made vertically or horizontally with equally good cosmetic results.

Do not incise through marking ink because some types of marker may cause tattooing. Put preoperative marks over the vein and incise alongside them. Bleeding may occur briefly but if troublesome will soon cease with pressure or elevation of the limb. Vein ends are not ligated; it is not necessary and in any case they are inaccessible.

With incisions up to 3 mm skin suture is not required. Permeable adhesive tape (such as Micropore) (2.5 cm) is used to close the wounds and to give a protective covering. If oozing threatens to lift the adhesive tape, make a slit along it over the incision to let the fluid escape.

Fig. 4.27 (a - t)   Surgical technique in the treatment of superficial vein incompetence.

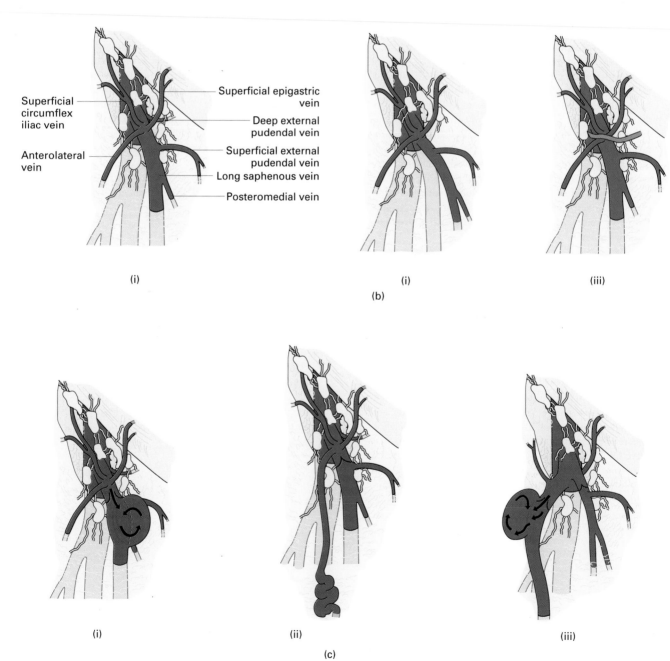

(a)

Superficial circumflex iliac vein

Anterolateral vein

Superficial epigastric vein

Deep external pudendal vein

Superficial external pudendal vein

Long saphenous vein

Posteromedial vein

(i)

(i)

(iii)

(b)

(i)

(ii)

(iii)

(c)

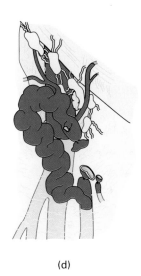

(d)

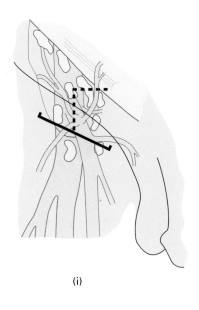

(i)

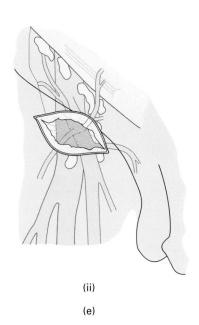

(ii)

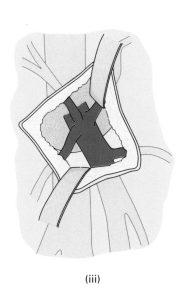

(iii)

(e)

Fig. 4.27 (continued).

(a) Planning the procedure before surgery. Preoperative 'marking out' of veins by an experienced person is essential to ensure easy identification of veins to be removed. There is no 'standard procedure'—the operation is planned individually for each patient.

(b) Flush ligation of long saphenous termination. Some anatomical points. (i) A typical arrangement of saphenous termination and its branches. (ii) There are many variants. A double long saphenous vein is shown here; either or both channels can be at fault. (iii) The superficial external pudendal artery may run over, as shown here, or under the saphenous vein.

(c) Some features commonly present. (i) Saphena varix—a saccule below an incompetent upper saphenous valve but often found beneath any incompetent saphenous valve in the thigh. (ii) An anterolateral branch may be the main pathway of incompetence and downflow in it may bypass a competent upper long saphenous vein. (iii) Saccules are often present on an incompetent anterolateral branch.

(d) 'Anatomical recurrence' caused by connection of surviving branches at the saphenous termination with an unstripped saphenous vein.

(e) Steps in the flush ligation of a long saphenous termination. (i) Incision centred 2 cm lateral to and below the pubic tubercle. (ii) Skin incision exposes the membranous layer of superficial fascia, which is incised separately. (iii) Fat is brushed downwards to expose the saphenous vein; the termination and its branches are cleared of fatty tissue.

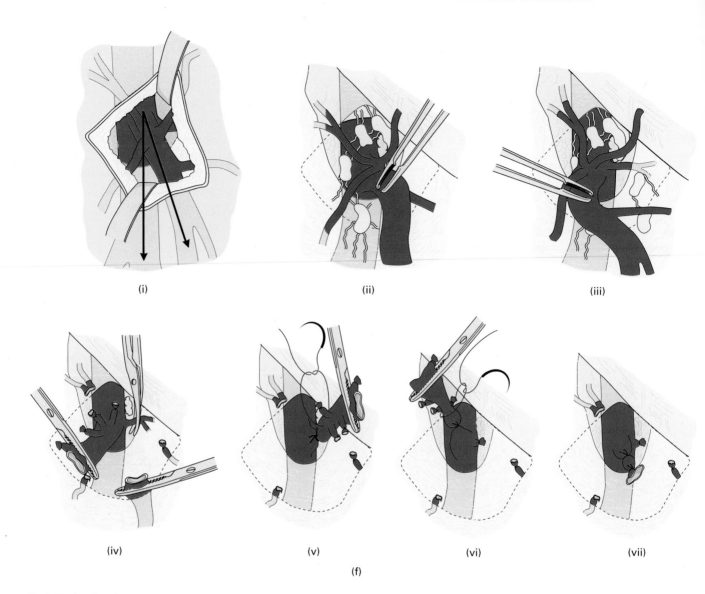

(i)   (ii)   (iii)

(iv)   (v)   (vi)   (vii)

(f)

Fig. 4.27   (continued).

(f) Checking the correct identity of the saphenous vein. (i) It is not axial to the limb but inclines to the medial aspect; several typical branches are always present at the true termination. (ii), (iii) The junction with the common femoral vein must be seen beyond doubt from both medial and lateral aspects. (iv) Once certain of its correct identity, the saphenous vein is divided and drawn forward to facilitate division of its branches. (v), (vi), (vii) When fully isolated, the saphenous stump is ligated flush with the common femoral vein and then again, more peripherally, with a transfixion stitch.

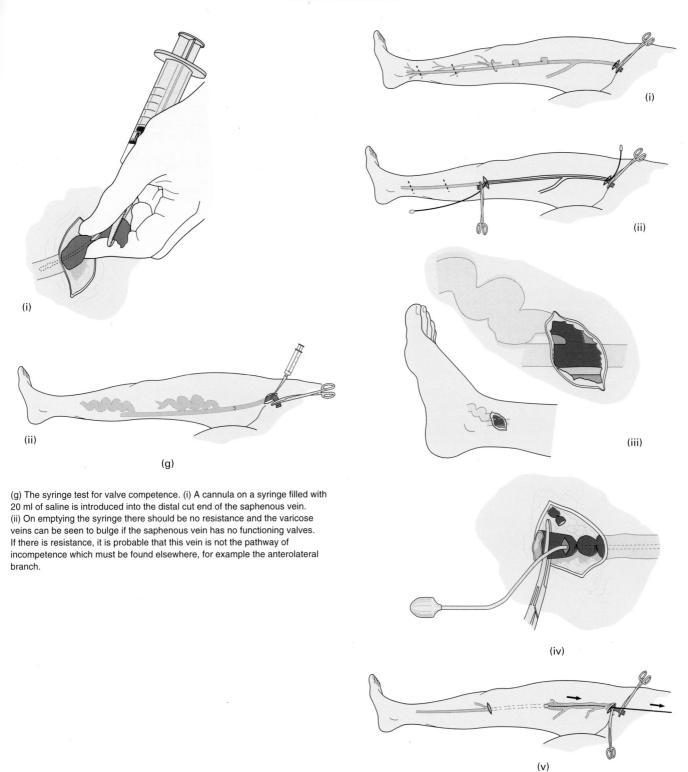

(g) The syringe test for valve competence. (i) A cannula on a syringe filled with 20 ml of saline is introduced into the distal cut end of the saphenous vein. (ii) On emptying the syringe there should be no resistance and the varicose veins can be seen to bulge if the saphenous vein has no functioning valves. If there is resistance, it is probable that this vein is not the pathway of incompetence which must be found elsewhere, for example the anterolateral branch.

Fig. 4.27 (continued).

(h) (*Above right*) When long saphenous incompetence has been confirmed, the vein should be stripped. The traditional method using a large-headed stripper is shown here. (i) The long saphenous vein is exposed just below the knee. Usually it is not necessary to strip below this level because the posterior arch vein is often the main pathway of incompetence and the long saphenous vein is not at fault. (ii) A stripper is passed up to the groin. (iii) If there are special reasons, this may be done from the ankle but here the saphenous nerve is endangered by its proximity. The position of the saphenous nerve is illustrated; note how close it is to the vein near the ankle. (iv) The vein is double ligated around the stripper to prevent invagination of the stripper head. (v) The stripper emerging from the groin is now pulled upwards to strip the vein. A controlled slow pull is best, with pauses when resistance and skin dimpling denote that a branch is about to be pulled off; this gives time for these veins to contract before avulsion and minimizes bleeding from them. *Note.* Many surgeons prefer to pass the stripper downwards and strip in this direction. This is equally good, but valve cusps may impede the stripper probe or it may enter side-branches.

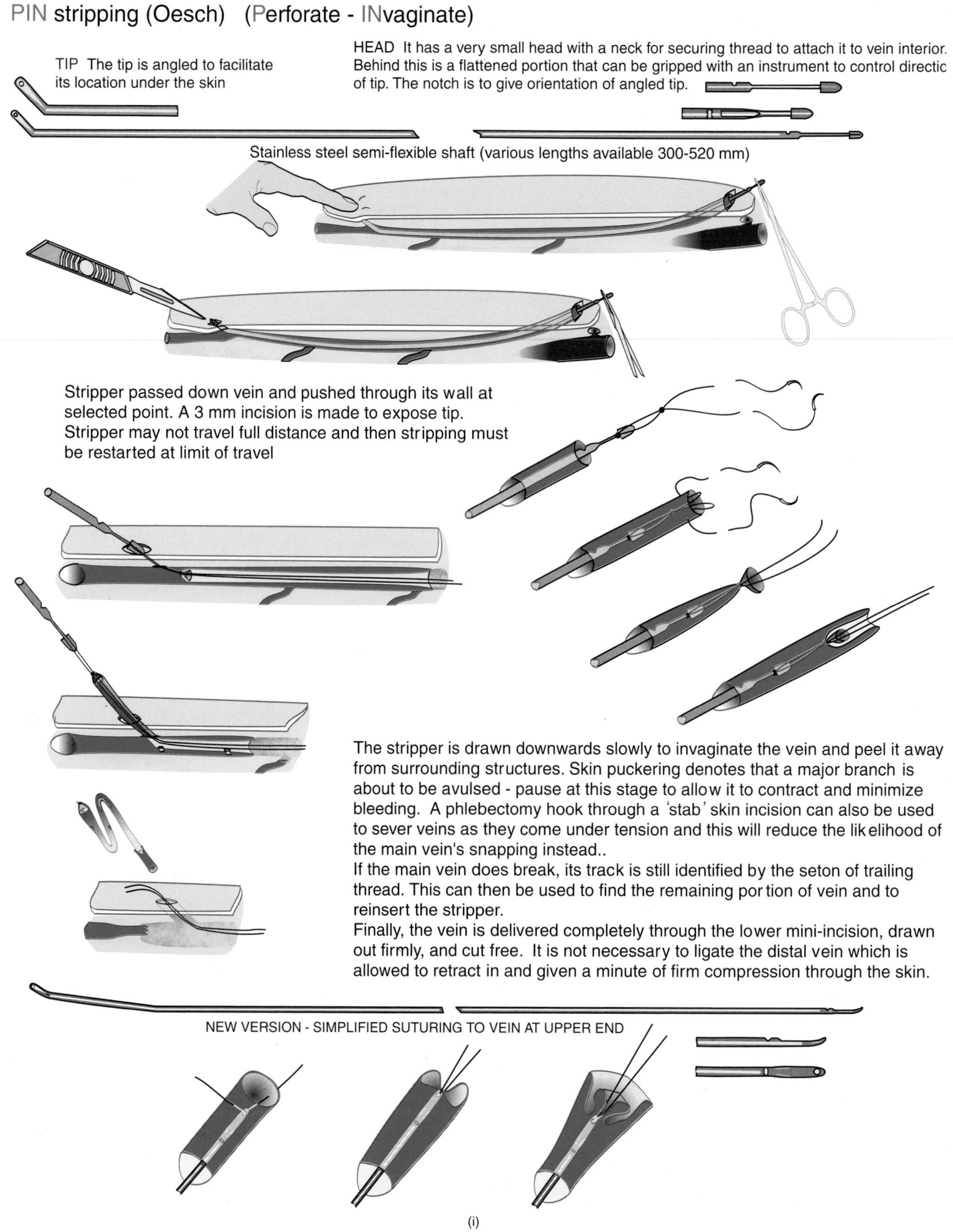

PIN stripping (Oesch) (Perforate - INvaginate)

TIP The tip is angled to facilitate its location under the skin

HEAD It has a very small head with a neck for securing thread to attach it to vein interior. Behind this is a flattened portion that can be gripped with an instrument to control directic of tip. The notch is to give orientation of angled tip.

Stainless steel semi-flexible shaft (various lengths available 300-520 mm)

Stripper passed down vein and pushed through its wall at selected point. A 3 mm incision is made to expose tip. Stripper may not travel full distance and then stripping must be restarted at limit of travel

The stripper is drawn downwards slowly to invaginate the vein and peel it away from surrounding structures. Skin puckering denotes that a major branch is about to be avulsed - pause at this stage to allow it to contract and minimize bleeding. A phlebectomy hook through a 'stab' skin incision can also be used to sever veins as they come under tension and this will reduce the likelihood of the main vein's snapping instead..

If the main vein does break, its track is still identified by the seton of trailing thread. This can then be used to find the remaining portion of vein and to reinsert the stripper.

Finally, the vein is delivered completely through the lower mini-incision, drawn out firmly, and cut free. It is not necessary to ligate the distal vein which is allowed to retract in and given a minute of firm compression through the skin.

NEW VERSION - SIMPLIFIED SUTURING TO VEIN AT UPPER END

(i)

Fig. 4.27 (continued).

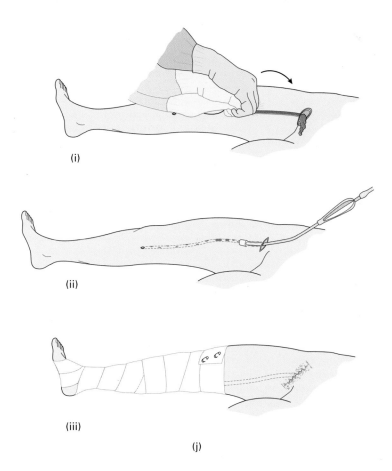

(i)

(ii)

(iii)

(j)

(j) Clearing haematoma; postoperative support. (i), (ii) At a late stage in the operation (to give time for haemostasis) haematoma in the track of the stripper is expelled by hand pressure and use of a sucker. ((iii) A crepe bandage or a light elastic stocking up to mid-thigh is sufficient support for the first 48 h; strong constrictive bandaging is most undesirable.

Fig. 4.27 (continued).

(i) (*Left*) PIN stripping technique. Many surgeons prefer the recently developed PIN stripping method for stripping veins. Originally designed for the short saphenous vein to protect the sural nerve whilst using very small incisions, it is now also used for the long saphenous vein and any other substantial branch. It gives excellent cosmetic results by minimizing incisions and allows the vein to be separated from nerves, such as the sural or saphenous, far more safely than with a conventional large-headed stripper. The absence of surgical dissection also avoids damage to lymphatics, which is sometimes a significant problem. There are many variants of this technique and in the instruments used, but the method illustrated here is based on that described by A. Oesch in *Phlebology*, **8**, 171–3 (1993) and G. Goren and A. Yellin in *Journal of Vascular Surgery*, **20**, 970–7 (1994).

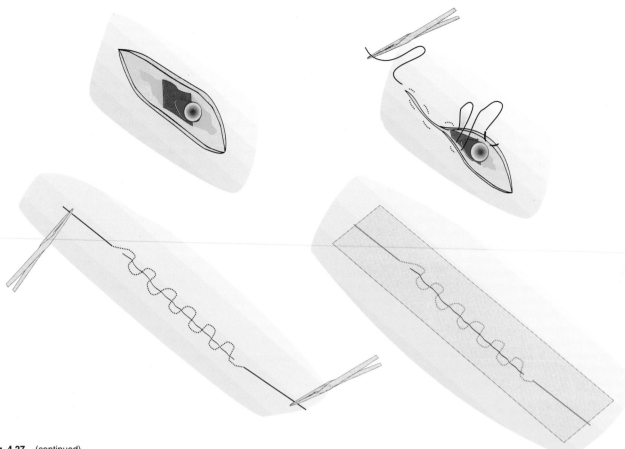

Fig. 4.27   (continued).

(k) Incisions in the groin and any others over 4 mm are best closed by a subcuticular stitch as shown in this illustration. A non-absorbable monofilament gives least reaction. This is unknotted, but the ends are left long so that they can be taped down with Micropore which also gives additional support to the incision. The stitch is withdraw 3–7 days later and Micropore is reapplied. With this method, the stitch does not cut into the skin; this minimizes wound reaction, is pain free, and gives the best cosmetic result (see also Box 4.12).

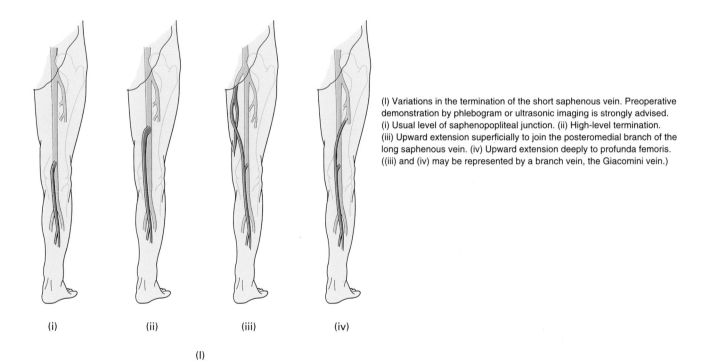

(l) Variations in the termination of the short saphenous vein. Preoperative demonstration by phlebogram or ultrasonic imaging is strongly advised. (i) Usual level of saphenopopliteal junction. (ii) High-level termination. (iii) Upward extension superficially to join the posteromedial branch of the long saphenous vein. (iv) Upward extension deeply to profunda femoris. ((iii) and (iv) may be represented by a branch vein, the Giacomini vein.)

(i)   (ii)   (iii)   (iv)

(l)

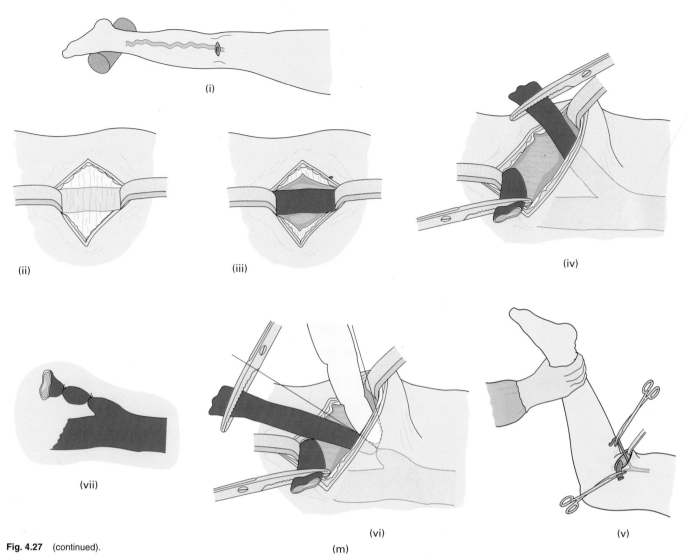

(i)

(ii)   (iii)   (iv)

(vii)   (vi)   (v)

Fig. 4.27 (continued).   (m)

(m) High ligation of the short saphenous vein. (i) The patient is positioned face down, or nearly so, in a fashion that allows bending of knee. (ii) Transverse skin incision, at a level indicated by ultrasonic imaging or phlebography, exposes the deep fascia. (iii) Incision in the deep fascia. The short saphenous vein usually directly underlies it and is easily seen. Too deep a dissection may expose the popliteal vein and lead to a bad error if this is assumed to be the saphenous vein! If the popliteal artery can be felt immediately under the vein exposed, then this is likely to be the popliteal vein. Do not proceed! Passing the probe end of the stripper up the saphenous vein from mid-calf can be a great help if identification is difficult, but is not infallible because it can occasionally enter the deep vein lower down.
(iv)–(vii) When certain of identity, the saphenous vein is divided and followed upwards as far as possible to its junction with the popliteal vein where it is doubly ligated and the excess removed. Flexing the knee facilitates access. The deep fascia should be sutured on closing.

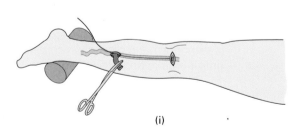

(i)

(n) Traditional stripping of the short saphenous vein. (i) A stripper is passed up from the point where the lowest varicosity takes off. (ii) Exposing the saphenous vein in the lower leg puts the sural nerve in danger as it is a sizeable structure applied closely to the vein. It must be identified and gently separated; the nerve has a distinctive vascular pattern on its surface. However, the PIN method (see Fig. 4.27(i)), which was originally designed for the short saphenous vein, is less likely to harm the vulnerable sural nerve and is cosmetically superior. This, or similar techniques, has gained widespread acceptance recently and become the preferred method.

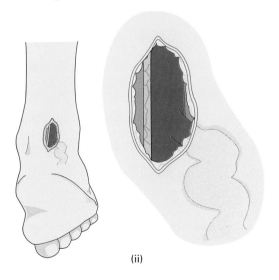

(ii)

Phlebectomy by stab incision and avulsion

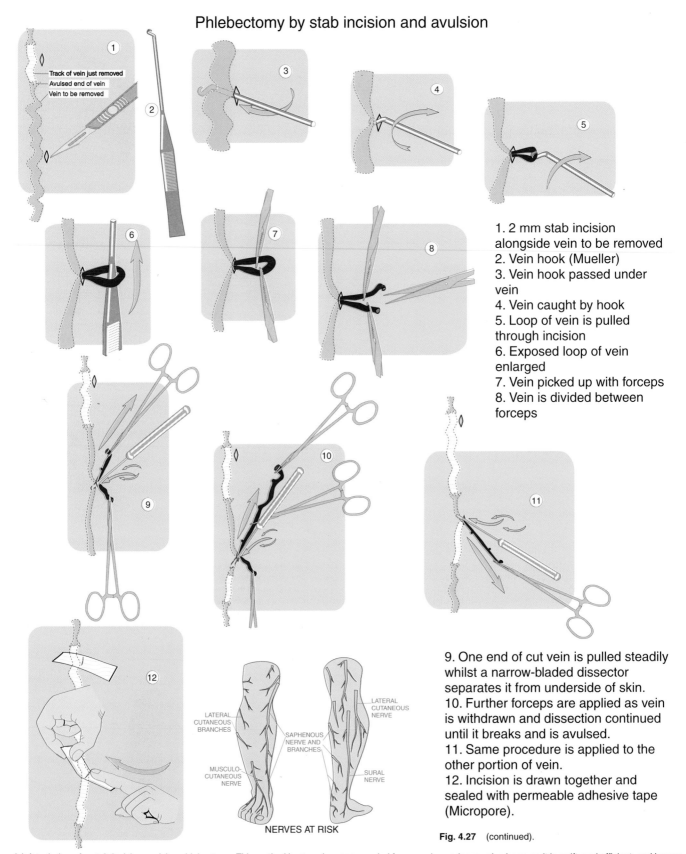

1. 2 mm stab incision alongside vein to be removed
2. Vein hook (Mueller)
3. Vein hook passed under vein
4. Vein caught by hook
5. Loop of vein is pulled through incision
6. Exposed loop of vein enlarged
7. Vein picked up with forceps
8. Vein is divided between forceps

9. One end of cut vein is pulled steadily whilst a narrow-bladed dissector separates it from underside of skin.
10. Further forceps are applied as vein is withdrawn and dissection continued until it breaks and is avulsed.
11. Same procedure is applied to the other portion of vein.
12. Incision is drawn together and sealed with permeable adhesive tape (Micropore).

Fig. 4.27 (continued).

(o) A technique for stab-incision avulsion phlebectomy. This method is strongly recommended for removing varicose veins because it is swift, and efficient, and leaves imperceptible scars. A Mueller hook is illustrated here but other patterns, or even a simple crochet hook, are also effective. The incision is repeated about every 8 cm along the varicose vein to be removed. These small incisions may be vertical or horizontal. Do not incise through marking ink because with tattooing is possible with some types of marking pen. Avoid the ankle region because important sensory nerves lie very near the surface and are easily caught. Bleeding may occur briefly, but if troublesome will soon cease with pressure or elevation of the limb. In this procedure the avulsed vein ends are not ligated; it is not necessary and in any case they are inaccessible. With incisions up to 3 mm, skin suture is not required. Permeable adhesive tape (2.5 cm) is used to close the wounds and to give a protective covering. If oozing threatens to lift the adhesive tape, make a slit along it over the incision to let the fluid escape.

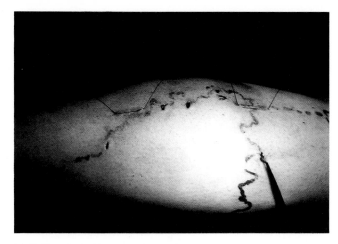

(p) (i) The main incisions used for stripping a short saphenous vein have been closed with subcuticular stitches (use of the PIN method would not have required this); several stab incisions already used can be seen.

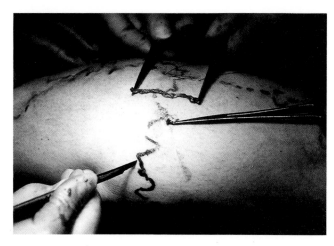

(p) (ii) The portion of vein just removed from a stab incision is displayed.

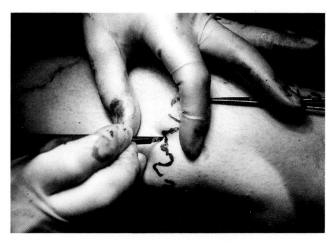

(p) (iii) A further stab incision (about 2 mm across) is made.

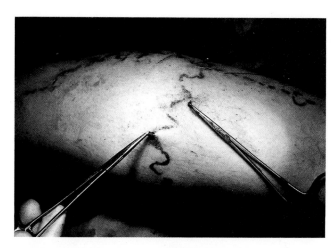

(p) (iv) The underlying vein is picked up and teased out.

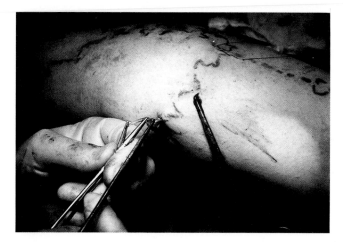

(p) (v) By pulling gently on the vein and pushing tissue away from its base with the points of closed artery forceps, more and more of its length is freed.

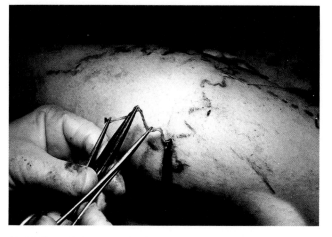

(p) (vi) The entire length, back to the previous stab incision, has been delivered and removed. This process can be repeated through further stabs as far as desired.

Fig. 4.27 (continued).

(p) Photographs illustrating the stab incision and evulsion technique using mosquito artery forceps. In fact, the vein is coaxed and teased out rather than simply pulled upon, and the aim is to remove several centimetres from each stab incision.   *Continued*

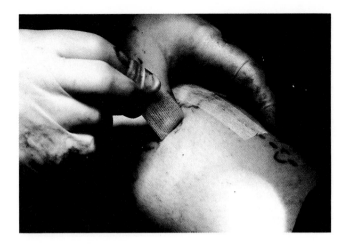
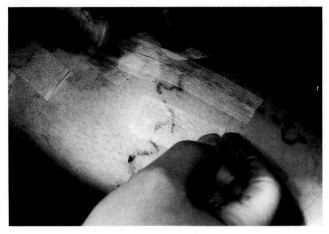

Fig. 4.27   (continued).

(p) (vii), (viii) Closure with Micropore sterile tape, without any stitch, is usually sufficient. In the background subcuticular stitches, held in place only by adhesive strips (to allow expansion of tissues with oedema), can be seen at the main incisions.

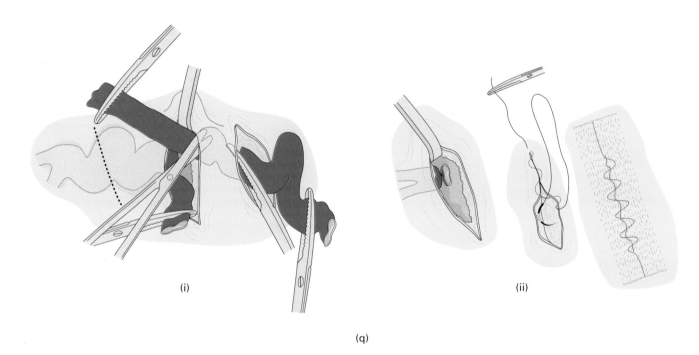

(i)   (ii)

(q)

(q) Not all varicosities can be dealt with by the stab–avulsion method and will need a small incision and dissection of the veins. (i), (ii) Massive varicose veins adherent to the skin, through long neglect or previous surgery, can be removed by making small oblique incisions and tunnelling between them. Always use a subcuticular stitch to close these incisions. An unknotted monofilament, taped down with Micropore and withdrawn at 7 days, is ideal and avoids ugly cross-hatching of the scar.

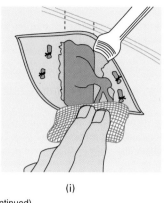

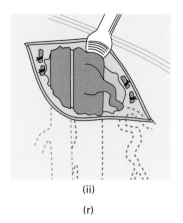

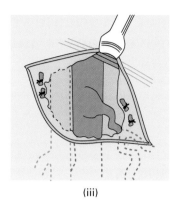

(i)

(ii)

(iii)

Fig. 4.27 (continued).

(r)

(r) Recurrence from a long saphenous stump. Preliminary phlebography or ultrasonic imaging is essential. Scar tissue with varicose veins embedded in it can make operation difficult; lymphatics abound and damage to these may cause a lymph fistula. Use a transverse incision to skin but deepen this by a longitudinal incision to minimize injury to lymphatics. Three approaches are available. (i) Directly following local varicosities to the stump. These fragile veins amongst scar tissue break easily, but bleeding can be controlled by local pressure allowing progress elsewhere. It can prove difficult and the two approaches, shown in (ii) and (iii), skirting the scar tissue may be preferable. (ii) The common femoral artery is exposed first and dissection is then moved medially to expose the neighbouring common femoral vein which is followed to the saphenous stump. (iii) The inguinal ligament is exposed first and then the common femoral vein, which is followed down to the stump.

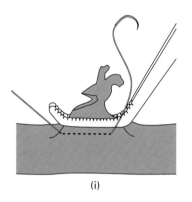

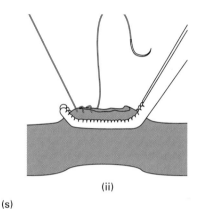

(i)

(ii)

(s)

(s) Removing the saphenous stump and repair of deep vein. (i), (ii) Operation to remove a saphenous stump may involve repair of the deep vein. A suitable vascular clamp should be at hand and is invaluable if the need arises, as in the examples illustrated. Remember that using a sucker to clear a field of copious bleeding can soon exsanguinate the patient. Never continue using the sucker regardlessly—stop haemorrhage by finger pressure on a tight gauze pad and pause to think out another approach. One of those described above can allow the femoral vein to be exposed and a side-clamp applied from a different direction.

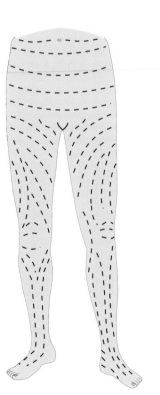

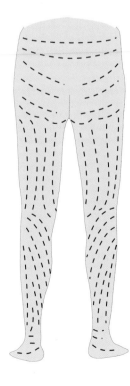

(t) When larger incisions are necessary. Lines of skin cleavage along which incisions over 3 mm should be made to give optimal cosmetic result Do not spoil this by creating the cross-hatched scar caused by conventional stitching. Use subcuticular stitches or, with small incisions, adhesive strips. Adapted from H.T. Cox, *British Journal of Surgery*, **29**, 234 (1941).

Treatment of varicose veins with venotensive changes and ulceration

When the characteristic skin changes of venous hypertension are evident and particularly when ulceration is present, care must be taken to be sure that the cause is simple incompetence in superficial veins and not a post-thrombotic deep vein impairment (Fig. 4.28). Surgery to the veins that is appropriate for the former may well be wholly inappropriate for the latter. Once unequivocal evidence has been obtained that the cause is superficial incompetence and the pathway of this has been accurately defined, treatment can be carried out as described above. The presence of venotensive changes indicates a severe state of incompetence probably best treated by surgery because the large incompetent veins likely to be present may soon reopen after sclerotherapy and more lasting benefit will be given by surgical removal of the source and pathway of incompetence, including the varicose veins themselves.

If the skin is unbroken, or even when a substantial 'clean' ulcer is present, there is no reason why surgery should not be performed without any preliminary treatment. However, if infection, such as cellulitis or an ulcer discharging pus, is present, the patient should have a short period of treatment in hospital with the limb elevated and systemic antibiotics should be given. This is maintained until the ulcer enters a healing phase, i.e. its base is covered with 'healthy' granulation tissue, pus is no longer being formed, pathogenic organisms such as *Staphylcoccus aureus* or *Streptococcus viridans* have been eliminated, and the skin edges slope smoothly to a thin grey line of regenerating epithelium extending on to the granulation tissue. At this stage, when the ulcer is 'clean', there is no need to delay surgery by waiting for the ulcer to heal completely; healing can continue concurrently with the patient's postoperative mobilization once the cause for venous hypertension has been removed. This policy would not be appropriate where superficial vein incompetence is accompanied by the more fundamental problem of primary valve deficiency (valveless syndrome – see Chapter 5) because here the benefits to be expected of surgery may be so marginal that the ulcer could fail to heal without continued elevation.

Recurrent varicose veins

Undoubtedly, there is an appreciable recurrence rate for varicose veins and other expressions of superfical vein incompetence treated by sclerotherapy or surgery. The recurrences created by surgery can sometimes be more formidable than the original state. The causes of such failure in treatment can be summarized as follows.

Persistent varicose veins

Here it is soon apparent that the varicose veins have survived treatment. This may be due to one of the following factors.

- Misdiagnosis of the original state where in fact the enlarged veins were, for example, not simple varicose veins but due to deep vein impairment.

- Incorrect identification of the source and pathway of incompetence.

> **Box 4.14   Surgery when venotensive changes and ulceration are present**
>
> There are two major causes of venotension and ulceration:
>
> (1) superficial vein incompetence — usually suitable for surgical treatment
> (2) deep vein impairment, usually post-thrombotic syndrome — surgery is not usually appropriate and may be harmful to important collaterals.
>
> **Diagnosis of superficial vein incompetence must always be proved beyond doubt when ulceration is present** by the selective Trendelenburg test, Doppler flowmetry showing downward flow after exercise, photoplethysmography or other form of plethysmography showing temporary restoration to near normal with selective occlusion of the pathway of incompetence, and, if necessary, demonstration of normal deep veins by imaging technique.
>
> Surgery need not be delayed waiting for an ulcer to heal, provided that it is clean and in a healing phase, a shown by epithelial ingrowth from its edges, and no bacterial pathogens are present. If the cause of the ulcer is superficial incompetence, it should heal progressively after operation and skin grafting is not necessary. (There are borderline cases with a poor musculovenous pumping mechanism where continued conservative treatment may be needed after surgery (see Chapter 5)).

- Two separate sources feeding the same varicose veins were present originally and too limited a procedure has been carried out.

- Removal of the pathway of incompetence and/or the varicosities has been inadequate and the remaining veins fill easily from a secondary source or by reflux through an enlarged perforating vein. This may respond to sclerotherapy or require a further operation to complete the first procedure.

True recurrence

The varicose veins first disappear but then reappear in the same distribution within a year or two. The following reasons may account for this problem.

Inadequate removal of the source   This will usually be due to failure to ligate a saphenous termination flush with the deep vein. The branches that survive re-establish the source. This is most likely to happen when the original main pathway of incompetence, usually a saphenous vein, has not been removed.

Failure to remove or obliterate the main pathway of incompetence   It has already been pointed out that if a grossly incompetent saphenous vein is left intact, it will act as a conduit directly communicating with the low-pressure areas below the venous pumping mechanisms (the original key failure). During exercise, such as walking, the upper end of this large vein will then be at low pressure in close proximity to the relatively high deep vein pressure in the saphenous stump. This is a strong inducement for a vascular connection to be established from the high pressure vein to

Fig. 4.28 Treatment of ulceration in superficial vein incompetence.

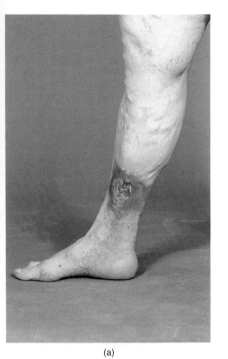
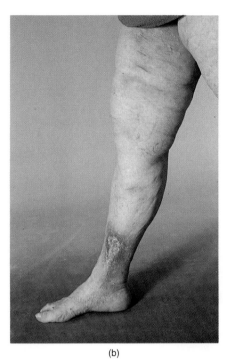

(a)   (b)

(a) This ulcer, in a middle-aged woman, was caused by massive incompetence in the long saphenous vein.
(b) The ulcer, now healed, 2 months after surgery with immediate postoperative mobilization. It remained well healed when seen a year later.

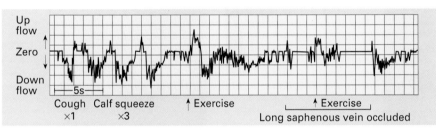

(c)

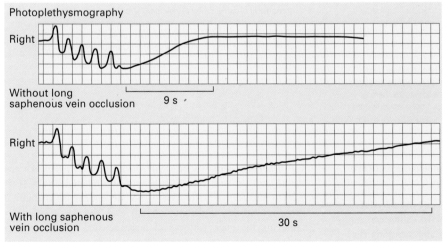

(d)

(c), (d) Preoperative findings. All clinical tests strongly confirmed the diagnosis. The Doppler flowmetry recordings reproduced here show downflow in the long saphenous vein after exercise, characteristic of simple incompetence; the photophlethysmograms show refilling within 9 s, but this was restored to a normal 30 s when the long saphenous vein was temporarily occluded by fingertips.

Fig. 4.29 Recurrence at site of previous saphenous ligation.

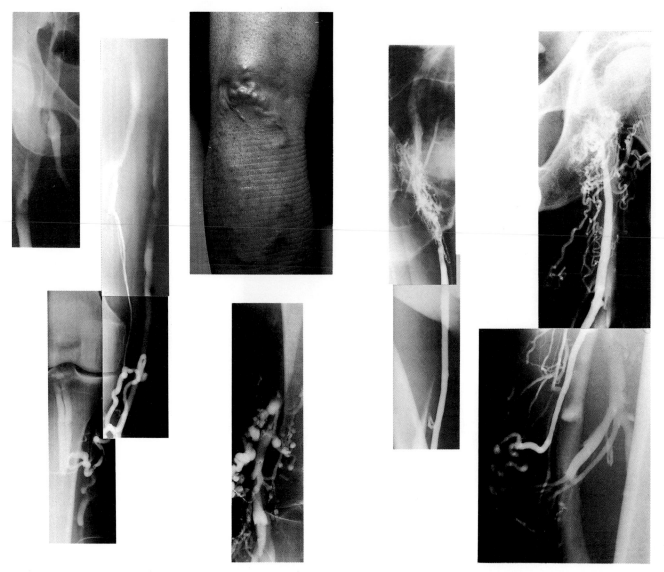

(a) Anatomical recurrence: a renewed source from existing branches connecting with the original pathway of incompetence. (i) After long saphenous high ligation. A composite phlebogram showing a narrowed saphenofemoral junction with an otherwise intact but incompetent saphenous vein running down to the calf and filling varicosities (and gastrocnemius veins) there. A previous operation had removed only the superficial component of a double saphenous vein and had left the true termination narrowed but intact. (ii) Clinical appearance and (iii) phlebogram of a recurrence after 'high' ligation of the short saphenous vein. A large varicosity arises from a surviving branch on the stump. This was confirmed at surgery which gave a good result.

(b) Non-anatomical recurrence by revascularization of a long saphenous stump. Two examples are shown in different patients with reconnection between stump and an unstripped vein by a newly formed plexus of veins. (i) Connection with an unstripped incompetent long saphenous vein. (ii) Connection with a retained incompetent anterolateral branch.

the low-pressure vein. Two types of venous connecting network may be formed.

1. Anatomical reconnection, based on surviving side-branches of a saphenous stump (Figs 4.29(a) and 4.29(d) (i)). This can be avoided by flush ligation with the deep vein and stripping the saphenous vein down to knee level.

2. Non-anatomical reconnection (revascularization or neovascularization). In recent years it has been repeatedly shown that, even when the saphenous vein has been ligated and divided above

any branches, a plexus of small veins may form between the stump and an unstripped, incompetent saphenous vein (Fig. 4.29(b) and (c)). This process is not dependent on anatomical branches of the saphenous stump and can be avoided by removing the main pathway of incompetence, whether this is saphenous vein or an enlarged branch, such as an anterolateral branch in the thigh. In the treatment of simple varicose veins it should be a fundamental principle that when the source of incompetence is surgically ligated the main pathway of incompetence should also be removed.

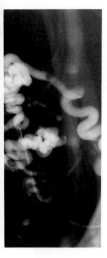

Fig. 4.29 (continued).

(c) Non-anatomical revascularization at other sites of ligation. In this example, outflow has been re-established to the original pattern of varicose veins after ligation of a perforator in midthigh.

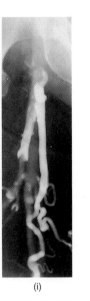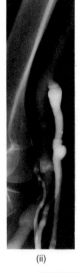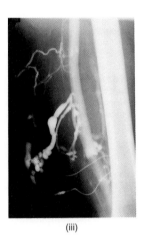

(i)   (ii)   (iii)

(d) Recurrence from a latent second source. Phlebograms after previous surgery to the long saphenous veins. (i) A small anatomical recurrence due to an incompetent anterolateral long saphenous branch is present. (ii) However, the major cause for renewed varicosities is from the short saphenous vein shown here. This became obvious only after the dominant long saphenous downflow had been reduced by previous operation. Surgery to both veins brought this elderly patient relief from long-standing discomfort. (iii) Phlebogram in another patient showing a typical mid-thigh perforator that has taken over remnants of the long saphenous system.

A latent second source has become active and surviving varicose veins have been taken over by this For example, if varicose veins are not removed at the time of long saphenous ligation and stripping, they form a ready-made vacant pathway of incompetence which may be 'acquired' by a mildly incompetent short saphenous vein. This new source soon enlarges with the stimulus of unrestricted downflow (Fig. 4.29(d) (ii)). Alternatively, some other source, such as a mid-thigh perforator, may take over in similar fashion (Fig. 4.29(d) (iii) and see Fig. 4.12(b)). The possibility of a second source opening up in this fashion is considerably reduced if the varicose veins are effectively removed surgically or obliterated by sclerotherapy at the first procedure, since otherwise they are a con-

stant and visible invitation for an incompetent vein at higher level to send an ever-increasing flow down to them. A second operation can give a good result provided that every effort is made to ensure accurate location of the source and, if there are any doubts, to confirm this by functional phlebography and varicography, or by ultrasonography.

A minority of recurrent varicose veins will arise in the states, described in Chapter 5, of either primary valve deficiency or weak vein syndrome In the latter, varicose veins may proliferate within a few months after a good initial result. The surgeon should not conclude too quickly that treatment cannot succeed, perhaps condemning the patient to a lifetime of strong elastic stockings, but should assess the case in detail by ultrasonic imaging and, if necessary, phlebography. This may show that there is an opportunity for carefully planned surgery based on accurate information, and this can be very successful.

Many varicose veins are labelled 'recurrent' when, in fact, they are due to a different set of veins unrelated to the originals For example, several years after successful treatment of long saphenous varices a new set of varicose veins arising from the short saphenous vein may appear. This may reflect widespread weakness in veins and valves, prone to incompetence and varicosis, but is not a contraindication to further treatment.

Box 4.15 'Recurrent' varicose veins

There are several categories within the loose description 'recurrent':

- residual or persistent, evident immediately post-operatively
- recurrence after an interval because of inadequate removal of source or pathway of incompetence
- a new source has been acquired by original varicose veins which have not been removed.

Cause
Hurried inadequate treatment, insecurely based on an unproven source, is a major factor in 'recurrent' varicose veins. The source and pathway of incompetence must always be conclusively demonstrated by clinical tests and backed by Doppler flowmeter studies or ultrasonic imaging before surgery.

Treatment

- Minor residual varicose veins can be treated by sclerotherapy.
- Major residual, persisting, or new varicose veins. These must have a detailed investigation to determine their *source*, and whether it is a persistent or a new one, by ultrasonic imaging or functional phlebography. Further surgery should not be proceeded with until this basic information has been satisfactorily demonstrated and an appropriate operation planned. Without this full understanding, an increasingly difficult problem may be created.

Compression sclerotherapy in the treatment of residual and recurrent veins after surgery

Residual varicose veins due to incomplete surgery or small veins that appear after an interval are often best treated by compression sclerotherapy. There is a good prospect of response so that it is well worth a trial. This is no more than a completion of the original treatment, particularly when extensive varicosities have made complete elimination impractical at one operating session and survivors declare themselves later. Here, sclerotherapy is particularly valuable, but in most cases adequate removal at surgery by multiple small incisions (Fig. 4.27(o) and p)) makes this additional treatment unnecessary. In order to reduce time on the operating table, some surgeons have a deliberate policy of doing no more than 'high ligation and strip', leaving the varicose veins for treatment by sclerotherapy later; however, this is tedious for the patient and misses an ideal opportunity to complete treatment by a single procedure.

Treatment of major recurrences of varicose veins

Large recurrent varicose veins are often among the most difficult to treat. Previous surgery will have fragmented the anatomy of the superficial veins so that the new patterns are far less predictable. Some of the worst recurrences occur in the groin or behind the knee, over the site of saphenous ligation; there may be a history of several unsuccessful attempts to remove these, but such attempts have been followed by early reappearance, perhaps even larger and more uncomfortable than before. Such veins are unlikely to give more than a temporary response to sclerotherapy, and surgery may be the only answer despite the previous failures. The problem is compounded by the fact that several sources of incompetence may be present and the patient may suffer from a degree of weak vein syndrome. Nevertheless, with careful mapping out and study of flow patterns by Doppler flowmeter and ultrasonic imaging, it is usually possible to understand the overall arrangement of the varicose veins and the likely sources of flow down them from the deep veins. Guided by this information, a combination of functional phlebography and varicography can give a good display of the key features, the sources, and the pathways of incompetence upon which surgery can be based. No surgery should be considered without this detailed information, and only a surgeon experienced in its interpretation and in carrying out such operations should embark on it; it is probable that exposure of the deep vein through dense scar tissue, traversed by large fragile varicosities, will be needed in order to attain complete elimination of a leaking saphenous stump (Fig. 4.30) and this may involve repair to the deep vein (Figs 4.27(r) and 4.27(s)). Any lesser effort is likely to produce yet another failure when in fact a most satisfying result may be attainable. An example of the intricate patterns that may be encountered is given in Fig. 4.12. Such cases are not rare and require special skill and perseverance. If weak vein syndrome is a factor, it may be wise to back up successful surgery with long-term use of elastic support up to the knee.

Having emphasized the difficulties of this aspect of venous surgery, it must be stressed again that the best opportunity to carry out successful surgical treatment of varicose veins is at the first operation. The principles to be used in minimizing massive recurrence have been outlined in this section.

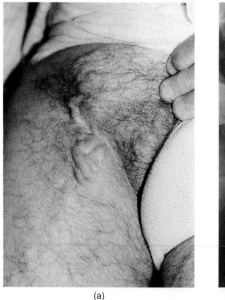
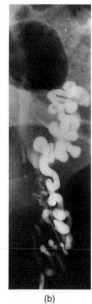

(a)   (b)

Fig. 4.30   Repeated failure to eliminate a saphenous recurrence; the importance of preoperative assessment. (a) These varicose veins reappeared in the groin after three previous operations to remove them. Large varicose veins ran from the groin down the length of the limb and required a heavy full-length elastic stocking to control them. (b) Phlebogram showing the origin from a shallow saphenous stump. Surgery exposing the common femoral vein allowed this to be closed off by direct suture of the deep vein (see Fig. 4.27 (s)). The stump was negligible in size but gave considerable outflow through a venous plexus believed to be formed by revascularization. Surgery for this type of recurrence requires careful preparation including phlebography. This patient was seen 3 years later and there was no evidence of any further recurrence.

Complications of varicose veins

Two specific complications may arise in varicose veins as distinct from the changes caused by venous hypertension.

Haemorrhage

Varicose veins lying directly beneath the skin commonly become adherent to it and may stretch it so much that it no longer provides adequate protective covering. Then, only the thinnest layer of skin and fragile attenuated vein wall retain the blood, which shows inky blue through the membranous covering. This state is most likely to develop in varicose veins on the foot, ankle, and lower leg, particularly in elderly patients. The vein may burst with minor trauma or spontaneously when the patient is up and about. The ensuing haemorrhage can be copious, but is easily stopped by finger pressure, or if the patient lies down with the foot elevated and a firm pad and bandage are applied. This can be an alarming experience for the patient, and although the aperture will be temporarily plugged with clot, it will soon bleed again (Fig. 4.31(a). There is little natural tendency for it to heal because the underlying vein remains open and the unsupported devitalized skin lacks the vascular base necessary for repair processes. Treatment must be completed by elimination of the affected varicosity, and in an elderly person this can often be most simply achieved by compression sclerotherapy. However, the problem is usually more than a local one, and whenever possible it is better to treat the accompanying superficial vein incompetence

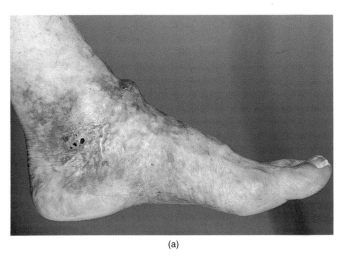
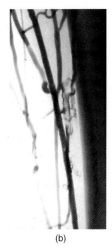

(a)   (b)

Fig. 4.31 Complications of varicose veins. (a) Haemorrhage. Large varicose veins and venotensive pigmentation near the ankle due to superficial incompetence in an elderly man. Just below the medial malleolus a scab can be seen marking the site of three episodes of severe haemorrhage; the veins nearby protrude through thin fragile skin. Urgent treatment was necessary and sclerotherapy, advised because of the patients's infirmity, proved successful. (b) Thrombosis. Phlebogram of an area of superficial thrombophlebitis in a varicosity. Opaque medium can be seen streaming round the thrombus, and Doppler flowmetry confirmed active downflow after exercise when standing. Use of a firm bandage to prevent such flow from causing a continuing build-up of thrombus is the basis of conservative treatment; this, combined with expression of clot through a stab incision, will bring immediate relief. Alternatively, appropriate surgery to the incompetent superficial veins may be carried out with excision of the thrombosed vein.

surgically and at the same time to excise the point of haemorrhage and its underlying varicose vein.

Veins liable to this complication can often be recognized and treated before haemorrhage occurs. Patients with such varicosities should be given clear instructions about how to control haemorrhage if it should occur before treatment.

Box 4.16   Haemorrhage from a varicose vein

Emergency treatment
- Lie patient flat
- Elevate limb
- Apply pad and firm bandage (check ankle pulses for arterial supply to foot)

Definitive treatment
- If elderly and infirm — limited sclerotheraphy to the vein causing bleeding since otherwise it will be a recurring problem.
- In most cases — treatment of choice is by surgery to eliminate the superficial incompetence causing varicosities and to excise the actual bleeding point with its underlying vein. An alternative is sclerotherapy as an immediate treatment and surgery if necessary later.

Phlebitis

Historical note

The term 'phlebitis' used to have a different and sinister significance before the introduction of asepsis towards the end of the nineteenth century. In the early part of that century surgeons thought of it as an inflammatory process in veins, with two types: one, fibrinous phlebitis, usually had a favourable outcome; the other, suppurative phlebitis, was likely to prove fatal. The fibrinous variety corresponds to present-day superficial or deep vein thrombosis, but it was not realized that in the deep vein it was far from benign and could cause death by pulmonary embolism until Virchow described this in the mid-nineteenth century. Even so, the dominant fear of the pre-Listerian surgeons was of suppurative phlebitis, which, as we now know, was a bacterial infective state filling a vein with purulent clot liable to enter the bloodstream, causing pyaemia with high fever, rigors, widespread abscesses, and, inevitably, death. It was a well-recognized complication of surgery at that time, particularly when veins were ligated (with non-sterile material in a septic operating field), trapping clot that suppurated and could only escape by entering the circulation. For this reason surgery to varicose veins was greatly feared. However, when the bacterial cause was understood, and with the development of aseptic surgery, it ceased to be a serious problem. For a long time the purely thrombotic form, whether in superficial or deep veins, was also assumed to be bacterial. With the realization that this was not so the terms 'thrombophlebitis', 'phlebothrombosis', or simply 'vein thrombosis' were introduced to emphasize their essentially thrombotic nature and to distinguish them from the very different infective suppurative type. It is important to realize that the latter is still a potential danger if ever the high standards of modern surgery should fail or when an uncontrolled infective cellulitis surrounding a vein creates a septic thrombosis within it. Fortunately, this is treatable with antibiotics and elimination of the source of infection, but surgery and medicine sometimes have to be practised in primitive conditions and the efficacy of modern methods should not allow past lessons to be forgotten. The old dragon of suppurative phlebitis has been subdued but not slain, and its retreat to the shadows uncovered another formidable dragon, deep vein thrombosis, which is damaging and dangerous and with which we continue to grapple (see Part II).

Superficial thrombophlebitis (phlebothrombosis)

Thrombosis in varicose veins is quite common and may be accepted as a complication without any very serious implications. However, when thrombosis occurs spontaneously in previously normal veins, it may well signify a serious background condition that is hitherto unsuspected. This includes malignancy (e.g. in the pancreas or bronchus), leukaemia or polycythaemia, vascular disease (particularly thromboangiitis obliterans), and disorders of blood clotting. Whether it appears as a single episode or recurring episodes in different parts of the body (phlebitis migrans), it is a clear indication for full medical screening to identify the cause. However, varicose veins in the lower limb can be regarded as sufficient explanation for local thrombosis without necessarily searching further for an underlying cause.

Thrombosis within a varicose vein, or any superficial vein, is accompanied by a tender swelling, often red and slightly warm to the touch. Until quite recently this was commonly regarded as an inflammation of the vein caused by infection. As explained above, the old term 'phlebitis' was retained until it was realized this was not so and that it must be distinguished from septic thrombosis in a vein secondary to a surrounding infection and which, by suppuration, is liable to cause a dangerous pyaemia. Now that it is recognized that the condition is a response to the thrombosis itself, the terms superficial thrombophlebitis or phlebothrombosis are used to denote this. Varicose veins are undoubtedly prone to thrombosis, partly because there are long periods of stasis in the unnaturally enlarged vein, for example when sitting, but also because production of fibrinolysin in the walls of a varicose vein is reduced. Even when quite a large thrombus has formed, blood continues to stream by it, continually depositing further thrombus so that the vein becomes progressively distended with clot. However, this does not completely occlude the vein, and studies by venography or by Doppler flowmeter show that, when the patient is upright and moving, blood continues to flow down the varicose vein, infiltrating its way round the clot and continually depositing further thrombus (Fig. 4.31(b). The vein becomes painfully overdistended and shows an inflammatory reaction. This gives the key to treatment, which is to apply external compression to prevent blood from continuing to flow through the affected vein. The process may limit itself to a few centimetres of vein or may go on extending progressively to involve a considerable area, perhaps the entire calf, when it may be mistaken for a deep vein thrombosis. It may extend into the saphenous vein and along its full length, and in these circumstances, may occasionally release a pulmonary embolus. Apart from this, it is seldom life-threatening although very troublesome to the patient.

Diagnosis

The tender red swelling on the leg with an indurated cord of thrombosed vein is characteristic. The diagnosis can usually be safely made on clinical grounds alone, but where deep vein thrombosis is seriously suspected, this should be checked by phlebography or ultrasonography rather than risk mistreating a life-threatening condition. Occasionally it is difficult to distinguish between superficial thrombosis in the long saphenous vein and a lymphangiitis, but the latter condition will lack the firm cord of thrombosed vein and will be accompanied by high fever unlike the low pyrexia that may be present in superficial phlebitis.

Treatment

Traditional conservative treatment is by applying a firm compression bandage (as in sclerotherapy). An anti-inflammatory agent such as indomethacin may be used to relieve pain, but antibiotics are not necessary. If the condition is unusually extensive, it may be advisable to put the leg in high elevation (but check for ankle pulses beforehand), with the patient encouraged in active movements and maintained like this until the condition starts to recede; at this stage mobilization is commenced in a firm support bandage. In most circumstances anticoagulants need not be used, but in extreme cases the condition will resolve more rapidly with a few days of heparin followed by oral anticoagulation for some weeks. If superficial thrombophlebitis extends above the knee to the groin, its extension into the common femoral vein with the threat of pulmonary embolus is possible, and anticoagulant treatment or surgery taking out the long saphenous vein, with careful thrombectomy to the common femoral vein, is indicated. (see Part II, pp.).

However, active intervention is often greatly to be preferred because it will bring immediate relief from pain and ensure a rapid recovery. If a substantial set of varicose veins are present and the circumstances allow it, the most effective course is to carry out the appropriate operation for this without delay and at the same time to excise the thrombophlebitic vein; this will be curative for the phlebitis and the varicose state that caused it. When this course is not possible, the simple procedure of evacuating the clot from the thrombosed vein is very effective and can be carried out under local anaesthesia by a single 2-mm skin incision into it. The clot is then extruded by firm finger pressure and a pad and bandage applied without skin suture. This gives complete relief and, provided that firm compression is maintained for several weeks afterwards, will cure the phlebitis so that the overall problem of widespread varicose veins can be tackled at a more convenient time.

Thrombosis in deep veins is described separately in Part II.

Box 4.17   Superficial thrombophlebitis

This is commonplace in varicose veins, but elsewhere, particularly if recurring at variable sites (phlebitis migrans), it may well signify hidden malignancy or a serious generalized disease such as leukaemia, polycythaemia, a blood clotting disorder or thromboangiitis obliterans (Buergers disease). **With an unexplained phlebitis, other than in pre-existing varicose veins, a full medical examination to determine its significance should be carried out.**

Varicose veins can be accepted as the cause unless veins elsewhere are involved, but do not entirely forget the other possibilities given above.

Local differential diagnosis
Inflammation due to sepsis, including lymphangitis. If very extensive, superficial phlebitis can be mistaken for a deep vein thrombosis. The usual investigations for venous disorder can be carried out and should confirm superficial incompetence and may even show Doppler downflow through the phlebitic vein with exercise.

Treatment
If obvious varicose veins are present and patient is otherwise fit, treat as follows.

- A firm bandage (as in sclerotherapy, to prevent further blood entering and clotting) and exercise. Antibiotics are not necessary and anticoagulants are only exceptionally required. Anti-inflammatory agents can be used to relieve discomfort.

or

- Evacuate clot through a stab incision and bandage firmly; this effectively relieves discomfort.

or

- At an early opportunity proceed directly to surgery treating the superficial incompetence fully and excising the phlebitic vein; this is the treatment of choice when circumstances allow.

5 Clinical patterns of venous disorder II
Syndromes of valve deficiency and weak vein walls

Valveless syndrome or primary valve deficiency

The spectrum of valve deficiency

The majority of patients with incompetence in the superficial veins, described in the Chapter 4, fall into a clearly defined group that responds well to treatment. However, there is a group, comprising about 8 per cent of venous disorders, in which a more widespread defect is present and treatment is far less satisfactory. There is no sharp demarcation between the two groups but, rather, a spectrum of defect with, at one end, well-defined superficial vein incompetence and, at the other, a widespread deficiency of functioning valves in both superficial and deep veins. This deficiency of valves in the deep veins (Fig. 5.1) must not be confused with the post-thrombotic state described later because the patients give no history suggesting previous deep vein thrombosis and, on phlebography, the deep veins are widely open without any evidence of post-thrombotic deformity or occlusion.

In the spectrum of valve deficiency, the 'well-defined' states at one end have a normal complement of valves in superficial veins but these are incompetent; moving along the spectrum, valves in both superficial and deep veins become increasingly deficient in number (Fig. 5.2). The absence of valves without any evidence of preceding thrombosis suggests an inborn error in valve development. This is supported by the not uncommon finding of incompetent superficial veins in early teenage boys and girls, and the occurrence of valveless deep and superficial veins in well-recognized states of congenital venous abnormality such as Klippel–Trenaunay syndrome. Deficiency of valves in the deep veins leads to ineffective venous pumping so that venous hypertension easily develops, particularly if the superficial veins also have gross incompetence. Patients with well-valved deep veins have a robust pumping mechanism which is not easily overwhelmed even by substantial superficial vein incompetence, and this may explain why many patients have large varicose veins without any evidence of venous hypertension. In contrast, other patients with similar varicosities show obvious venotensive changes and ulceration, possibly because they lie halfway along the spectrum of change, with poorly valved deep veins and a relatively weak pumping mechanism that is easily overwhelmed by superficial incompetence; surgery to the superficial veins can restore a precarious balance with healing of the ulcer, but some care is required to

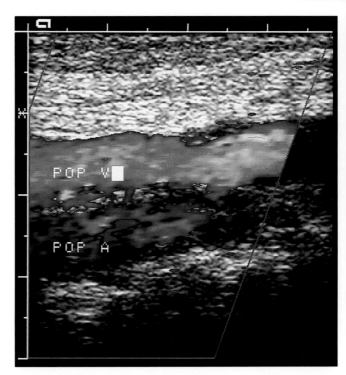

Fig. 5.1 The deep veins may show unexpected valve incompetence indicated here by heavy reflux (red) in an upper popliteal vein. Colour flow scanning picks this up very easily.

maintain this. At the far end, the predominant failure is in the deep veins and causes a pump insufficiency too severe to be remedied by removing incompetent superficial veins. These patients suffer from intractable ulceration that is not amenable to any form of surgery to the superficial veins (Fig. 5.3(a) (i)). For descriptive purposes this has been named the valveless syndrome here, but it is also known as primary valve deficiency and is, of course, one variety of chronic venous insufficiency (and see 'venous' oedema in Part III). The main features of this state are summarized in Box 5.1.

Clinical presentation of these cases is very similar to post-thrombotic syndrome and the diagnosis is usually made from phlebography or ultrasonography.

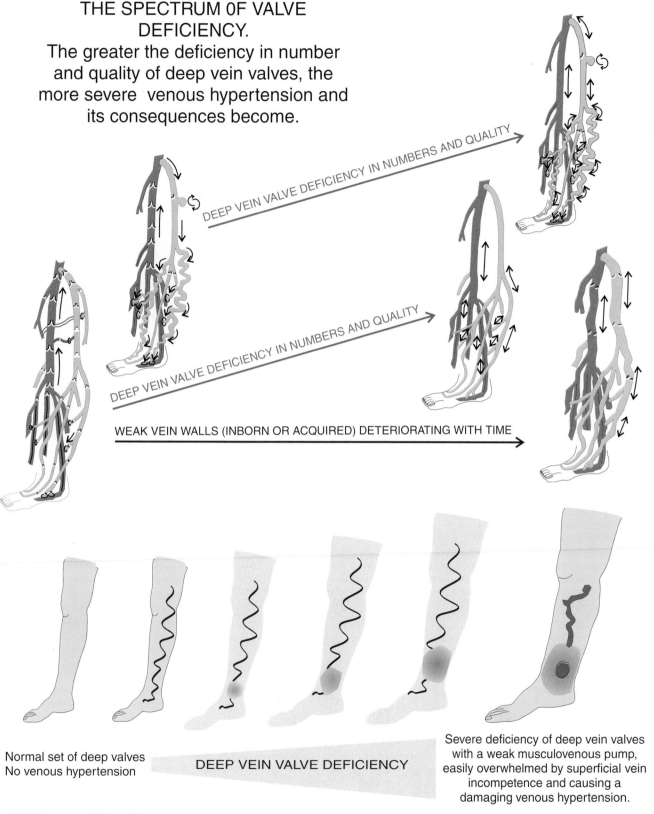

THE SPECTRUM 0F VALVE DEFICIENCY.
The greater the deficiency in number and quality of deep vein valves, the more severe venous hypertension and its consequences become.

DEEP VEIN VALVE DEFICIENCY IN NUMBERS AND QUALITY

DEEP VEIN VALVE DEFICIENCY IN NUMBERS AND QUALITY

WEAK VEIN WALLS (INBORN OR ACQUIRED) DETERIORATING WITH TIME

Normal set of deep valves
No venous hypertension

DEEP VEIN VALVE DEFICIENCY

Severe deficiency of deep vein valves with a weak musculovenous pump, easily overwhelmed by superficial vein incompetence and causing a damaging venous hypertension.

Fig. 5.2 The spectrum of valve deficiency. A small number of lower limbs without evidence of superficial vein incompetence have a deficiency of deep vein valves, ranging from mild to severe, and show a corresponding failure of the venous pumping mechanism. In patients with varicose veins due to superficial vein incompetence about 8 per cent have a similar deficiency of valves in the deep veins and according to the severity of this there is an increasing likelihood of venous ulceration which will fail to respond to surgical elimination of the incompetent superficial veins.

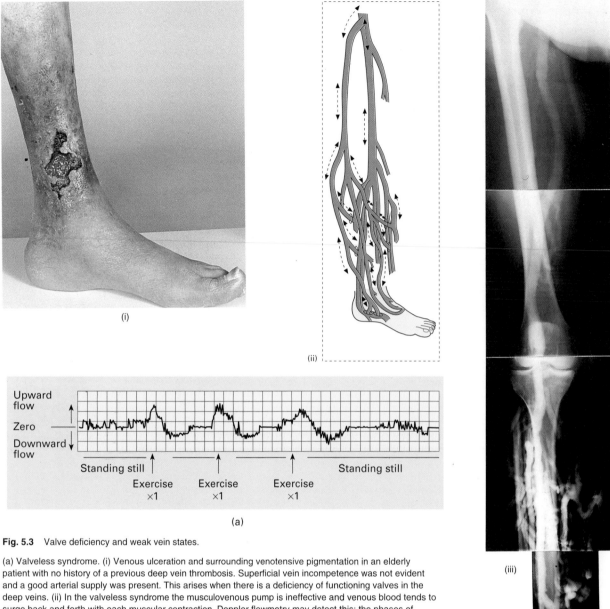

Fig. 5.3 Valve deficiency and weak vein states.

(a) Valveless syndrome. (i) Venous ulceration and surrounding venotensive pigmentation in an elderly patient with no history of a previous deep vein thrombosis. Superficial vein incompetence was not evident and a good arterial supply was present. This arises when there is a deficiency of functioning valves in the deep veins. (ii) In the valveless syndrome the musculovenous pump is ineffective and venous blood tends to surge back and forth with each muscular contraction. Doppler flowmetry may detect this; the phases of upflow and downflow with exercise are of equal duration and magnitude. (iii) Composite phlebogram in the valveless syndrome. Strong surge between tibial and superficial veins was evident on screening and, with a change of tilt from near-horizontal to near-vertical, opacified blood disappeared rapidly from higher levels as it shifted down valveless deep veins; no valves could be demonstrated.

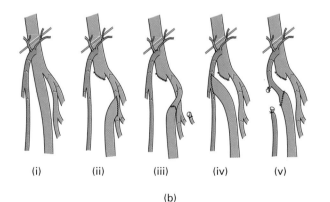

(b) Surgery for valve deficiency states. Transposition of a major vein to a well-valved channel nearby. (i) A valveless femoropopliteal state but with good valves in the long saphenous or profunda femoris veins offers several opportunities for transposition. (ii), (iii) End-to-side, or end-to-end, anastomosis with the profunda femoris vein or a tributary of it. (iv), (v) End-to-side, or end-to-end, anastomosis with the long saphenous vein.

(b)

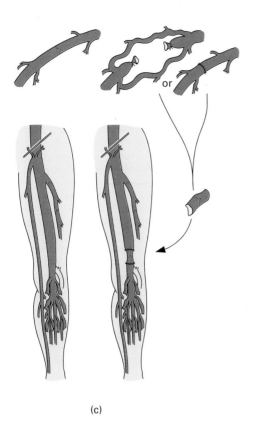

(c)

(c) Valve transplantation for femoropopliteal valve deficiency (Taheri). A good valve in the brachial vein is transplanted to the upper popliteal vein.

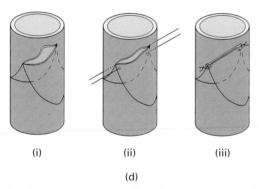

(i)   (ii)   (iii)

(d)

(d) Correction of prolapsing valve cusps (Kistner). The valve is exposed and the slack cusps are tightened by appropriate stitches.

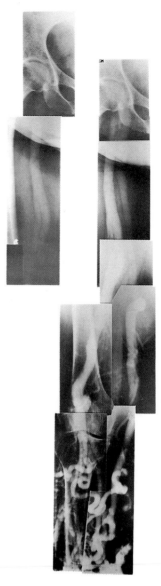

(e) Weak vein syndrome. Composite phlebogram in which superficial and deep veins show widespread weakening so that they have become massively enlarged, sacculated, or tortuous. This is accompanied by valve failure, caused by overexpansion of valve rings and separation of the cusps. Varicose veins in these patients are prone to massive recurrence after surgery.

Box 5.1 Features of valveless syndrome

- There is no history of a previous deep vein thrombosis.
- Gross saphenous incompetence is often present, or incompetence may come from multiple sources; obvious varicose veins are not necessarily present.
- Selective Trendelenburg test does not control enlarged superficial veins because of the incompetence in deep veins.
- Severe venotensive changes, often with ulceration, are present.
- Doppler flowmetry to enlarged veins shows surge back and forth with little purposeful movement in either direction (Fig. 5.3(a) (ii)).

- Photoplethysmography shows a short recovery time in keeping with an inadequate venous pump and incompetent valves; this is not improved by any manipulation of superficial veins.
- Phlebography: the deep veins are widely open throughout with no evidence of previous deep vein thrombosis and few, if any, functioning valves can be demonstrated in them (Fig. 5.3 (a) (iii)).
- Ultrasonography: this will confirm substantial reflux and lack of valves in the deep veins.

Treatment

Provided that phlebography has shown the deep veins to be widely open but valveless, it is permissible to remove enlarged and valveless superficial veins. In borderline cases, this reduction in the load on the pumping mechanism may restore it to an adequate performance. In more severe examples it brings little or no benefit and treatment will have to rely upon the conservative measures of elevation whenever possible and the use of external support by elastic stockings.

Surgical restoration of valve function

As incompetence in deep veins is the main problem, it may be possible to improve this by one of the following methods.

1. Transposition of a deep vein into a neighbouring vein that is well valved, for example implanting the upper end of a superficial femoral vein into the side of a valved profunda femoris vein nearby (Fig. 5.3(b)). This may be useful in congenital states of valve deficiency including Klippel–Trenaunay syndrome.

2. Transplantation of a suitable venous valve taken from elsewhere in the body and inserted as an autograft into an incompetent deep vein, for example using a valve from the brachial vein, or a saphenous vein of the opposite side, to transplant into the upper popliteal vein (Taheri's operation) (Fig. 5.3(c)). Again, this may be of help in inborn states of valve deficiency.

3. Repair of prolapsing valve cusps by valvuloplasty (Kistner's operation). This procedure tightens up selected valve cusps when incompetence is caused by excessive length with one cusp prolapsing beneath the other (Fig. 5.3(d)). A small number of patients with severe venous insufficiency have this form of incompetence in the femoropopliteal deep veins, and the procedure may be suitable them. The operation has yet to gain general acceptance although successful cases are reported.

4. Use of a tendon or silastic sling around the popliteal vein to act as a substitute external valve (Psathakis). This procedure has yet to be evaluated independently, and there is some indication that deep vein thrombosis and pulmonary embolism may be a problem. Until further evidence about its safety and success rate is available, it is not recommended.

Caution. These operations require an experienced surgeon.

Weak vein syndrome

This is a different state from that described above, although the two may coexist. The patients often have a strong family history of varicose veins and develop unusually large incompetent superficial veins leading down to equally large varicosities (Fig. 5.3(e)). With surgical treatment there is a strong tendency for further large recurrent varicosities to appear within a year or two. Gross examples are seen following inadequate surgery, for instance when the long saphenous vein has been ligated at too low a level or has not been stripped, and the source of the recurrent varicosities is from surviving branches in a saphenous stump, perforators in the thigh, or interconnections between the saphenous systems. It is possible that extrinsic factors play a part; for example some of the most severe cases are seen in people whose work involves prolonged standing and high consumption of alcohol, such as publicans and hoteliers. Clinical examination

and phlebography gives a strong impression that the veins lack inherent strength and easily overexpand. Indeed, this may be the primary problem because weak vein walls will allow valve cusps to separate and become incompetent; deficiency of valves does not seem to be a cause because an adequate number may be present but grossly incompetent. Histological studies commonly find some degenerative changes in the vein walls of patients with varicose veins, and in the state just described the primary defect may be an extreme form of this.

Box 5.2   Features of weak vein wall syndrome

This has some similarities with valveless syndrome but is due to lack of inherent strength in the walls of both superficial and deep veins. There may be an adequate number of valves but these are rendered ineffective by inadequate support from the vein walls.

Features
- Chronic venous insufficiency with venotensive changes which may be severe.
- Massive superficial (varicose) veins and oversized deep veins are widespread.
- Trendelenburg test is usually inconclusive.
- Doppler flowmetry is equivocal, but may show brief downflow and strong surge in superficial veins with exercise.
- Photoplethysmography shows a short recovery time in keeping with an inadequate venous pump and incompetent valves; this is not improved by any manipulation of superficial veins.
- Phlebography: The deep veins are widely open throughout, indeed baggy and oversized, but with no evidence of previous deep vein thrombosis. Although valves may be present, few, if any, functioning valves can be demonstrated (Fig. 5.3(a) (iii)).
- Ultrasonography: this will confirm substantial reflux and lack of functioning valves in enlarged deep veins.

Diagnosis and treatment

If there has been no previous treatment, all the usual features of simple incompetence will be found, including good control with a Trendelenburg test, although the veins are unusually large. This does not contraindicate surgery but rather is an encouragement for conscientious surgery; saphenous ligation must not leave any branches at the upper end, stripping of the long saphenous vein must be at least to upper calf, and all major varicosities must be removed.

If the patient presents with recurrent varicose veins, the massive size of these and their unusual pattern may be daunting. However, with careful mapping out and use of the Doppler flowmeter or ultrasonography, the source and pathway of incompetence may be identified. Further surgery must be carefully planned and this will require detailed phlebography to guide the surgeon. A good long-term result may be obtained but in the very nature of the condition further recurrence is possible and, as a last resort, strong elastic stockings will be required to control the varicose veins as a long-term policy.

Conclusion

The two states described above, i.e. the valveless syndrome and the weak vein syndrome, are ill-defined and poorly understood. However, it would be unrealistic in describing the venous disorders to give the impression that all categories are clear-cut and separate from each other. Certainly, most patients can be fitted into a well-defined category and rational treatment can be based upon this. In others, one of the ill-defined varieties just described may baffle the surgeon, or two separate categories of venous disorder may both to be present in the same limb and give a very confusing picture. In these circumstances clinical expertise alone is not sufficient and the extra information provided by ultrasonic imaging and phlebography must be called upon to make sure that the best decision is made for the patient. Care must be taken to exclude the next category, the post-thrombotic syndrome.

6 Clinical patterns of venous disorder III
Deep vein impairment: the post-thrombotic (post-phlebitic) syndrome

Deep vein impairment

Acute and subacute deep vein thrombosis

The most important form of deep vein impairment is, of course, active deep vein thrombosis because of its insidious onset, and its capacity to extend and possibly to give rise to life-threatening pulmonary embolism. The venous specialist must be familiar with acute deep vein thrombosis and this is considered in detail in Part II. However, it may well present unexpectedly at the vein clinic in subacute form, which may have caused no more than mild discomfort for some weeks and has been attributed to prominent veins on the leg. This subacute form, appearing unobtrusively in an otherwise active person, is not particularly rare, possibly related to a minor leg injury, and may continue to simmer indefinitely unless it is treated with anticoagulants. Each case will require careful screening for occult disease, such as malignancy or abnormality in blood clotting factors. On routine examination of the veins by Doppler flowmetry or ultrasonography, suspicion may be aroused by finding continuous upward flow in the long saphenous vein, accentuated by exercise, which is a strong indication that the deep veins may be obstructed, possibly by recent thrombus. Detailed examination by ultrasonography or phlebography (see Chapter 3) can soon clarify the diagnosis; this is discussed fully in the section on diagnosis in Part II.

Chronic deep vein impairment

Chronic venous insufficiency is caused by some form of impairment to the deep veins. Loss of valve function or obstruction to the lumen removes the essential ability to pump upwards against gravity. This may arise in several ways.

- An inborn or primary deficiency in the number and competence of deep vein valves. Also, weak vein walls may cause incompetence in valves by separation of their cusps; this may be inborn or by acquired degenerative change (incompetent valves and loss of pumping ability) (see Chapters 5 and 8).

- Post-thrombotic damage in the deep veins (incompetent valves, loss of pumping ability, and obstruction to venous return) (Fig. 6.1).

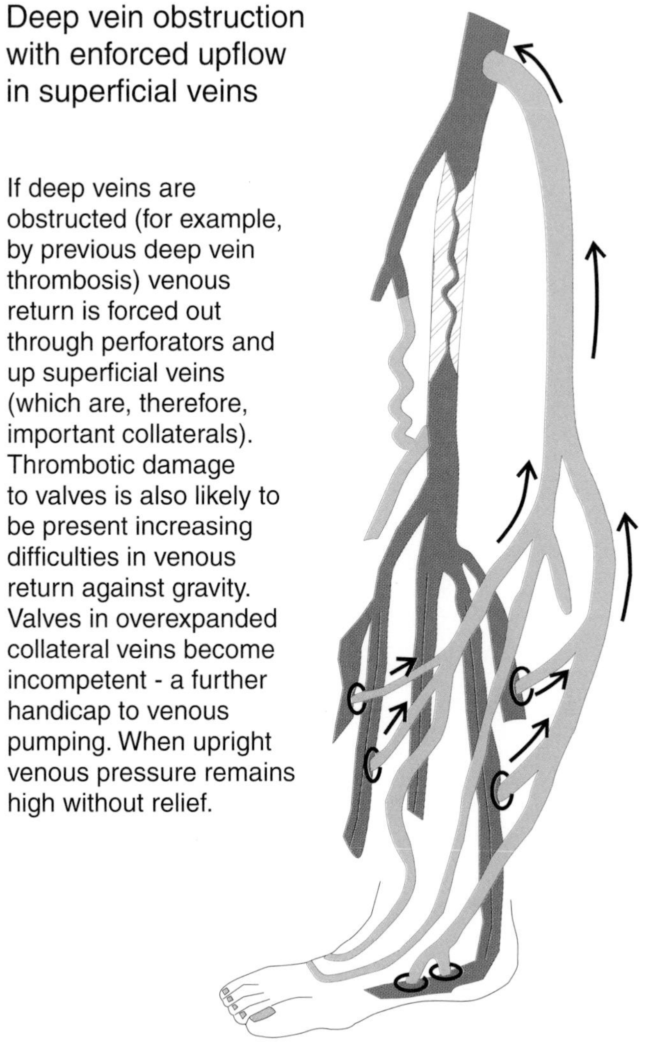

Deep vein obstruction with enforced upflow in superficial veins

If deep veins are obstructed (for example, by previous deep vein thrombosis) venous return is forced out through perforators and up superficial veins (which are, therefore, important collaterals). Thrombotic damage to valves is also likely to be present increasing difficulties in venous return against gravity. Valves in overexpanded collateral veins become incompetent - a further handicap to venous pumping. When upright venous pressure remains high without relief.

Fig. 6.1 Post-thrombotic syndrome with obstruction to a major deep vein and enforced collateral upflow in superficial veins.

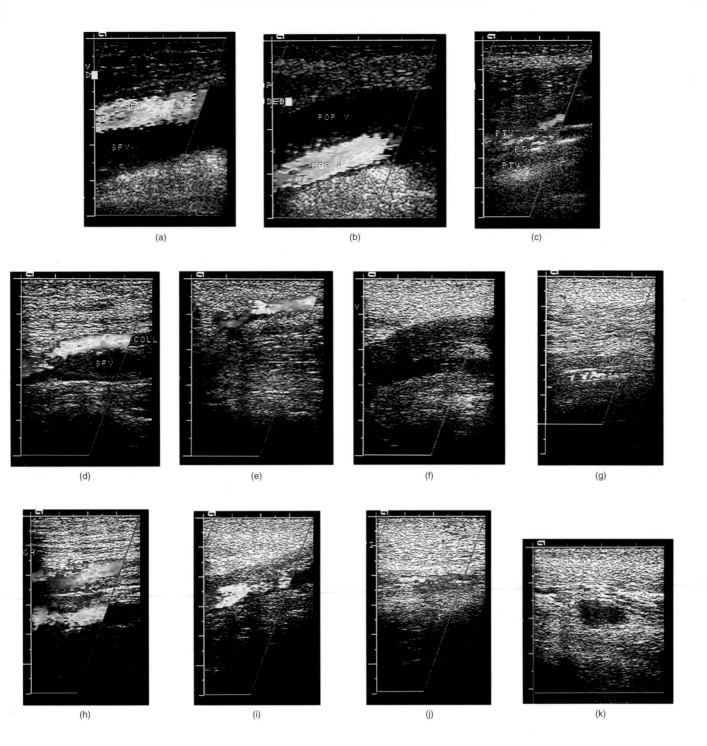

Fig. 6.2 Development of post-thrombotic syndrome. Three sets of ultrasonic colour flow scans taken at intervals over 6 months to show the changes following deep vein thrombosis, leading to lasting impairment of the deep vein pumping mechanism.

(a) Deep vein thrombosis is confirmed. The superficial femoral (deep) vein shows as a dark outline alongside the artery. It was found to be incompressible (did not narrow with pressure by probe) and there was no evidence of flow within it. The neighbouring artery shows normal flow.

(b), (c) Similar thrombotic changes extend through popliteal vein and one tibial vein.

(d)–(g) Four months later. The changes persist but collateral flow can be seen entering the superficial femoral vein by a branch vein and the short saphenous vein also shows some flow in a downward direction. One tibial vein remains occluded.

(h)–(k) Six months after onset. Patchy flow has now increased in the superficial femoral and popliteal veins, and the tibial vein appears open with flow distally. In (k) the outline of the gastrocnemius veins can be seen but they remain-occluded with thrombus.

   After 6 months recanalization is well established and is likely to continue but, at best, the vein lumen will be narrowed and irregular in many parts and the affected valves will not regain normal function. Thus recovery is only partial, with a persisting post-thrombotic syndrome which is likely to be quite severe (see also Fig. 10.5).

● External pressure on a main vein by neighbouring disease, for example a tumour (obstruction to venous return).

In this chapter we are mainly concerned with the most common variety, post-thrombotic damage.

Post-thrombotic syndrome

Thrombosis in the deep veins of the lower limbs (Fig. 6.2; see also Fig. 10.5) is a common complication in serious illness, pregnancy, following surgical operations, and after severe injury, particularly fractures of the lower limbs or pelvis. It may be localized to a small area or extend massively through both lower limbs; in its lesser forms it may pass almost unnoticed, but in its major form it causes severe illness and is a threat to life through pulmonary embolism (see Part II). In the affected limb(s) the severity of the resulting venous obstruction gradually subsides, due partly to absorption of thrombus and recanalization of the veins but also to the progressive enlargement of collateral veins, both superficial and deep, providing an alternative pathway of venous return. However, neither of these changes reflects a return to true normality, and venous flow in the limb is all too often permanently impaired with corresponding disability (Fig. 6.3(a)). The deep veins involved in this process will show the following changes in structure and function.

1. The vein may remain permanently obstructed, causing a persistently raised venous pressure beneath it and forcing other veins to act as collaterals (Figs 6.1 and 6.3 (b)).

2. The vein may recanalize but in this process it becomes severely deformed and the valves are rendered functionless (see Fig. 6.2). Not only does this channel offer resistance to venous return but it lacks one of the essential characteristics of a vein, i.e. properly functioning valves (Fig. 6.3 (c)). Thus the ability to pump is lost and heavy reflux occurs down the vein. It cannot make any contribution to venous return against gravity and by reflux it will actively invalidate any return achieved by neighbouring veins.

3. Collateral vessels formed from vasa vasorum, lesser deep veins, perforators, and superficial veins will undergo expansion with separation of the valve cusps so that the valves become disabled. Eventually large channels without effective valves are formed which compensate for obstruction in the deep veins but are unable to prevent heavy reflux of blood down their length when the patient stands (Fig. 6.3(d)). If only a small area is involved the effect may be insignificant, but when major veins are extensively involved, venous return, which is adequate when the patient is horizontal, will suffer from the compounded difficulties of defective pumping units, resistance to venous outflow from exercising muscles, and extensive loss of functioning valves in recanalized deep veins and collateral

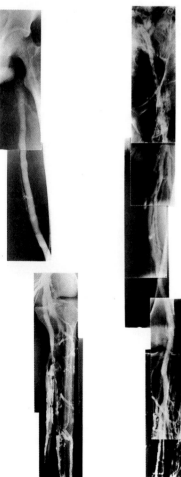
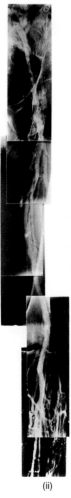

Fig. 6.3 Post-thrombotic states.

(a) The consequences of deep vein thrombosis in a young man. (i) A phlebogram taken at the time of a left deep vein thrombosis. The tibial veins are filled with thrombus (tram-line sign), and the common femoral and iliac veins fail to fill. (ii) Three years later the patient has post-thrombotic syndrome with pigmentation, swelling, induration, and ulceration. Phlebograms show unsatisfactory tibial veins and extensive deformity in the common femoral and external iliac veins. (iii) Photophlethysmography comparing the two sides. Left side (upper tracing) shows severely reduced refilling time at 8 s; the unaffected right side is normal at 25 s.

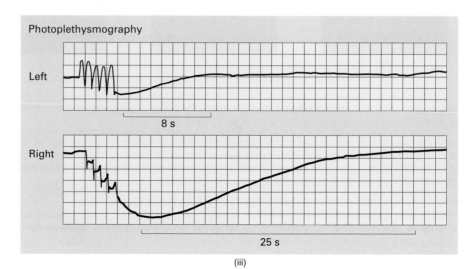

(i)   (ii)   (iii)

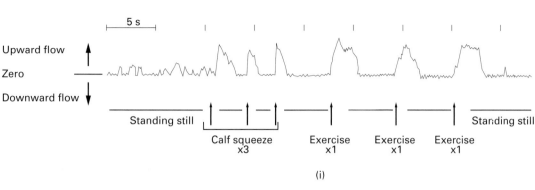

Upward flow

Zero

Downward flow

Standing still

Calf squeeze
x3

Exercise
x1

Exercise
x1

Exercise
x1

Standing still

(i)

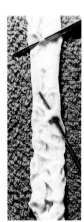

Fig. 6.3 (continued).

(b) Collateral flow in superficial veins compensating for deep vein obstruction. (i) A diagram of superficial veins taking the collateral flow past a deep vein obstruction. A Doppler flowmeter recording from the long saphenous vein of a patient with this condition shows upward flow, accentuated by exercise.
(ii) Composite phlebogram for a well-compensated post-thrombotic femoropopliteal obstruction, showing a short saphenous vein, and an upward extension of it, playing an important role in venous return. The long saphenous vein can be seen in the upper thigh also contributing to collateral return. This patient presented with slight swelling and prominent superficial veins some years after a fractured ankle and immobilization in plaster cast; conservative treatment was advised.

(ii)

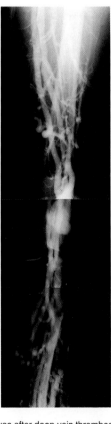

(c) Interior of a vein, recanalized after thrombosis. The lumen is irregular and deformed with synechiae stretching across it. A vein like this offers resistance to normal flow and lacks the valves essential to normal function.

(d) Loss of competent valves after deep vein thrombosis. A composite phlebogram in the post-thrombotic syndrome is shown. The normal pattern of principal deep veins cannot be recognized, but an enlarged short saphenous vein and an upward extension arising from a grossly tortuous vein in the popliteal fossa can be seen. No competent valves could be demonstrated at phlebography and the impression is of widespread veins capable of heavy reflux, although offering little resistance to venous upflow.

vessels. The reflux that this allows rapidly reverses any benefit from venous return against gravity achieved by neighbouring undamaged parts of the venous system. Normally, blood shifted upwards is held there by valves, but without functioning valves this key feature is lost and a complex but, in effect, continuous column of blood from foot to ankle is rapidly established on standing and exerts maximum venous pressure. This column moves up slowly by inflow across the capillaries, with peaks of upward movement from muscle activity but without any relief in its pressure by protective valves. On Doppler examination, actual reflux may only be seen when first rising from horizontal to upright while the high-pressure column of blood builds up. The net result is a sustained high venous pressure in the limb, unrelieved by exercise, when the patient is up and about. This leads to venous congestion and oedema, with the characteristic changes of venous hypertension, pigmentation, induration of superficial tissues (dermatoliposclerosis), and, eventually, ulceration near the ankle (see post-thrombotic syndrome in Part III). These long-term consequences of deep vein thrombosis are known as the **Post-thrombotic or post-phlebitic syndrome** and can give rise to severe disability in the limb. This is the most common cause of chronic venous insufficiency, but it is important to realize that similar venotensive changes can be caused by gross incompetence in the superficial veins, a state usually curable by surgery in contrast with the post-thrombotic state which can be ameliorated but seldom cured (Fig. 6.3(e)).

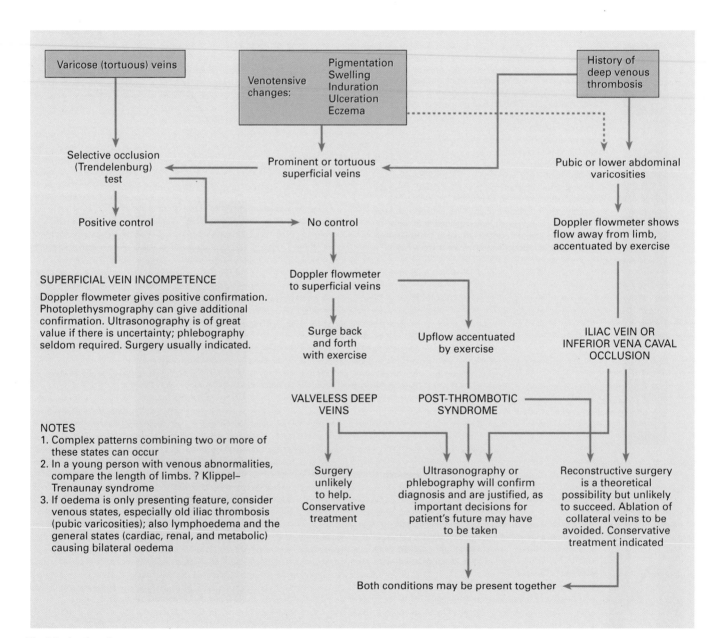

Fig. 6.3   (continued).

(e) Diagram of diagnostic pathways when venotensive changes are present. Treatment depends on the state causing venous hypertension and accurate diagnosis of this is essential. This requires more than clinical examination, and special investigation will be necessary.

Fig. 6.3   (continued).

(f) (Right) Patterns of post-thrombotic occlusion and some of the superficial veins used as collateral channels. In tibiopopliteal and femoropopliteal occlusion, long and short (and upward extension from it) saphenous veins and their branches are of paramount importance. In iliac vein occlusion, superficial veins (branches of external pudendal and superficial epigastric veins) cross the pubic region to the opposite side; many collateral deep veins within the pelvis will also be present. Demonstration of these veins, enlarged and tortuous, on phlebography is important diagnostically.

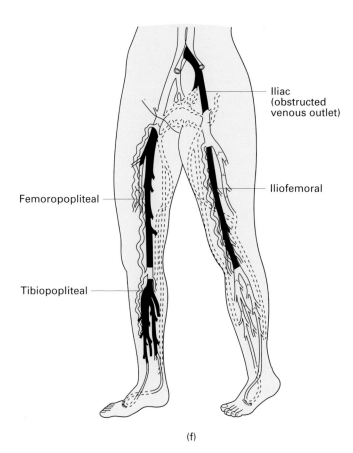

Iliac
(obstructed
venous outlet)

Iliofemoral

Femoropopliteal

Tibiopopliteal

(f)

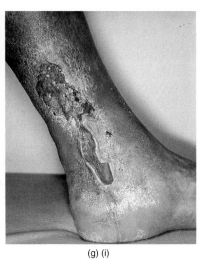

(g) (i)

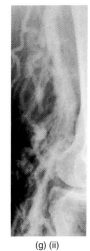

(g) (ii)

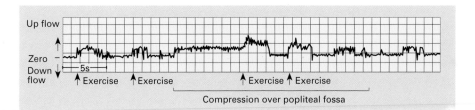

Up flow

Zero

Down
flow

5s

↑Exercise   ↑Exercise   ↑Exercise ↑Exercise

Compression over popliteal fossa

(g) (iii)

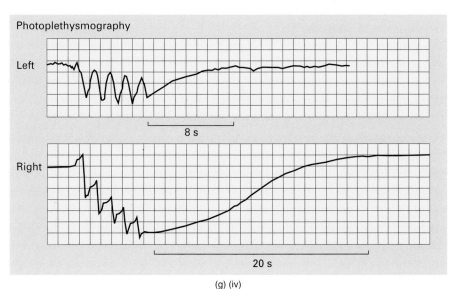

Photoplethysmography

Left

8 s

Right

20 s

(g) (iv)

(g) Chronic ulceration in severe post-thrombotic syndrome due to trauma, with occlusion of left popliteal vein. (i) Clinical appearance, showing the ulcer surrounded by typical pigmented liposclerotic changes (see Fig. 9.2 (d)) for response to treatment). (ii) Phlebography was unable to demonstrate any filling in the popliteal vein but gastrocnemius veins and an unidentified tortuous vein substitute for it. (iii) Doppler flowmetry in the remnants of the left long saphenous vein. Exercise, or compression of the popliteal fossa (containing many collateral veins, shown on the phlebogram), accentuates upflow; there is no downflow. (iv) Photoplethysmography. On the left side, the response to exercise is poor and the refilling time is abnormally brief at 8 s; on the right side, the refilling time is normal at 20 s.

There is great variation in the extent of changes that such a limb will show depending upon location, extent, and importance of the veins involved. Several patterns can be recognized, but one or more of these may be present in the same limb (Fig. 6.3(f)).

1. Tibiopopliteal   Here the deep veins below the knee are mainly affected. Small areas of thrombotic damage may give rise to perforating veins forcibly ejecting blood outwards, but more diffuse patterns can disorganize the massive pumping mechanisms in the muscles below the knee sufficiently to create severe venous hypertension and all its complications (see Fig. 6.3(g)). The deep veins in this region are so numerous and complex that it is often difficult to define the defect precisely or to demonstrate it satisfactorily on phlebography or ultrasonography. Moreover, it may be difficult to say whether the state found is due to episodes of deep vein thrombosis, possibly multiple and silent, or whether there is a diffuse valveless state due to an inborn weakness or deficiency in the valves which has become progressively more severe as the years pass. As with all forms of deep vein impairment, the superficial and deep veins in the foot may respond to the excessive venous pressure by becoming greatly enlarged to form a venous pool in which blood is sequestered as the foot is raised from the ground but forcibly ejected upwards when it is put down again. This shift back and forth to the foot can only be an added burden on the already damaged pumping mechanism.

2. Femoropopliteal   This is a common and more easily recognized form of post-thrombotic state (Figs 6.1 and 6.3(b) (ii)). There is likely to be significant venous obstruction, with permanent swelling below the knee and all the undesirable effects of venous hypertension because the superficial veins, forced to act as collaterals, will ensure that venous hypertension is shared by the surface tissues. Added to this are all the undesirable effects of reflux in open but valve-damaged deep veins, and in veins enlarged as collaterals, both superficial and deep, when the patient stand is standing. The result is a continuous column of venous blood, uninterrupted by effective valves and at high venous pressure.

3. Iliac   The left common iliac vein is particularly vulnerable to thrombosis because it may be narrowed by the right common iliac artery passing over it. Thrombosis in this vein often fails to recanalize so that the venous outlet to the limb remains permanently obstructed (obstructed venous outlet syndrome). If the limb below this is otherwise virtually undamaged, it may cause little more than slight swelling and the development of tortuous collateral veins crossing from the left to the right side of the pelvis, usually visible as varicosities in the pubic region (Fig. 6.4). Beneath this it is possible for a typical long saphenous incompetence to develop, taking its source from the pubic collateral veins, as described under the complex patterns referred to below. If this is not recognized, surgery to the saphenous system may damage important collateral veins in the groin.

4. Iliofemoral   Iliac thrombosis is often accompanied by simultaneous thrombosis in the femoral and popliteal veins to give an iliofemoral post-thrombotic syndrome with a particularly severe pattern of venous hypertension combining the worst features of obstruction to the venous outlet, impaired pumping mechanism, and heavy reflux in recanalized deep veins and overdistended collateral veins (Figs 6.4(d)–6.4(h)), causing rapid build-up of a continuous column of venous blood at sustained high venous pressure.

Fig. 6.4 (a-h)   Post-thrombotic iliac vein occlusion.

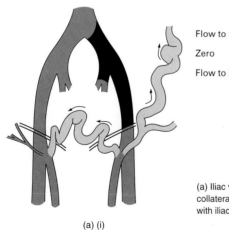

(a) (i)

Flow to right

Zero

Flow to left

←— 5s —→

Standing still

Exercise ×5

Standing still

(a) (ii)

(a) Iliac vein occlusion and superficial collateral veins. (i) Diagram of superficial veins likely to be involved. Many collateral veins also cross over deeply within the pelvis. (ii) Doppler flow recording from a pubic varicosity in a patient with iliac occlusion. The predominant direction of flow is away from the occluded side and it is accentuated by exercise.

Complex states

These can occur if the great pumping units in the muscles of the leg are substantially undamaged and are able to reduce venous pressure in the ankle and foot successfully. In these circumstances it is possible to find the long saphenous vein acting as a collateral but giving off branches which set up a simple pattern of incompetence by allowing downflow to the low-pressure areas in the lower leg and foot, or pubic collaterals may act as a source for incompetent downflow in the limb on the opposite side. This has been described earlier and is illustrated in Fig. 4.13. Such contradictory flow and counterflow is not uncommon and all too easily confuses the diagnosis.

Special investigations in deep vein impairment

In all the states just described, plethysmography will show a poor response to exercise and a shortened refilling time (Figs 6.4(f) (iv) 6.4(g) (iii)); volumetric methods measuring expelled volume will find this substantially reduced. These findings cannot be restored to normal by any manipulation of superficial veins. Functional phlebography or ultrasonography will confirm and define the state of the deep vein and valves. It is essential to obtain this evidence before deciding that no cure is available, and only conservative management can be employed.

Prevention of post-thrombotic syndrome

Needless to say, with such a formidable catalogue of disability as the long-term effects of deep vein thrombosis, every effort must be made to avoid the occurrence of this complication in patients under medical and surgical care. Much can be done to minimize its occurrence and this is discussed in Part II, pp. 197–199.

If deep vein thrombosis should occur, a full length graduated compression stocking should in worn over the following two years as this will help to minimize eventual post-thrombotic damage.

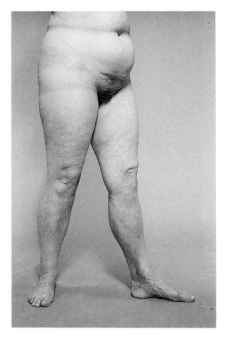

(b) Unsuspected iliac vein occlusion. This patient, aged 58, complained of swelling, pigmentation, and a small ulcer in the left lower leg. The history included a hysterectomy 5 years previously without known complication. However, pubic varicosities, in keeping with left iliac occlusion, were present as shown in this illustration. This is an important factor to be weighed in deciding treatment.

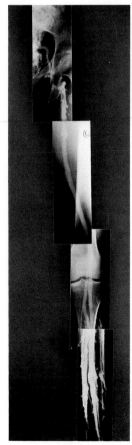

Fig. 6.4 (continued).

(c) Minimal disturbance with isolated occlusion of the iliac vein. This patient noticed swelling of the left lower limb soon after the birth of twins 4 months previously and anticoagulant treatment had been maintained since then. Examination showed only 2 cm of swelling at calf level but no enlarged veins or obvious pubic varicosities. (i) Photoplethysmography showing a virtually normal refilling time. (ii) Phlebography showing occlusion of the left iliac vein with a large collateral vein running across the pelvis; the deep vein system below the inguinal ligament appears undamaged in keeping with the normal photoplethysmogram (see (i)).

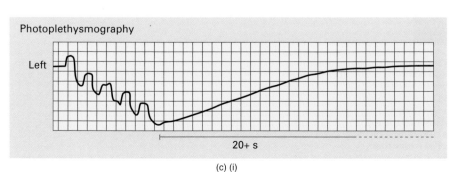

(c) (i)

(c) (ii)

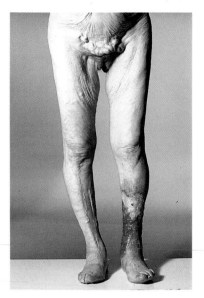

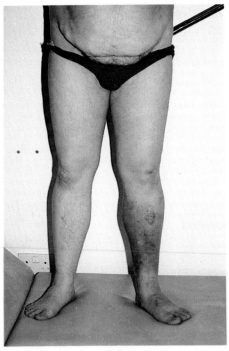

(f) (i)

Fig. 6.4   (continued).

(d) The consequences of severe iliofemoral occlusion. In this elderly patient there is a huge chronic ulcer on the leg, with overall swelling of the limb. The massive pubic veins are clear evidence of iliac occlusion and part of a compensatory mechanism that should not be disturbed.

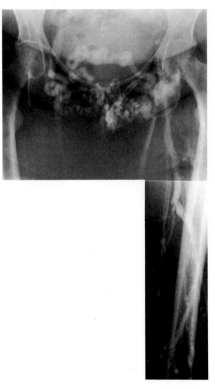

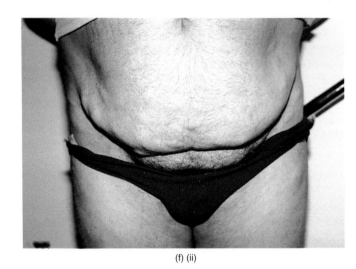

(f) (ii)

(f) Iliofemoral post-thrombotic state due to injury.

(i), (ii) This man, aged 20, had sustained a fractured pelvis 2 years previously. The left limb is swollen up to the groin, with induration and pigmentation in its lower part; large pubic varicosities are seen in the lower abdominal folds of fat.

(e) Late consequences of iliofemoral thrombosis seen on phlebography. This patient gave a history of 'white leg' of pregnancy 30 years previously. The left iliac veins are occluded and extensive pubic varicosities can be seen compensating; the superficial femoral deep vein is occluded and venous return from below this occlusion is by the profunda femoris vein and the long saphenous vein. Apart from mild swelling, this limb had given little trouble and her present complaint was of recurring phlebitis in varicose veins of the right limb due to long saphenous incompetence on that side arising from the pubic varicosities (see Fig. 4.13 (b) (i) (ii)).

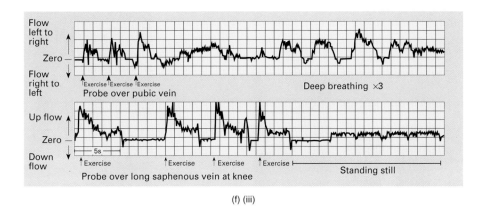

(f) (iii)

Fig. 6.4   (continued).

(iii) Doppler flowmetry recordings from pubic varicosities with predominant flow from left to right accentuated by exercise, and from the long saphenous vein with strong upflow with peaks caused by exercise movements.

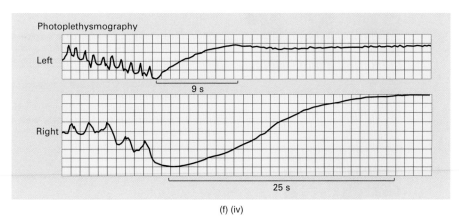

(f) (iv)

(iv) Photoplethysmograph. On the left side refilling time is only 9 s but on the right side it is normal at 25 s.

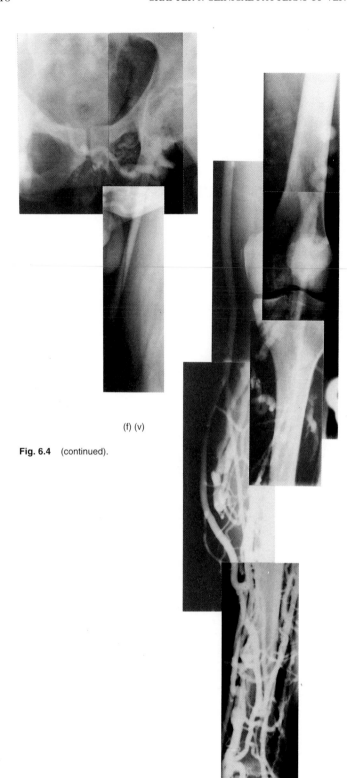

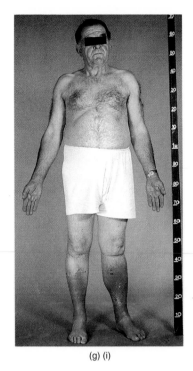

(g) (i)

(g) Severe iliofemoral post-thrombotic syndrome after multiple fractures in a road traffic accident.

(i) The patient's left limb is swollen up to the groin and heavily pigmented below the knee. The right side is also pigmented but without obvious swelling.
(ii) Doppler flowmetry and photoplethysmography showing all the features of deep vein impairment on both sides.
(iii) Doppler flowmetry and photoplethysmography showing all the features of deep vein impairment on both sides.
(iv) Phlebograms showing left iliac obstruction with collaterals crossing the pelvis and extensive failure in filling of deep veins on both sides.
(v) Phlebograms showing extensive failure in filling of deep veins of leg and thigh on both sides.

(f) (v)

Fig. 6.4 (continued).

(v) Composite phlebogram showing the features of deformed and occluded deep vein at all levels, including the iliac veins; the pubic and long saphenous veins, and an upward extension of the short saphenous vein, form prominent collateral pathways of venous return.

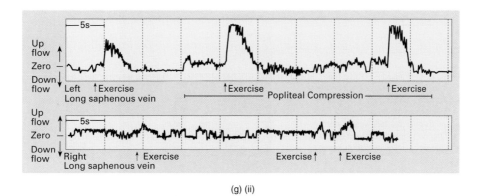

(g) (ii)

Fig. 6.4 (continued).

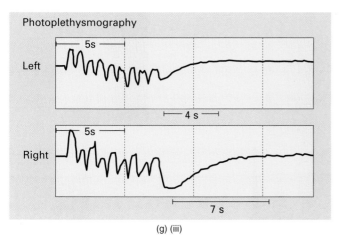

(g) (iii)

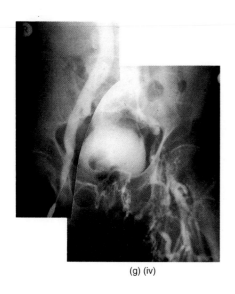

(g) (iv)

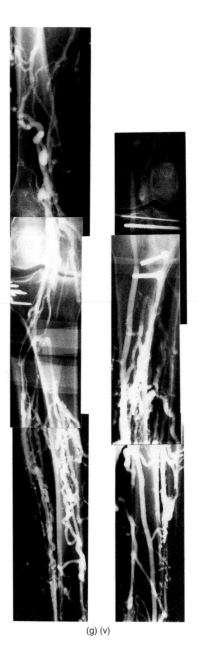

(g) (v)

Fig. 6.4 (continued).

(h) Iliofemoral post-thrombotic syndrome is the most common cause of severe disability from chronic venous insufficiency. Two further examples are illustrated here by composite phlebograms.
(i) This patient sustained deep vein thrombosis following fractured hip and prosthetic replacement. The long saphenous vein shows preferential collateral upflow and the deep veins are either severely deformed or fail to fill.
(ii) This patient was known to have had a left deep vein thrombosis 3 years previously. Preferential collateral upflow is shown in the long saphenous vein which is interrupted in its upper part; a major role in venous return has been assumed by the short saphenous vein and an upward extension from it, winding round the posterior thigh to join remnants of the long saphenous vein. The iliac veins are occluded and pelvic collateral veins cross the pelvis.

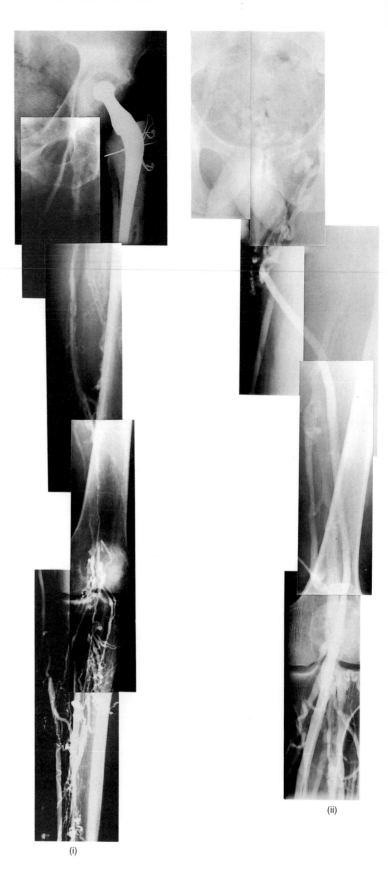

(i)

(ii)

Box 6.1 Late consequences of deep vein thrombosis

In some, nearly complete resolution occurs, particularly in the calf. However, in many there is persisting fibrotic damage in varying degree:

- deformed, narrowed, or totally occluded lumen
- damaged valves—fibrotic, thickened, and ineffective

This leads to a combination of occlusion and, in veins that are still open, incompetence.

The occlusion leads to the development of compensatory collateral channels:

- in neighbouring deep veins, often lesser branches, and in the vasa vasorum
- in superficial veins by outflow through perforators

These overexpanded veins often become incompetent by separation of valve cusps. On standing, the combined incompetence in deep and superficial veins causes a rapid build-up of sustained full (ankle to heart) venous pressure, unrelieved by exercise, exerted by a continuous valveless column of blood. This is a direct cause of venotensive skin changes and eventually ulceration in the leg. All this is aggravated by a surge of high pressure in the superficial veins with each footstep as the venous pool on the underside of the foot is forcibly thrust upwards when compressed by body weight.

In practice, Doppler flowmetry on the standing patient will show continuous upward flow in the superficial veins, accentuated by exercise movements. Reflux may not be seen except at the actual moment of rising from a horizontal to an upright position.

Microvascular changes

The high venous pressure leads to increased capillary filtration of fluid and proteins into the extracellular space. This is aggravated by white cell trapping and release of cytotoxins which further increase capillary permeability. The ultimate effect is reduced nutritional exchange, particularly to the skin.

Conservative treatment

Treatment by surgery can, at best, give only limited benefit to a post-thrombotic syndrome and the mainstay of treatment will be by conservative means. The worst manifestations of post-thrombotic syndrome are essentially due to venous hypertension, but even partial reduction of its effects brings great benefit. This can be achieved in two ways.

Warning

The requirements of conservative treatment for venous ulceration are in direct conflict with those of ischaemia due to arterial occlusion. The treatment described below involves elevation or compression bandaging of the limb. In an ischaemic limb this will severely aggravate its state and even cause its loss. If there is any doubt, the limb should not be raised above the horizontal and no form of compression bandage used until it has been proved that an adequate arterial supply is present.

Elevation of the limb above the horizontal

In this position, venous return occurs by gravity without requiring any pumping mechanism. During elevation, with the feet above heart level, venous pressure in the extremity falls away and the higher the elevation the more complete this will be (Fig. 6.5(a)). When the limb is maintained in this position (Figs 4.21(g) and 4.21(h)), all the adverse changes will steadily recede. However, it is clearly not practical to keep a patient indefinitely immobilized in this fashion, and so, as a compromise, there will be an initial period of continuous elevation in order to allow the worst lesions, such as ulceration, to heal. This is followed by increasing mobility alternating with spells of elevation. Eventually the proportion of the day to be spent in elevation, necessary to keep the limb healthy, will be learnt and the patient will have to try to arrange his or her life within this limitation. Certainly this must include the great advantage given by 7 or 8 h continuous elevation overnight. Usually it is possible, and this measure alone may be sufficient to maintain the limb in a reasonable state. If the patient becomes careless about spending sufficient time in elevation, deterioration of the limb soon gives a sharp reminder. Each patient will have to learn his or her own requirements in this respect. A programme of this sort, particularly during the time of continuous elevation, will bring the serious disadvantages of prolonged immobility unless this is counteracted by a firm policy of exercise. The time of continuous elevation to heal an ulcer must never be referred to as 'bed rest' but, instead, the patient must be urged to exercise his or her limbs and body repeatedly during the day, in fact 'activity elevation'. In addition, getting up for a few minutes active walking each hour will not harm the ulcer provided that the exercise time is strictly limited, but will prevent the patient from developing weak muscles and stiff joints. An initial period of instruction is necessary so that these principles are fully understood. The patient will then know how to control the health of the limb. This regimen is by far the most effective aspect of conservative treatment and, although it puts quite severe restrictions on the patient's way of life, this is a price most are prepared to pay to avoid the discomforts of uncontrolled venotensive changes. Clearly, in some patients the necessity to earn a living will prevent their following the programme that they know to be necessary, but even here ways of managing may be found. An example is that of a chef who worked every summer at a high salary in a top hotel, enduring steady deterioration in his limb as the season passed, but who then spent the winter in Mediterranean sunshine giving the limb proper care. He knew exactly how to heal the ulcer when opportunity allowed.

Even slight elevation above the horizontal overnight is of great value and must be continued if there is any hint of recurrence. This may have to be continued indefinitely.

Improving the efficiency of the damaged pumping mechanism by the use of external support

The ability to pump blood upwards against gravity is impaired in a post-thrombotic limb by the following factors which may be influenced, harmfully or beneficially, by external compression.

Occlusion or severe deformity in major veins causes obstruction to venous return. Numerous lesser veins will dilate to provide a compensatory collateral mechanism, but little can be done to assist this process which is a response to the venous changes in the limb.

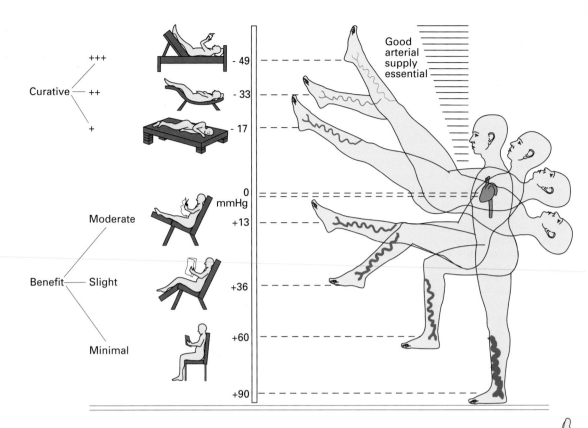

Fig. 6.5 Conservative management in post-thrombotic syndrome (chronic venous insufficiency).

(a) Elevation of the limbs is by far the most important measure. This is only truly effective when the limbs are raised above the level of the heart because then there is no venous pressure in the extremity. This diagram shows various positions of elevation related to heart level and the resulting venous pressures in the lower leg. Elevation is only curative (e.g. in healing an ulcer) when the limb is well above heart level and maintained there for prolonged periods with minimal interruption. Lesser elevation brings some benefit and may be sufficient to protect a healed ulcer from recurrence. Always assess arterial supply before advising a policy of elevation.

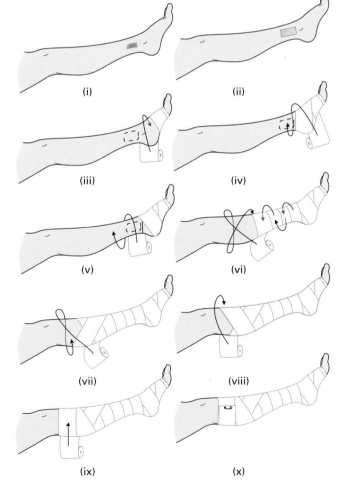

(b) External support by bandage. In severe cases this may be necessary and a careful system of even application is essential, as illustrated here. This is best done with the limb horizontal or higher. The method shown is suitable for applying inelastic compression by paste bandage which is to remain in place for many days.

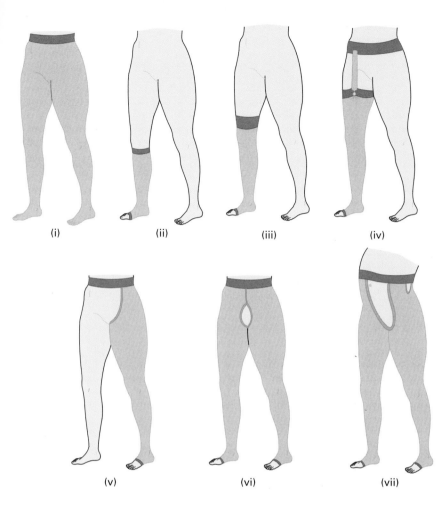

Fig. 6.5 (continued).

(c) Styles of graduated elastic stocking commonly used. (i) Tights: widely used in lighter weights. (ii) Below knee: this requires a well-rounded calf or use of one-way-stretch material to avoid riding down. (iii) Above knee (lower thigh): only suitable for a slim limb since otherwise it may not stay up. (iv) Thigh length (half or mid-thigh): requires suspenders. (v) Thigh length with waist attachment for support: used in special problems when extra-strong support is needed. (vi) Waist length for special bilateral problems requiring maximal support. (vii) Maternity stocking, as support tights or 'panty hose' stocking with adjustable top.

(i) (ii) (iii) (iv)

(v) (vi) (vii)

However, the superficial veins play a large part, and any form of external compression, particularly elastic compression, can impair this important mechanism. In superficial incompetence, firm compression of the superficial veins brings great benefit by preventing heavy downflow in them, but in post-thrombotic syndrome similar pressure in the upper calf or thigh can cause increased discomfort and deterioration in the limb by impeding collateral return. For this reason elastic support used in post-thrombotic syndrome must be carefully graduated to avoid compression where the main collaterals lie.

There is valvular incompetence because of the widespread loss of effective valves, both in recanalized deep veins and in overexpanded lesser deep veins and superficial veins now acting as collaterals. No conservative measure can adequately restore valvular competence in these limbs. Any external compression designed to reduce reflux in these valveless veins may also impair their vital function of venous return, and the advantages gained in controlling reflux will be lost by the disadvantages of restricting collateral return. Again, notice how this contrasts with superficial incompetence where elastic compression to the incompetent superficial veins brings no disadvantage because these veins are not acting as avenues of venous return. The elastic stocking, so successful in superficial incompetence, may be completely inappropriate to the post-thrombotic syndrome and this is a fundamental distinction between the two conditions.

Widespread overexpansion of the superficial and deep veins in the leg and foot is created by the sustained high venous pressure and, in effect, forms a large venous pool which constantly handicaps the venous pumping units that have survived undamaged. On muscle relaxation these healthy pumping chambers will be immediately flooded by blood from the unwanted venous pool and much of their effort is wasted on reducing a pool which has inexhaustible replenishment from above. When the foot is raised, blood which should be available to the pumping units cascades down to the underside at the very moment that it should be entering the venous pumping chambers; on return of the foot to the ground the blood is forced up again, giving a surge of high venous pressure in the lower leg. Reducing the venous pool by external support to the foot and lower leg, strong enough to resist the venous pressures, can take away this undesirable element and bring some relief to the overburdened pumping mechanism. Here external support can be of real benefit, but if it is inexpertly applied it can impede collateral return as explained above. It is quite wrong to believe that crude compression is a virtue in the post-thrombotic limb—it must be used with discernment and then may bring benefit.

External support can assist in other ways. In venous hypertension much of the damage is from excessive capillary filtration of fluid and unwanted proteins into the extracellular space. The cumulative effect of this interferes with nutrition, particularly to the skin which leads to ulceration. External support limits the capacity of the extracellular space so that pressure within it soon rises to a level opposing further capillary filtration. Another factor may be improved flow in capillaries narrowed by external support so that white blood cell trapping is reduced and its cytotoxic effect on capillary permeability is lessened.

Box 6.2   Basic principle of conservative treatment

Elevation and external compression conflict strongly with requirements of an ischaemic limb—**always check adequacy of arterial supply.**

Elevation

In a limb raised above horizontal, the venous pressure drops to zero and healing of venotensive changes starts. The higher and more prolonged the elevation, the more effective it will be. Elevation above the horizontal in bed overnight is a great opportunity for 8 h of continuous benefit and should always be employed. However, the patient must not be inactive since this will cause weak muscles and stiff joints; a programme of exercises and short hourly 'walk-abouts' must be followed. This is not 'bed rest' but 'activity elevation'!

The time of being up and about is increased as healing progresses to find the optimum without causing deterioration. The patient must discover this tolerance limit and keep within it. It is important for the patient to learn this if recurrence is to be prevented. Elevation overnight is a most valuable contribution to the limb's well-being and should continue throughout, perhaps indefinitely.

External support

Undue external pressure can impede collateral flow. Note the contrast between the effect of external pressure in superficial vein incompetence and in post-thrombotic occlusion.

- Superficial vein incompetence (usually with varicosities): external pressure prevents potentially damaging downflow in superficial veins and therefore is beneficial.
- Post-thrombotic syndrome: external pressure will tend to impede the important compensatory mechanism of collateral flow in superficial veins and may actually be harmful.

In post-thrombotic syndrome actual reflux mainly occurs when first rising from horizontal to vertical and a short phase of reflux, rapidly filling the veins to capacity, is soon followed by continuous collateral upflow which must not be hindered.

How then can external support bring benefit to deep vein impairment?

Benefit comes in three ways:

- By limiting the venous pool in the overdistended veins of the leg and foot. Reducing the venous pool reduces the burden on the pumping units so that their efforts are more effective. The venous pool of the foot is also reduced and the surge upwards at each foot step is less, so that these peaks of high pressure are minimized.
- By limiting overdistension of undamaged veins, valve cusps are brought together and function is improved.
- By resisting capillary exudate and encouraging lymphatic return of oedema fluid.

Controlled trials in moderate to severe post-thrombotic syndrome and other forms of deep vein insufficiency have shown that elastic compression at the ankle between 30 and 40 mmHg produces most benefit.

Furthermore, external support is believed to promote lymphatic drainage with increased removal of fluid and unwanted proteins from the extracellular space.

Two main forms of external support can be used:

- inelastic containment
- elastic compression by stocking or bandage

Inelastic containment

This is the principle used in the paste bandage. This form of external support is often more successful than any other type in the ambulatory treatment and healing of a venous ulcer, and this is particularly true in post-thrombotic syndrome. Although these bandages are combined with various medical ingredients, it is the mechanical properties of the bandage when it is properly applied, rather than the ingredients, that make it so successful. In its basic form it is a 7.5-cm cotton bandage impregnated with zinc oxide paste. This is applied from the toes up to the knee whilst the limb is well elevated so that the veins are completely empty (Fig. 6.5(b)). Care is taken to lay it on in a series of overlapping loops so that at no point is it tight or exerting a constricting effect. In this way it will set to form a strong inelastic shell encasing the elevated limb. When the patient stands, overfilling of enlarged veins will be immediately resisted by the shell, but venous pressure at any point will not rise above the hydrostatic pressure between that level and the heart. The tension exerted by this external support is determined by the fluid, the venous blood, contained within it and gives a perfect graduation of pressure, decreasing up the limb. The large venous pool in the foot and lower leg is held to a minimum and the efforts of functioning pumping units are proportionately more effective. The veins and capillary beds are prevented from excessive distension by the external support, but at no point is the external pressure greater than that in the superficial veins so that collateral upflow will not be impeded.

The effect on the microvascular circulation is as follows. Tissue within an unyielding containment will be subjected to the venous pressure at that level (around 100 mmHg at the ankle). This will reduce the capillary-to-tissue pressure gradient, so that capillary filtration is lessened and the accumulation of fluid and protein in the extracellar space is reduced. Also, pressure by the containment bandage, fluctuating with movement to give a massaging effect, will promote lymphatic return. Limitation of capillary filtration and increased lymphatic sweeping out of extracellular fluid and proteins is a very positive benefit. It is also possible that pressure upon the dilated capillaries of venous hypertension, by narrowing them and improving flow, diminishes white cell trapping and its harmful effects on capillary permeability.

When the patient walks, venous pressure around the ankle will be reduced to the lowest levels attainable in that limb; when the patient is at rest, with the leg horizontal or elevated, there is no residual pressure from an inelastic external support to impede arterial inflow. In contrast, an elastic support will give sustained compression between 20 and 40 mmHg or more of residual pressure, a significant handicap to arterial perfusion.

Although it provides the most effective form of external support, the paste bandage has the disadvantage that it cannot be taken off and put on again at will. Once applied, it will usually be left in place for up to 3 weeks and it cannot satisfactorily be replaced by the patient. This requires some skill, which is not always easy for others in the family. For this reason it tends to be used only during the time necessary to heal an ulcer and has the great advantage that it allows this to continue while the patient is up and about. Once the ulcer has healed, the external support can be changed to a more convenient elastic stocking which may be sufficient to help prevent recurrence.

Certain types of elastic stocking, skilfully fitted, can come near to giving the same effect as a paste bandage. A strong one-way-stretch elastic stocking up to the knee, fitted accurately to give a snug fit but no compression when the limb is elevated, will immediately resist any expansion of the veins when the patient stands; this comes quite near to the principle of inelastic containment whilst having the advantage of being easily removable. Its elasticity is used to give accurate conformity with the limb and to allow it to be pulled on and off over the prominence of the heel, but, as it is one-way-stretch, it does not suffer from down-pull. Skilled fitting of this sort is not always available, and the tendency is for the patient to be directed towards the convenience of easy fitting using a two-way-stretch stocking. Because of the need for the latter to grip the calf in order to resist down-pull, it is not suitable to provide inelastic containment. Strong elastic webbing bandage laid lightly around the elevated limb, without any compression, can also be used to give a form of inelastic containment, but this form of bandage is so often misused (see box 6.3) that it is best avoided unless the circumstances ensure proper use.

Elastic compression

A large variety of elastic stockings of various strengths are available. These may or may not envelop the toes, and extend from the foot up to the knee or to the thigh; depending on the strength required, they may be fashioned as stockings or tights (Fig. 6.5(c)). The compression they give is graded so that light support gives 14–17 mmHg compression (class I in the United Kingdom), medium support gives 18–24 mmHg compression (class II), and strong support gives 25–35 mmHg compression (class III) at foot and ankle level. Above this level the stocking is designed so that the compression tapers off in parallel with the lessening venous pressure up the length of the limb when the patient is standing. In this way heavy compression in, say, the thigh, and constriction of venous outflow, is avoided. In most countries clear standards are laid down, and in the United Kingdom the Drug Tariff of the National Health Service gives strict specifications for the various classes of graduated compression hosiery together with indications related to the severity of venous disorder and other conditions for which they are suitable. The manufacturers keep within these specifications and have succeeded in evolving knits that give compression with relatively little downward pull, but nevertheless the majority available are two-way stretch and will require support either by gripping the calf or, at higher levels, by suspenders or as tights. In post-thrombotic syndrome the high venous pressures quickly generated when the patient is standing will require controlling with a relatively strong stocking giving 25 to 35 mmHg compression in foot and ankle. This has been found to be optimal but is really insufficient to resist full venous pressure; however, the stronger the stocking the higher is the residual elastic compression when the limb is elevated and no longer needs compression. When a limb is raised above horizontal or when the patient is lying flat there is no significant venous pressure in the limb, and external support, inelastic or elastic, serves no useful purpose. However, an elastic support will continue giving residual compression, and this can be most undesirable by reducing arterial flow in the impoverished tissues near the ankle in post-thrombotic syndrome; for this reason it is best removed at night.

The importance of avoiding an elastic stocking which may impede collateral return through superficial veins has already been emphasized above. Many patients with post-thrombotic syndrome try various forms of elastic support but find that they actually increase their discomfort and abandon their use. A stocking that brings comfort to the patient is likely to be beneficial, but one causing discomfort may actually be doing harm. The patient must not be coerced into wearing stockings if the benefits are not apparent. With an active ulcer which is extremely tender and is discharging purulent fluid, an elastic stocking is not in any way suitable; it will cause too much pain and within a short time will be saturated with exudate. An ulcer at this stage requires a spell of elevation to bring it to a healing phase, followed by ambulatory treatment in a paste bandage and, finally, healing maintained by a skilfully fitted elastic support and policy of elevation whenever possible. In the post-thrombotic limb it is often a matter of trial and error to see if the patient can be suited. In simple incompetence of the superficial veins (primary varicose veins), where all that is required is firm compression to stop the downflow in the incompetent veins, the fitting of elastic stockings is far less critical and often an ulcer will heal with their use. However, this is the very variety of venous disorder where surgery or sclerotherapy is highly successful, and it should not be necessary to condemn these patients to the undoubted nuisance of permanent elastic support.

Conclusions

1. An active expression of venotension, such as a purulent ulcer, requires an initial phase of treatment in elevation to give the sustained reduction in venous pressure necessary to bring the ulcer to a healing phase.

2. This may be followed by use of ambulatory external containment (paste bandage). However, elevation between walks is still essential.

3. When the ulcer has healed, good condition without recurrence may be maintained by an elastic stocking and a policy of elevation whenever possible, certainly including elevation overnight. Some patients may prefer elastic bandages with geometric stretch indicator patterns, but care and a perceptive patient is needed.

4. This is not an easy field, and success is only possible with careful instruction of the patient whose conscientious co-operation is essential.

Box 6.3   External support

There are two methods:
(1) inelastic containment, as in the paste bandage.
(2) elastic compression by stocking or elastic bandage.

Inelastic containment
This is applied, usually as an inelastic paste bandage, to the foot and leg whilst in elevation to form a semiflexible container, enveloping but not compressing the limb. When the limb is lowered the container immediately limits filling of the veins, but the venous pressure under it will never rise above that within the veins themselves. Therefore the container does not exert any pressure beyond the hydrostatic pressure generated by the veins themselves and flow is not impaired.
Advantages   This does provide the most effective and safest way of improving venous return in the upright position and allows the patient to be mobile.
Disadvantages   Requires skilful application, which is not easy for the patient, and therefore is usually left in place for up to 3 weeks.

Elastic compression stocking
This is very effective in controlling incompetence in superficial veins by preventing downflow in them. Here, fitting a stocking is less exacting than in post-thrombotic syndrome where skilled fitting is required. For post-thrombotic syndrome the pressure exerted up the length of the stocking must be carefully graduated so that it never exerts a constricting effect; it should be maximal at the foot and ankle (up to 40 mmHg) and taper off up the limb. Manufacturers conform to strict guidelines to ensure that this is so.

Disadvantages   When lying down, external compression is not necessary but an elastic stocking gives a residual elastic compression (difficult to avoid) which can impede arterial flow when this is poor. However, as the stocking is removed overnight this need not be a problem.

Advice
It is difficult to predict when elastic compression is going to benefit the patient and it is not always easy to obtain an ideal fitting. The only way to resolve this is to give a trial to a stocking with the best available fitting. The benefits can then be judged by the patient. It should only be used if the benefits (comfort, healing, and prevention of recurrence) are apparent to the patient, who should not be allowed to be too easily discouraged by the undoubted nuisance of a stocking and must give it a fair trial.

Categories of elastic stocking (United Kingdom National Health Service Drug Tariff given in parentheses; all figures rounded off to the nearest whole number)

Class I: light support. Exerts (14–17) 18–21 mmHg pressure at ankle. Suitable for early varicosities from superficial vein incompetence.
Class II: medium support. Exerts (18–24) 25–32 mmHg pressure at ankle. Suitable for moderately severe superficial vein incompetence with varicose veins and the prevention of ulcer from this. Also for control of mild oedema.
Class III: strong support. Exerts (25–35) 36–47 mmHg pressure at ankle. Indicated for post-thrombotic venous insufficiency and prevention of ulcer recurrence in this condition. Also for gross oedema.
Class IV: extra-strong support. Exerts over 59 mmHg or more at ankle. Used for control of lymphoedema, extensive congenital angiomatosis, or multiple arteriovenous fistulas.

See Fig. 6.5(c) for the various styles (below knee, thigh length, etc.) of stocking available.

Elastic compression bandages
The danger with these is that unskilled application can result in excessive and damaging levels of pressure if layer after layer is strongly applied. However, elastic bandages are available with patterns imprinted on them which give an indication of the pressure being exerted by their shape which varies with the amount of stretch and force used (Thuasne geometric two-way stretch bandage).

Another approach is the short-stretch bandage which has limited elastic stretch and beyond this behaves as a non-stretch bandage. This device allows a limited elastic compression to be applied and easy recognition when this has been reached so that further tightening can be avoided; of course, the cumulative effect of multiple layers must be avoided. When used with the maker's recommendations, it can safely achieve a degree of inelastic containment.

These improved versions are certainly permissible when used with proper instruction, and many patients prefer to adapt them to their individual requirements and comfort in preference to a stocking. They do allow a near-inelastic containment if put on lightly with the leg in elevation so that little pressure is exerted then, but immediately resist overfilling of veins when the leg is down.

Advice
If a discerning patient cannot accept an elastic stocking, use of an elastic compression bandage, self-applied, may be more successful. The patient learns by experience when the bandage is 'right' and uses the adaptability of bandaging to obtain an optimal fit and compression that a fitted stocking may not be able to provide. This approach is only possible with an astute patient, but is safe since excessive pressure causing pain is unlikely to be used.

Continued

Box 6.3   *Continued*

In active ulceration
1. The initial step must be to obtain a 'healthy' ulcer in the healing phase by a period of 'activity elevation'.
2. Following this, inelastic containment by paste bandage, applied by a skilled nurse (self-application is not easy), is usually the most effective and comfortable policy, and allows increasing ambulation
3. When the ulcer is healed, elastic support and a policy of elevation whenever possible, including overnight, is used to prevent recurrence.

See also gravity counteraction policy in Box 9.3.

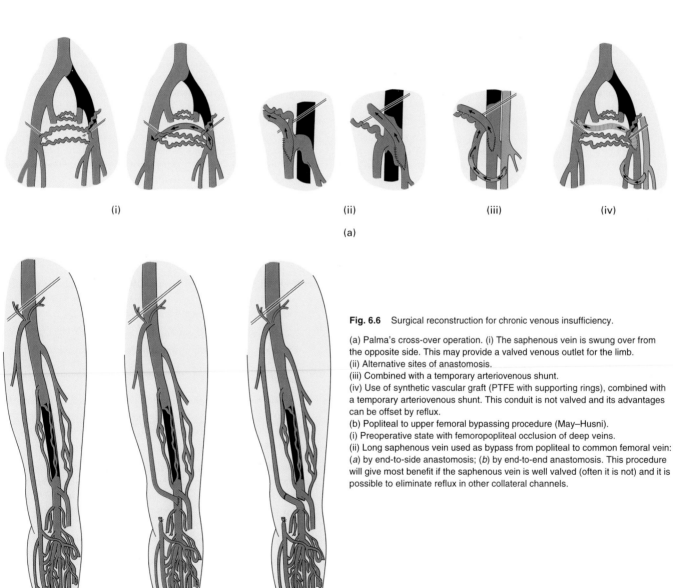

(i) (ii) (iii) (iv)

(a)

Fig. 6.6 Surgical reconstruction for chronic venous insufficiency.

(a) Palma's cross-over operation. (i) The saphenous vein is swung over from the opposite side. This may provide a valved venous outlet for the limb.
(ii) Alternative sites of anastomosis.
(iii) Combined with a temporary arteriovenous shunt.
(iv) Use of synthetic vascular graft (PTFE with supporting rings), combined with a temporary arteriovenous shunt. This conduit is not valved and its advantages can be offset by reflux.
(b) Popliteal to upper femoral bypassing procedure (May–Husni).
(i) Preoperative state with femoropopliteal occlusion of deep veins.
(ii) Long saphenous vein used as bypass from popliteal to common femoral vein: (*a*) by end-to-side anastomosis; (*b*) by end-to-end anastomosis. This procedure will give most benefit if the saphenous vein is well valved (often it is not) and it is possible to eliminate reflux in other collateral channels.

(i) (ii*a*) (ii*b*)

(b)

Surgery to the veins in post-thrombotic syndrome

In this condition enlarged surface veins are usually acting as collaterals to underlying occluded deep veins. Not infrequently, in these circumstances a saphenous vein may have several competent valves along its length and therefore is a most valuable valved pathway of venous return that must be preserved. However, more often phlebography or ultrasonography will have shown that it has no competent valves and it is tempting to consider its surgical removal in order to eliminate at least one cause of rapid build-up of venous hypertension by reflux along its length. However, this will also be destroying an important compensatory collateral mechanism, and the disadvantages of this may outweigh the advantages of eliminating the component of incompetence. Moreover, Doppler flowmetry may show continuous upflow, accentuated by exercise, without reflux, except briefly when the patient first stands. This implies that it is an important collateral which must not be removed without good evidence of alternative pathways of venous return. Phlebography may have supplied this, but useful confirmatory evidence may be obtained by phlethysmography during exercise with and without selective occlusion of the saphenous vein in question; occlusion may cause deterioration in the ability of the limb to reduce venous pressure by exercise and gives clear warning that the vein should not be removed. In true post-thrombotic syndrome there are few circumstances in which removal of the superficial veins will bring benefit. One such circumstance may be when there is an intractable ulcer directly overlying an enlarged perforator carrying collateral outflow, demonstrated by phlebography or ultrasonography. Elimination of this may redistribute collateral outflow and reduce the intensity of venous hypertension overlying the perforator, and so enable the ulcer to heal. The use of phlethysmography with selective occlusion of the veins concerned, as just described, may support this procedure, but without some such evidence it is not justifiable to remove enlarged superficial veins or perforators indiscriminately.

Surgical reconstruction of veins and valves

In post-thrombotic syndrome the real requirement is the replacement of occluded veins and valveless channels with good well-valved veins. However, our ability in this respect is extremely limited, but the following procedures may occasionally prove helpful.

Palma's operation

This is appropriate for the relief of oedema in post-thrombotic occlusion of an iliac vein, usually the left side, when the deep veins below the inguinal ligament are relatively undamaged. The long saphenous vein of the opposite limb is divided in the lower thigh and mobilized to swing it across to the affected side for anastomosis with the common femoral or profunda femoris vein (Fig. 6.6(a) (i)–(iii)). If successful, this acts as an additional collateral vein providing a substantial venous outlet for the limb. Swelling may be considerably reduced, but severe venotensive changes such as ulceration near the ankle are unlikely to be improved because these are the result of thrombotic damage at lower levels in the limb. A corresponding procedure using a PTFE vascular graft with external supporting rings, running extraperitoneally between the femoral vein on the affected side and the lower external iliac vein of the opposite

side, and supported by a temporary arteriovenous fistula, has given a number of reported successes (Fig. 6.6(a) (iv)). During the acute stage of severe iliofemoral thrombosis with an imminent threat of pulmonary embolus, direct thrombectomy with a temporary arteriovenous fistula may be indicated (see the section on therapy for deep vein thrombosis in Part II), but this is not appropriate for the chronic occlusive stage just described.

Popliteal to upper femoral vein bypassing (May–Husni operation)

This is designed to relieve the effects of deep vein obstruction in lower or mid-thigh. The long saphenous vein of the same limb is anastomosed to the lower popliteal or posterior tibial vein in order to provide a more effective outflow from the deep veins below the knee and take it upwards to re-enter deep veins in the groin above the obstruction (Fig. 6.6(b)). This will be particularly effective if the saphenous vein is well valved and a number of successes have been reported. However, this vein is often already acting as an effective collateral so that the rearrangement brings little improvement and, of course, it does not eliminate the heavy reflux in naturally occurring deep and superficial collateral veins throughout the limb which are so often grossly incompetent. This operation may be supported by a temporary arteriovenous fistula to ensure that the new venous channel is well distended with continuous flow and does not thrombose in the early postoperative healing period.

Restoration of valve function

If incompetence in a deep vein is the main problem, the following possibilities can be considered (see Figs 5.3(b)–5.3(d)).

- Transposition of a deep vein into a neighbouring vein that is well valved, for example implanting the superficial femoral into a valved profunda femoris vein alongside, as described earlier. This is seldom applicable in post-thrombotic syndrome.

- Transplantation of a suitable venous valve taken from elsewhere in the body. This is most unlikely to be appropriate in thickened, deformed post-thrombotic veins or in the multitude of collateral veins.

- Repair of prolapsing valve cusps (Kistner's operation) is not in any way appropriate in post-thrombotic syndrome where the valve cusps are thickened, deformed, and adherent to neighbouring vein wall.

- Various procedures with synthetic vein grafts, often supported by temporary arteriovenous fistulas, are under trial in the lower limb, but these suffer from the serious defect that they are not valved (Fig. 6.6(a) (iv)). Attempts to evolve synthetic vein grafts for use in the lower limb are severely limited at present by the inability to provide any satisfactory valve mechanism.

- External valves. A sling may be used around a vein to act as a substitute valve. Psathakis has reported favourable results in over 200 patients using a tendon or silastic sling attached to flexor tendons of the knee and placed around the popliteal vein in patients with venotensive changes, including many with post-thrombotic syndrome, thought to be due to reflux in this vein. The theory is that when the flexor muscles contract whilst walking the sling tightens around the vein and prevents reflux in it. Its efficacy and the possible incidence of thromboembolism await independent evaluation.

Operations reconstructing the veins in post-thrombotic syndrome are very limited, with few suitable cases, and are best left to the experts specializing in this field.

Surgical injury and trauma to major veins

Surgery involving the deep veins in the lower limbs or abdomen can produce special problems if injury to a large vein causes severe haemorrhage. Box 6.5 considers some aspects of this, and Figs 6.7 (a) and (b) illustrate the principles to be used in controlling haemorrhage and repairing the vein.

Accident trauma to a limb may cause injury to a major artery and vein. A scheme of action to meet such an emergency is outlined in Box 6.6 and illustrated in Figs 6.7 (b) and (c).

Box 6.4   Surgical possibilities in post-thrombotic syndrome

Providing a new valved venous channel of venous return to overcome obstruction
Iliac vein obstruction: Palma's operation using the long saphenous vein swung over from the opposite side (Fig. 6.6(a) (i)–(iii)).
Mid-femoral vein obstruction: May–Husni operation using long saphenous vein of same limb to bypass the obstructed vein (Fig. 6.6(b)).
Comment these two methods give the opportunity of substituting healthy valved vein in place of an obstructed or severely deformed vein and, in suitable cases, can be successful.

Restoration of valve function
Recognized methods for achieving this are as follows.

● Transposition of obstructed or incompetent vein into a neighbouring well-valved vein (Fig. 5.3(b)).
● Transplantation of a valved vein from elsewhere into the incompetent deep vein (Fig. 5.3(c)).
● Repair of incompetent valves (Fig. 5.3(d)).

Comment these methods are seldom suitable for the deformed fibrotic post-thrombotic vein but are of value in non-thrombotic chronic deep vein insufficiency, where the veins have a more normal texture, such as primary deep vein valve deficiency (see Chapter 5) and the congenital venous disorders (see Chapter 8).

Using a valveless conduit to overcome obstruction in iliac veins
In iliac vein occlusion with severe obstructive symptoms a synthetic vascular graft of PTFE with supporting rings may be used to open a bypass between the femoral vein of that side to the external iliac vein of the opposite side. This is usually accompanied by a temporary arteriovenous fistula giving full distension and swift flow to counteract thrombosis in the early stages (Fig. 6.6(a)(iv)).
Comment This may give a good measure of relief from oedema and is valuable in this respect but, being valveless, cannot provide a true cure in a limb that has widespread post-thrombotic damage. The great need in venous surgery at present is an acceptable vein graft that is well valved.

Constructing an external valve
A sling of neighbouring tendon placed around the popliteal vein to provide a form of valve has been suggested for popliteal vein incompetence (Psathakis).
Comment Very few cases of post-thrombotic syndrome are suitable for this, and its effectiveness and safety (with respect to local thrombosis and pulmonary embolism) have yet to be satisfactorily proved. It is not recommended.

Caution. The operations given above require an experienced surgeon.

Box 6.5   Control of haemorrhage from major deep vein (Fig. 6.7(a) and Fig. 6.7(b))

DO NOT persist in trying to see the bleeding point by using the sucker. **This can swiftly and silently exsanguinate the patient.** If a sucker is used ask the anaesthetist to watch its container and call out the score! Venous pressure is easily controlled by light pressure with fingers or a gauze pad. Do this immediately and take time to think out the best strategy to meet the situation. In many cases with a small wound the vein will seal itself within a few minutes, but in others proceed along the following lines.

- Find a way to control the haemorrhage that gives sufficient view to expose the vein above and below the bleeding point. This may be achieved by direct pressure to the actual point of bleeding by an assistant's single fingertip or a small swab in Allis forceps or similar. Clear the veins on either side sufficiently to apply soft-faced vascular clamps to them.
- Alternatively the bleeding point may be straddled by an assistant using two fingers, or by a two small swabs on forceps placed on either side of the bleeding point. This will allow either direct application of an instrument (Allis forceps may be very suitable) to the rent in the vein, or the application of vascular clamps to the vein on either side or the injury.
- Repair a local injury with a continuous stitch. If the vein is completely divided, clean and trim the ends, and anastomose them by interrupted stitches (8 to 12 in all is usually sufficient). A continuous stitch without interruption in the thin walls of a vein may allow the vein ends to separate when the clamps are removed and cause a drawstring effect at the anastomosis which collapses and ceases to function.
- If the deficiency of vein is too great to allow the ends to come together (over, say, 1 cm), a portion of saphenous vein must be collected and used to construct an autograft that matches the damaged vein. **The alternative of sacrificing the vein by ligating its ends should not be done lightly without careful thought as to the consequences,** which may be severe disability due to venous outlet obstruction and exceedingly difficult to repair later on.

Haemorrhage from a major vein during surgery

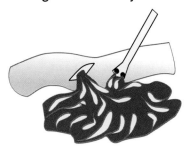

Do not use prolonged suction to find bleeding aperture in vein. This can swiftly exsanguinate the patient!

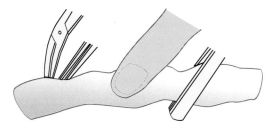

Place a finger over bleeding point and dissect vein above and below so that vascular clamps can be applied

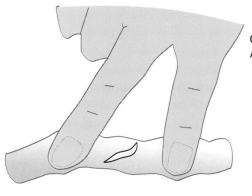

OR
Assistant straddles bleeding point with fingers

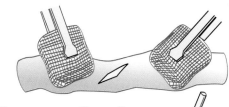

OR
Assistant applies pressure with small gauze swabs held in Allis forceps.

OR
Isolate the bleeding point with a metal (Shen's) ring or similar shape improvised from malleable wire

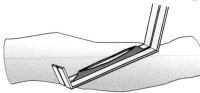

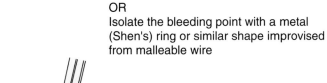

This may allow clear vision to apply a side-clamp or Allis forceps so that the vein may be sutured.

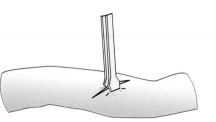

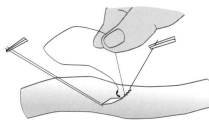

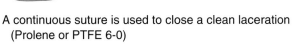

A continuous suture is used to close a clean laceration (Prolene or PTFE 6-0)

(a)

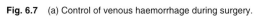

Fig. 6.7 (a) Control of venous haemorrhage during surgery.

End-to-end anastomosis of a major vein

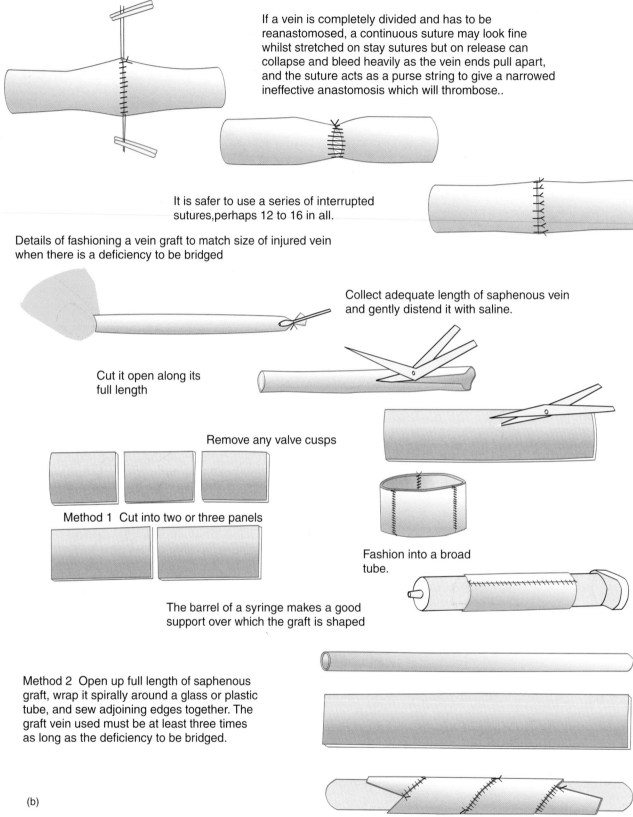

If a vein is completely divided and has to be reanastomosed, a continuous suture may look fine whilst stretched on stay sutures but on release can collapse and bleed heavily as the vein ends pull apart, and the suture acts as a purse string to give a narrowed ineffective anastomosis which will thrombose..

It is safer to use a series of interrupted sutures, perhaps 12 to 16 in all.

Details of fashioning a vein graft to match size of injured vein when there is a deficiency to be bridged

Collect adequate length of saphenous vein and gently distend it with saline.

Cut it open along its full length

Remove any valve cusps

Method 1 Cut into two or three panels

Fashion into a broad tube.

The barrel of a syringe makes a good support over which the graft is shaped

Method 2 Open up full length of saphenous graft, wrap it spirally around a glass or plastic tube, and sew adjoining edges together. The graft vein used must be at least three times as long as the deficiency to be bridged.

(b)

Fig. 6.7   (b) Anastomosis of a major vein and use of autologous vein graft.

External trauma causing simultaneous injury to artery and vein

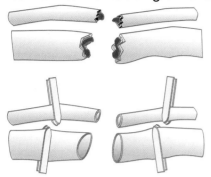

Extract clot carefully before applying clamps.
Trim away devitalized tissue to give clean ends

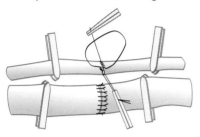

Anastomose the vein first and then
the artery.

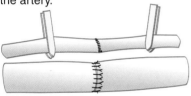

Remove clamps from the vein first

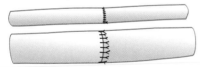

Then release the artery: this prevents
a phase of excessive venous
engorgement

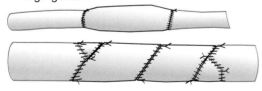

If there is a deficiency in the artery - use a
reversed saphenous vein graft to bridge gap
If there is a vein deficiency - fashion a graft
of matching size from saphenous vein.

(c)

SO-CALLED 'ARTERIAL SPASM'

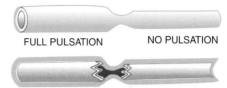

FULL PULSATION   NO PULSATION

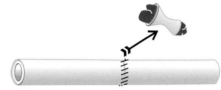

ADVENTITIA ANDMEDIA ARE INTACT BUT THE BRITTLE INTIMA
HAS FRACTURED AND THE GAP FILLED WITH THROMBUS.
SPONTANEOUS RE-OPENING OF ARTERY IS NOT POSSIBLE.

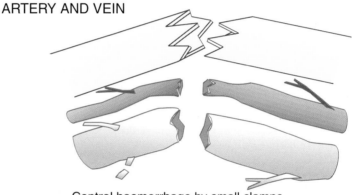

DAMAGED PORTION OF ARTERY IS EXCISED TO GIVE CLEAN ENDS AND
THEN REANASTOMOSED OR, IF GAP TOO GREAT, BRIDGED WITH A
REVERSED GRAFT OF SAPHENOUS VEIN

WHEN A MAJOR FRACTURE IS ALONGSIDE A SEVERED ARTERY AND VEIN

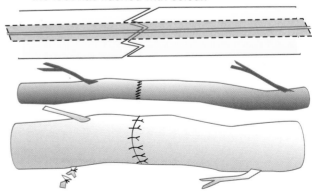

Control haemorrhage by small clamps
Orthopaedic surgeon reduces and stabilizes
fracture (internal pin ideal)
Repair vein then artery and release vein first.
Check for a good pulse in distal artery, that
the vein anastomosis has a well-filled shape, and
the foot has flushed with colour.

Fig. 6.7   (c) Repair of injury to artery and vein, and when a major fracture is also present.

Box 6.6   Injury to arteries and veins of the lower limb (Figs 6.7(b) and 6.7(c))

This book is mainly concerned with disorders of veins but it seems appropriate to outline briefly the recognition and management of arterial and venous injury.

Closed injury to artery and vein

The history will usually give the force and locality of injury, and the patient will complain that the foot feels cold and numb. On examination it is pale and cold to touch, or may show blanching on elevation; ankle and/or popliteal pulses are not palpable. On Doppler flowmetry pulses are either very reduced or absent.

Never make a diagnosis of 'arterial spasm' and adopt a waiting policy—this can easily lead to unnecessary loss of the limb; a critical ischaemia moves to irreversible changes within a few hours. A narrowed artery after injury, seen on an arteriogram or at open surgery, is due to torn intima and local occlusion by thrombus; this cannot recover spontaneously and survival of the limb depends on the adequacy of the collateral circulation. At this stage there may be little to indicate the state of the vein. Time is not favourable, and irreversible extensive death of tissue can occur within 6 h.

Thus, when critical ischaemia following closed injury is diagnosed:

● An arteriogram is an urgent necessity to localize the position and extent of the injury.
● If this confirms a local block, surgical exploration must be carried out immediately.
● When a portion of narrowed artery is found—*THIS IS NOT SPASM BUT DUE TO FRACTURED INTIMA.* Open the artery to confirm this.
● On confirmation, excise the damaged portion, clear away any entangled adventitia to give clean ends, and remove clot from within both portions of artery. Check for good pulsatile flow from the proximal part and backflow from the distal artery. If need be use a balloon catheter of suitable size *with care*; harm can be done by rough repeated usage or rupturing the artery by overdistension.
● *If the main vein has been damaged or ruptured it must be repaired* since otherwise the limb may be unnecessarily left with a severe and persisting post-thrombotic syndrome. Repairing the vein only takes a few minutes, and failure to do so is a bad error. Excise the vein ends and clear away clot; check for freedom from clot and distal return flow by sharp firm pressure on limb below the injury. Reanastomose the vein ends using interrupted sutures, because a continuous suture on a large vein may pull apart and collapse the vein ends by a purse-string effect.
● Open up the vein circulation before the arterial circulation, since otherwise there will be severe venous engorgement. If all is well, the vein will swell up within a few seconds of releasing the artery to give an even full-sized vessel and well-shaped anastomosis.

In open injury and when accompanied by a major fracture of bone

An orthopaedic colleague must be called in. All the same vascular principles given above apply, but as soon as haemorrhage has been controlled the fracture must be stabilized, usually by some form of pinning, before repairing the blood vessels. Therefore the sequence is as follows.

● Control haemorrhage from major vessels.
● Reduce and stabilize the fracture.
● Clean and repair the vein and instil weak heparin saline solution.
● Clean and repair the artery. This may require excision and reanastomosis or, if torn across, excise back to clean artery ends and remove all clot; check that strong pulsatile flow comes from above and backflow from below.
● Release the vein circulation and then the arterial circulation.
● Check that there is good pulsation, that the injured main vein has good contour, and that the foot flushes with colour.

7 Clinical patterns of venous disorder IV
Role of the perforator

The diagnosis of 'incompetent perforator' is made frequently, but often incorrectly. The following summary may help to put this into better perspective (Fig. 7.1).

Inward flow to deep veins

Inward flow from the superficial to deep veins is normal but it is greatly enhanced in superficial vein incompetence as part of the retrograde circuit of gravitational downflow (see Fig. 4.1). This is an essential feature of the most common venous disorder, superficial vein incompetence, but the perforator is not at fault—it is perform-ing its normal function in an exaggerated fashion (Fig. 7.2(a)). However, in many patients, there may also be a brief outward surge as the muscles contract or the foot is placed to the ground, alternating with the predominant downward and inward flow (Fig. 7.2(b)). This represents a degree of incompetence in one or more perforators, probably because they have been overenlarged by heavy inflow from the varicose veins, but this is not the primary fault. However, it can certainly be an aggravating factor if venotensive changes are present, and, after surgery to the varicose veins, it may become the source of downflow to the foot. For these reasons an enlarged perforating vein showing surge is best eliminated at surgery when it is detected.

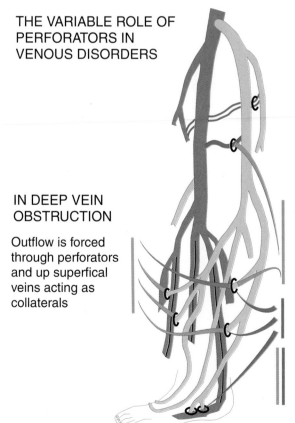

THE VARIABLE ROLE OF
PERFORATORS IN
VENOUS DISORDERS

Fig. 7.1   The varying roles of perforating veins.

IN SUPERFICIAL VEIN
INCOMPETENCE

Incompetent
perforators can act
as a source for
gravitational
downflow in
superficial veins

Perforators provide
points of inflow to
deep veins

Surge will occur when
local incompetence
in deep veins and
perforator(s) is present

IN DEEP VEIN
OBSTRUCTION

Outflow is forced
through perforators
and up superfical
veins acting as
collaterals

Fig. 7.2   Role of the perforator.

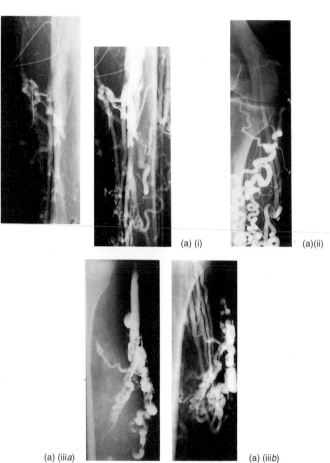

(a) (i)   (a)(ii)

(a) (iii*a*)   (a) (iii*b*)

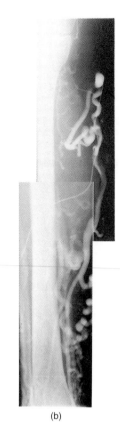

(b)

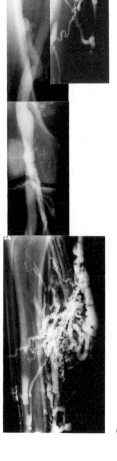

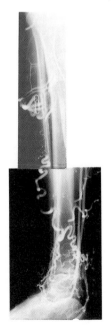

(a) Inward flow. (i) Inward flow from superficial varicosities in lower leg filling deep veins progressively through a pair of perforating veins. (ii) Direct entry of flow from calf varicose veins into gastrocnemius venous sinuses. (iii) Flow from long saphenous varicosities into multiple gastrocnemius venous sinuses: (*a*) before exercise; (*b*) after one exercise movement. As a single static picture, this can be misinterpreted as gastrocnemius vein incompetence, but for a full explanation of events in this illustration see Fig. 7.2 (c) (i)

(b) Surge between tibial deep veins and overlying superficial varicose veins. The dilated vein and the underlying perforator, near the centre of picture, showed a strong surge of flow, back and forth, with each movement during functional phlebography.

(c) Perforating vein outflow as a source of downflow in incompetent superficial veins. (i) Composite phlebogram of the veins partly shown in Fig. 7.2 (a) (iii). The main origin of superficial downflow is from a mid-thigh perforator running to a portion of unstripped long saphenous vein in the thigh. (ii) Perforator outflow as a source of superficial incompetence may occur at any level from groin to lower leg. In this phlebogram, a pair of perforators are the source of outflow from anterior tibial veins to a varicose vein running down to the foot; a paperclip marks the point at which finger pressure controlled the vein.

(c) (i)   (c) (ii)

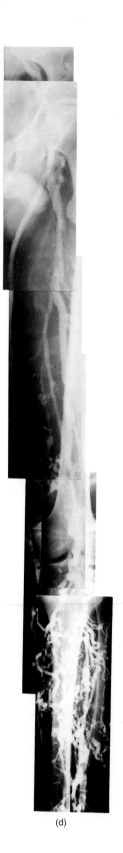

(d)

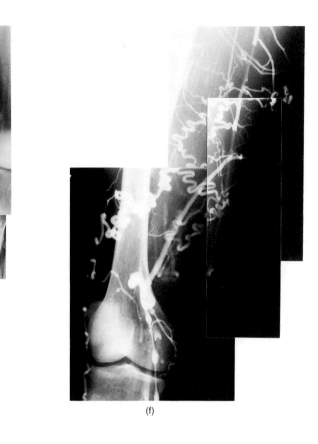

(e)

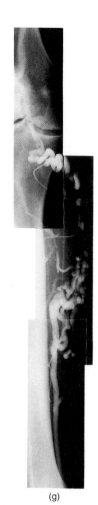

(f)

(g)

Fig. 7.2 (continued).

(d) Perforator outflow as part of a collateral mechanism. In this composite phlebogram, previous thrombosis has severely damaged the principal deep veins so that superficial veins are forced to act as collaterals up the length of the limb. The disorganized state of the leg veins is evident, with outflow from deep vein remnants at multiple points; this is well seen in the pair of dilated and tortuous perforating veins overlying the lower fibula.

(e) Gastrocnemius vein incompetence and perforator outflow from a gastrocnemius venous sinus. This occurs as gravitational outflow when the muscle is relaxed or as forcible outward pumping on contraction. An example found at functional phlebography is shown here. Ultrasonographic colour imaging is probably the most effective way of demonstrating this.

(f) Unexpected superficial interconnection mimicking a true perforator. In this composite phlebogram, a pseudoperforator, the source of incompetence in mid-thigh, is shown to arise from an upward extension of the short saphenous vein, running upwards posteriorly to join the long saphenous vein in mid-thigh. The commencement of this upward extension is dilated and tortuous, but the short saphenous vein below this shows a series of effective valves.

(g) Interconnection in the upper calf between the two saphenous systems may be mistaken for a perforator. In the composite phlebogram shown here, a substantial varicose branch of the short saphenous vein sends incompetent flow to remnants of the long saphenous system.

Source of superficial incompetence and gravitational downflow

The upper termination of the long and short saphenous vein (Figs 4.19(b) and 4.19(c)), the mid-thigh perforating veins (Fig. 4.29(d) (iii) and Fig. 7.2(c) (i)), and veins connecting between the pelvis and upper thigh (Fig. 4.10) are all examples of perforating veins which commonly become incompetent and act as the high-level source for a pathway of simple incompetence. In similar fashion, a perforator on the leg below the knee may act as a source of downflow to the foot (Fig. 7.2(c) (ii)). All the above are certainly 'incompetent perforators', and it is unfortunate that this term is also used to refer to heavy outward pumping through perforating veins below the knee, particularly near the ankle.

Outward and upward pumping through low-level perforators

Outward pumping may occur as part of a surge back and forth accompanying simple varicose veins as described above (Fig. 7.3). Of far greater importance is its occurrence in the post-thrombotic syndrome as part of a collateral mechanism in venous return past occluded deep veins (Figs 1.13, 6.3(b), and 7.2(d)). Here the perforator is playing a compensatory role, and this must be recognized because it may be an important channel of venous return although inadvertently bringing high venous pressure to the vulnerable surface layers. There must not be an automatic response to remove an outward pumping perforator in the leg, but instead the cause must be understood and its importance in collateral function assessed. Surgical removal of this vein may sometimes be justifiable; for example, in post-thrombotic syndrome heavy collateral flow may be concentrated through one perforator and increase local venous pressure so much that ulceration occurs over it. It is possible that removing this perforator will cause redistribution of collateral flow

and dissipate the raised venous pressure over a wider area elsewhere in the leg. In this way the high venous pressure is no longer concentrated in one small area and the ulcer heals. The decision to do this rests on the adequacy of alternative collateral pathways shown by radiography or ultrasonography, and the demonstration that recovery times at plethysmography are improved or, at least, not made worse by temporary occlusion of the perforator by finger pressure.

Incompetent gastrocnemius and soleal veins are perhaps the best examples of localized incompetent perforators capable of allowing passive reflux but forcibly ejecting blood to the surface on muscle contraction (Fig. 7.2(e)). These are increasingly being recognized and diagnosed by phlebography or ultrasonography. Suspicion of their presence is usually aroused by unusual discomfort, venotensive changes, and a pattern of radiating varicosities on the calf. Surgery ligating such veins in popliteal fossa, carefully selected by phlebography or ultrasonography, may prove very successful but does require experience.

Pseudoperforators

Certain arrangements of veins may be mistaken for direct leakage from the deep veins. In the mid-thigh, an upward extension of the short saphenous vein (Giacomini vein) may join the posteromedial branch of the long saphenous vein. In this way incompetence with its source in the short saphenous vein can give rise to long saphenous varicosities and may only be recognized when surgery ligating the long saphenous vein fails; even then it may be regarded as a mid-thigh perforator (Figs 4.12(b) and 7.2(f)). In the upper calf a branch from an incompetent short saphenous vein may run across to the inner aspect and appear to be a true deep vein perforator (Fig. 7.2(g)). An incompetent long saphenous vein, or its posterior arcuate branch, may run down to the lower leg in concealed fashion and give off a large branch running to the surface near the ankle, where it is interpreted as coming from a perforator.

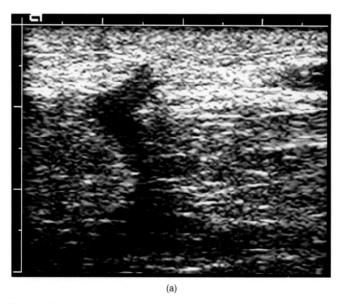

(a)

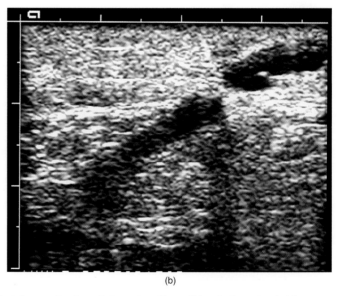

(b)

Fig. 7.3 Two duplex scan views obtained by slight repositioning of the probe, showing a large perforating vein 5 cm above the medial malleolus and underlying an ulcer. It can be seen arising from a tibial vein and traversing the deep fascia, which shows as a layer of increased density, to join a superficial vein. Substantial incompetence in the superficial veins was also present, and this perforator showed heavy surge back and forth when the leg was compressed intermittently nearby. The combination of superficial and perforator incompetence is the probable cause of the ulcer, and surgery removing the defective veins should give a good result.

Box 7.1 Role of the perforator

Over 60 perforators are present in each lower limb. All except the smallest are valved and only allow flow inwards from superficial to deep veins. Each is associated with its own area of superficial veins demarcated by valves. Small unvalved perforators may play a role in equalizing pressure from deep to superficial veins. Perforators are involved in a wide range of venous disorders, but this is usually incidental and not the main point of failure.

A hollow palpated in the horizontal leg does not necessarily indicate an enlarged and incompetent perforator aperture in the deep fascia. It is more likely to be a hollow in subcutaneous tissue normally filled by a large varicosity; there may or may not be an associated enlarged perforator with this.

The arrangement of deep fascia at a perforator opening may play a part in controlling flow through it, acting as a gate.

Inward flow to deep veins
This occurs endlessly in the normal state when upright and moving about.

In *superficial vein incompetence and its varicosities* inward flow through perforators occurs as the final part of the pathway of incompetence (the points of re-entry). Here they carry on exaggerated load in the normal direction. (These need not necessarily be eliminated in treatment of varicose veins.)

In some cases, excessive enlargement of a perforator by heavy inward flow causes it to become incompetent and allow a surge of outflow at the moment of muscle contraction. However, the dominant flow is that of superficial incompetence–down and inwards. (These are best eliminated in treatment.)

As a source of outflow to superficial veins by gravitational downflow

- Via the saphenofemoral and popliteal junctions–these are in essence special perforators and the cause of most varicose veins (treatment must eliminate these.)
- Via perforators at all levels, from pelvis, thigh, popliteal fossa, and lower leg, particularly in recurrent varicose veins. (Treatment must eliminate these.)

There are special cases, such as a gastrocnemius perforator which may allow either forceful outward pumping or simple gravitational outflow from the popliteal vein via a gastrocnemius vein and venous sinus. (Treatment may involve gastrocnemius ligation.)

Outward and upward pumping
This occurs in two forms.
- *In primary (inborn) deep vein valve deficiency*, as a surge back and forth with each muscle pump contraction; this may be combined with superficial vein incompetence. (Elimination can be attempted but elastic support may be the only way to help.)
- *In deep vein obstruction and widespread valve damage, particularly post-thrombotic syndrome*. The lack of normal venous outlet forces return by collateral channels, including perforators whose valves are either damaged by thrombosis or have broken down under venous pressure to become part of an important compensatory mechanism. Such perforators must not be indiscriminately destroyed as this may do harm. However, in some cases, such as when an intractable ulcer overlies it, elimination (possibly by endoscope) may redistribute the collateral circulation to a wider area and allow healing of the ulcer. Careful testing to simulate this, by plethysmography or ultrasound, and to demonstrate no adverse effect is essential beforehand. As stated earlier, direct communication with a pumping chamber, such as a gastronemius vein sinus, can cause forceful outward pumping demonstrable on ultrasonography. This may be suitable for surgery which will involve careful selection of a gastrocnemius vein for ligation.

Pseudoperforators
Intercommunication between the saphenous systems can give misleading effects. For example, short saphenous incompetence, via a Giacomini vein appearing in mid-thigh, may be diagnosed as a profunda femoris or femoral vein perforator when the true origin is the short saphenous vein.

8 Congenital venous disorders

Venous anomalies in the lower limb

The venous system is subject to many minor aberrations such as duplicated deep veins, differing levels of short saphenous termination, or the presence of unusually large interconnecting branches between long and short saphenous systems in the thigh. All these variants originate in the embryo during development of the venous system and, if the valves are inadequate, may account for unusual sources of incompetence, but most are harmless and need not be detailed here. However, one particular abnormality deserves special mention. This is the persistence of the lateral vein of the lower limb to form a massive valveless channel running superficially up the outer side of the leg and thigh, and terminating either in the profunda femoris or by running with the sciatic nerve into the pelvis to join the internal iliac vein (Figs 8.1, 8.2(a), and 8.2(b)). The importance of this is that there may be a concurrent failure in the development of the normal deep vein system so that the large superficial channel forms the main venous return of the limb and inept surgical removal may cause considerable embarrassment to venous return. Gross anatomical aberrations of superficial veins should always bring to mind the possibility of a corresponding failure in the deep veins which should be checked by phlebography before attempting any treatment.

Abnormal development of capillaries and veins

Localized vascular malformations

These take the form of angiomas of capillary or cavernous varieties. The former are made up of multiple enlarged capillaries and venules to give a dark red blemish (strawberry naevus), often present at birth and disappearing within a year or two. The cavernous angioma forms a protuberant swelling composed of large irregular blood-filled spaces. It usually proves persistent and may show apparent enlargement in childhood. Often it affects no more than skin and subcutaneous tissues, but it may extend deeply, lying in and amongst muscle (Fig. 8.2(c)). The boundaries of these lesions are not clearly defined but may be sufficiently limited to allow surgical removal. Surgery may require considerable skill, as these angiomas cross anatomical boundaries and involve important structures which will

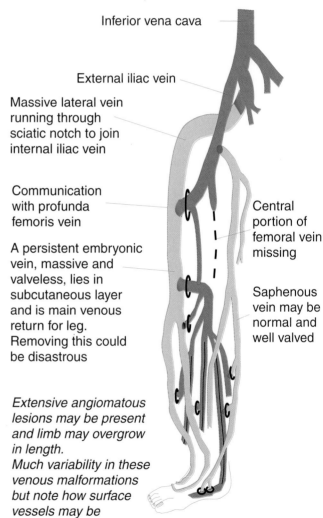

Congenital defects
Anomalous development of veins
Main characteristics of major limb involvement shown.

Inferior vena cava

External iliac vein

Massive lateral vein running through sciatic notch to join internal iliac vein

Communication with profunda femoris vein

Central portion of femoral vein missing

A persistent embryonic vein, massive and valveless, lies in subcutaneous layer and is main venous return for leg. Removing this could be disastrous

Saphenous vein may be normal and well valved

Extensive angiomatous lesions may be present and limb may overgrow in length.
Much variability in these venous malformations but note how surface vessels may be essential for venous return.

Fig. 8.1 Congenital venous anomalies. Lateral vein of thigh with partial failure in development of major deep veins.

require separating from the main mass by sharp dissection; the fringe of angioma that has to be left behind is usually unimportant. A small angioma can be treated by sclerotherapy or by laser.

Fig. 8.2 Congenital vascular malformations in the lower limbs.

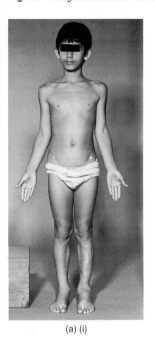

(a) (i)

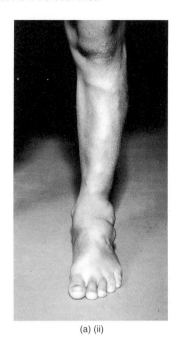

(a) (ii)

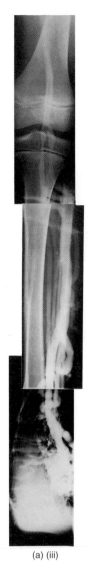

(a) (iii)

(a) Venous anomaly: persistence of lateral vein in leg. (i), (ii) This boy presented with a massive and tortuous superficial vein on the outer aspect of his left foot and leg. A branch runs across the upper tibia to join an enlarged long saphenous vein. The lower limbs are of equal length. (iii) Phlebogram showing the lateral vein joining deep veins just below the knee and also sending branches across to the medial aspect of the leg. The deep veins appear slender and possibly valveless. Much more detailed information on the adequacy of the deep veins would be required before considering surgery.

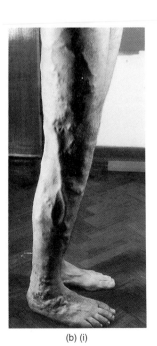

(b) (i)

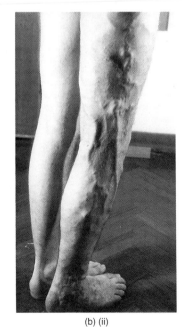

(b) (ii)

(b) Persistence of the lateral vein of thigh in a young man with Klippel–Trenaunay syndrome. Two views of the right limb are shown with enlarged superficial veins (phlebectasia) running into a large persistent lateral vein. This terminated by joining the profunda femoris vein in the upper thigh and substituted in part for underdevelopment of the deep veins. The right tibia showed 2 cm of lengthening compared with the normal left limb.

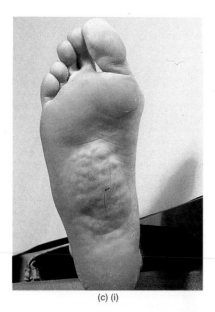

(c) (i)

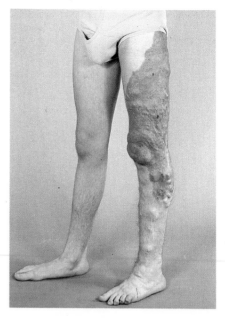

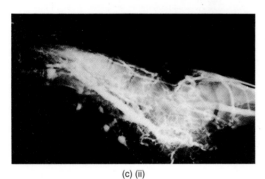

(c) (ii)

(c) Localized cavernous angioma. (i) A large cavernous angioma causing discomfort under the foot of a young man. (ii) Angiogram in venous phase showing venous caverns in the sole of the foot and enlargement of plantar vein. It was possible to excise this angioma, and, although extensions through the plantar aponeurosis were not pursued, a good result was obtained.

(d) Extensive venous angiomatosis (phlebangiomatosis and phlebectasia) without bone change. This 15-year-old boy had been followed over the previous 10 years. Massive superficial phlebangiomatosis involves the skin of upper calf, knee, and thigh; below this level extensive phlebectasia was present in the subcutaneous layers. Both limbs were of equal length; in the absence of any change in bone length this cannot be regarded as a full Klippel–Trenaunay syndrome. Various attempts at treatment by sclerotherapy and surgery met little success, largely limited by the vulnerability of the angiomatous skin which necrosed easily with any interference. The patient chose to avoid complex plastic surgery, preferring to wear strong elastic support to restrain excessive bulging of the abnormal vessels on standing. He was fully active in all sports including football.

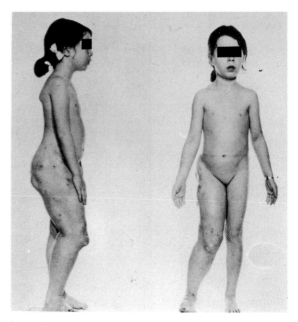

Fig. 8.2   (continued).

(e) Klippel–Trenaunay syndrome in a child. Extensive phlebangiomatosis with considerable bone lengthening (hypertrophy) is shown, and it is probable that the lymphatic system is also affected.

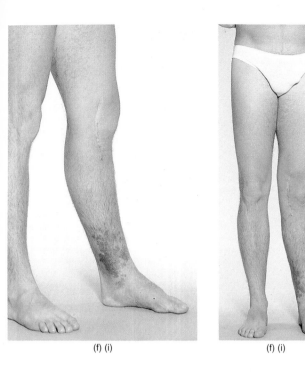

(f) (i)   (f) (i)

Fig. 8.2   (continued).

(f) Klippel–Trenaunay syndrome in a young man. From childhood onwards the left limb had shown obvious enlargement in girth and, increasingly, in length. Epiphysiodesis had been carried out to control the overgrowth in length. The patient had played hockey at national level but in his early twenties developed discomfort and pigmentation in the lower leg, typical of venous insufficiency. Doppler flowmetry showed continuous upflow in superficial veins in keeping with deep vein deficiency (hypoplasia), and photoplethysmography indicated impairment of the venous pumping mechanism. Phlebography was not carried out as the patient was travelling from abroad, but his condition was explained to him, with advice on the general care of venous insufficiency and encouragement to keep active.

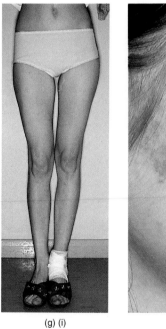
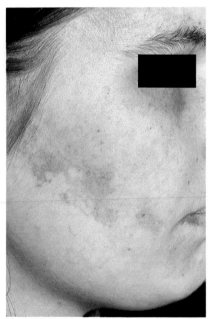

(g) (i)   (g) (ii)

(g) Klippel–Trenaunay syndrome in a young woman. This patient came for treatment of pigmentation and recurring ulceration at the left ankle, typical of venous hypertension. (i) The left limb was found to be 3 cm longer than the right. This photograph shows inequality in limb length, causing a tilted pelvis and different knee levels. (ii) Vascular markings were present elsewhere, here shown on the face. (iii) Venotensive pigmentation and healed ulceration seen at the left ankle. Phlebography showed extensive hypoplasia of deep veins, giving warning that interference with superficial veins could be harmful; conservative treatment succeeded in controlling the ulcer. There was no evidence of arteriovenous fistula.

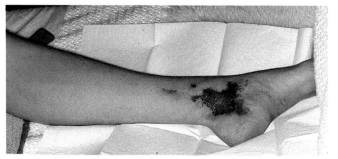

(g) (iii)

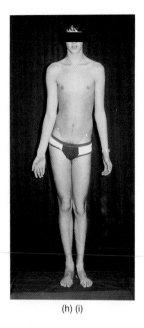

(h) (i)

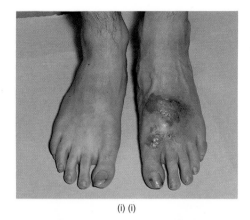

(i) (i)

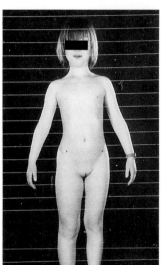

(h) (ii)

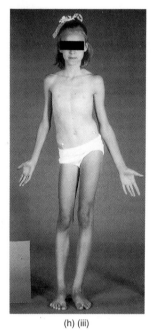

(h) (iii)

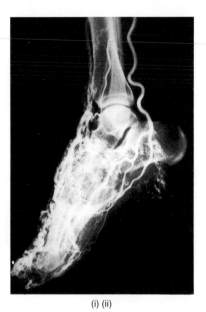

(i) (ii)

(i) Localized congenital arteriovenous fistulas. (i) The foot of a boy aged 12 is shown. It is slightly enlarged and the veins are prominent; on the dorsum are areas of pigmentation and threatened ulceration, typical of venous hypertension. All the clinical features of multiple arteriovenous fistulas were present and angiography confirmed that these ramified through the foot so that local surgery was not feasible. A watchful policy, with strong external elastic support, was advised; an amputation through normal tissue in the lower leg may become necessary eventually but only when circumstances make this essential.
(ii) Arteriogram of a similar arteriovenous lesion in a young woman.

(h) Limb hypertrophy with overlengthening of bone without vascular change.
(i) Segmental (one limb only) hypertrophy of right lower limb. Note tilted pelvis and differing knee levels. (ii) Gross segmental hypertrophy in right lower limb of a child. (iii) Hemihypertrophy in a girl aged 9, showing overall enlargement and lengthening of one half of the head, trunk, and both limbs on one side. None of these patients showed evidence of vascular abnormality.

Fig. 8.2   (continued).

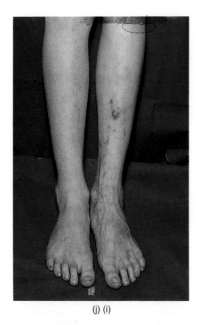

(j) (i)

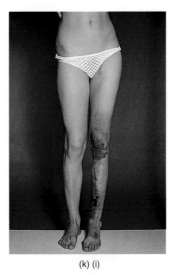

(k) (i)

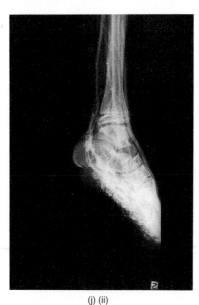

(j) (ii)

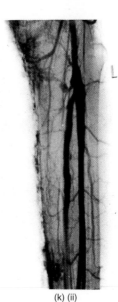

(k) (ii)

(k) Multiple congenital arteriovenous fistulas involving an entire lower limb and neighbouring pelvis in a young woman aged 18 (Parkes–Weber syndrome). (i) General view showing extensive pigmentation and ulceration from the knee downwards. Severe pelvic tilt due to 4 cm overlengthening of the limb is evident, and the left knee is 2 cm higher than the right because of tibial overgrowth. All the clinical features of diffuse arteriovenous fistulas were present, including cardiac hypertrophy and Branham's sign. (ii) Portion of arteriogram for this patient to show the distinctive spongework of multiple fistulas on the inner aspect of tibia. In the upper part, a large feeding artery can be seen running to an extensive area of fistulas. At a later stage, this artery was occluded by a Gianturco coil and this healed an overlying ulcer. This patient successfully went through two pregnancies without any apparent deterioration. For some years the ulceration has been controlled by strong elastic support, and this conservative policy will be followed as long as possible.

(j) Multiple arteriovenous fistulas in the foot and leg of a boy aged 9 (Parkes–Weber syndrome). (i) The features are essentially similar but more extensive than those in the preceding figure. The left tibia was 2 cm longer than the normal side, with a corresponding increase in the foot size. (ii) Arteriogram showing rapid perfusion into the vascular spongework of the foot and transit to the venous system.

Fig. 8.2 (continued).

Congenital defects
Multiple arteriovenous fistulas

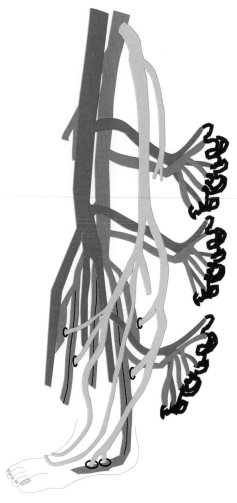

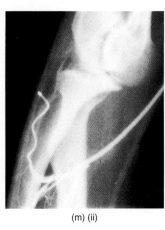
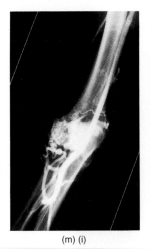

(m) (i)

(m) (ii)

(m) Treatment of localized arteriovenous fistula by transluminal occlusion of its feeding artery. (i) Angiogram of fistula at the elbow of a young woman. The feeding artery to the fistulous area is clearly seen. (ii) Angiogram immediately after insertion of a Gianturco coil introduced by arterial catheter; all blood flow through the fistula has ceased. When reviewed 1 year later only a slight thickening was present with no evidence of persisting fistula.

Features:
Multiple sponge-like communications between a series of large arteries and veins.
Massive hypertrophy of main arteries leading to the fistulas
Overgrowth of bones in region of fistulas
Loud arterial bruits
Pulsatile flow in veins (Doppler)

(l) Features of extensive multiple congenital arteriovenous fistulas in the lower limb.

Fig. 8.2   (continued).

Extensive venous angiomatosis and angiodysplasia

Cavernous angiomatosis may occur as a congenital defect extensively over a lower limb or elsewhere in the body (Fig. 8.2(d)). It is most obvious when the skin is involved, as a dark purple irregular compressible swelling, but it often pervades the underlying layers extending into muscle and bone beneath. In the worst examples, this grossly abnormal venous state may be accompanied by severely defective deep veins which are either absent or lacking valves. A

massive persistent lateral vein, referred to above, may be present. In such limbs venous return against gravity is likely to be severely defective, and by the time that adult life is reached venous hypertension causes a strong tendency to ulceration. Lymphatic abnormality may accompany these extensive venous aberrations (see congenital vascular syndromes in Part III).

Box 8.1   Features of congenital venous abnormality

Venous dysplasia comes in several forms and varies from being localized to extensive throughout the limb. It may have any or all of the following components.

Phlebectasia Enlarged and irregular superficial and deep veins.

Phlebangiomatosis Areas of cavernous angiomas—a diffuse alteration of capillary beds, venules, and small veins into large irregular blood-containing spaces. In the skin this gives a striking blue-red discoloration and raised irregular surface (birthmark). It also may involve deep layers including bone without apparent defined boundaries.

Hypoplasia (underdevelopment) and **agenesis** (complete failure to develop) of veins, including major anatomical pathways normally present.

Mixed angiodysplasia, where other congenital malformations, such as spina bifida or incomplete development of a limb, are also present.

Arterial dysplasia, particularly giving rise to arteriovenous fistulas.

Lymphatic dysplasia is commonly combined with venous lesions but obscured by them

A curious feature is that any of the above features may be combined with increased growth of bone causing **lengthening of the limb.**

Box 8.2   Major venous anomalies

1. Persistence of an embryonic axial vein. A well-recognized example is the lateral vein which run up the outer side of the limb subcutaneously as a large valveless channel either terminating in the profunda femoris or continuing up and through the sciatic notch to join the internal iliac vein. Numerous phlebectactic branches join it

2. These anomalous veins may take over the functions of the normal major veins which fail to develop so that the limb in dependent on the abnormal valveless channels for return of venous blood. Removal of these can be catastrophic and may lead to loss of the limb.

3. In varying degree there also may be areas of angiomatosis which may be extensive. The skin is likely to be involved, with much disfigurement.

4. In some limbs there is increased bone growth with lengthening of the limb. The combination of venous vascular changes and overgrowth of limb length is know as the Klippel–Trenaunay syndrome.

Note. Arterial dysplasia with arteriovenous fistulas (also with lengthening of the limb) is considered to be a separate phenomenon and its many different features are considered below.

Klippel–Trenaunay syndrome

The extensive venous abnormality just described is often, but not always, accompanied by overgrowth in the bones to give increased length in the limb and this special variety is known as the Klippel–Trenaunay syndrome (Figs 8.2(e)–8.2(g)). Because of the close association of severe venous malformation with overgrowth of the bones, any patient showing venous abnormality or angiomatosis should be examined for a change in bone length. This change is usually made obvious by careful clinical examination comparing measurements between the bony points on the two limbs, or simply by inspecting the patient in a standing position and looking for inequality in the levels of the corresponding bony prominences. Measurement by radiography is only necessary if study of progressive change over the years is required.

The significance of bony overgrowth in a limb (limb hypertrophy)

Overlengthening of a limb may arise without any other abnormality and will then usually be seen in an orthopaedic clinic (Fig. 8.2(h)), but it is often found as a previously unnoticed accompaniment of gross vascular abnormality, as in Klippel–Trenaunay syndrome. Even if obvious vascular changes are not present, the possibility of deep vein abnormality, perhaps with large valveless channels causing venous hypertension and eventually ulceration in the limb, must be borne in mind. The association with a large superficial lateral venous channel and defective or absent deep veins has already been mentioned above. Another cause of overlengthening of bones is the presence of multiple arteriovenous fistulas (Parkes–Weber syndrome), but this condition should be regarded as separate from the venous states just described (see below). When bony overgrowth is found by a venous clinic it is important to place the young patient under orthopaedic care. Inequality in the length of the lower limbs with tilting of the pelvis should be compensated for by raising the shoe on the normal side since otherwise it may cause arthritis of the spine at an early age. Surgical correction of the bone length, either by epiphysiodesis whilst the bone is still growing or, better, by bone shortening as a young adult, may be necessary if the vascular state allows this.

Relationship between congenital arteriovenous fistulas and Klippel–Trenaunay syndrome

It is well known that extensive congenital arteriovenous fistulas will cause overgrowth of bone in the vicinity. This leads to speculation that occult arteriovenous fistulas may account for bony overgrowth in the Klippel–Trenaunay syndrome. This has not been demonstrated reliably and, although there are cases where both states undoubtedly coexist, the current view is that the two conditions have no direct relationship.

Treatment of angiomas, angiomatosis, and Klippel–Trenaunay syndrome

Small lesions may be treated by laser therapy but others, if not too extensive, may be treated by sclerotherapy or by appropriate plastic surgery. It should be noted that the skin involved in angiomatous change may easily necrose if it is raised or undermined.

Klippel–Trenaunay syndrome

Repeated sclerotherapy may bring considerable improvement in the cutaneous lesions. In some cases surgical excision and provision of skin coverage by a vascularized flap from the opposite limb may prove possible in order to give good skin coverage over, for example, the knee joint. However, the difficulties in doing this must not be underrated; it is seldom possible to progress beyond the angiomatosis, and numerous vascular apertures may bleed copiously from the fringe that remains. Raising flaps of heavily involved skin may result in extensive necrosis and problems in skin coverage. Tissues involved in angiomatosis do not respond in a normal fashion if surgery is required, and such problems are best left to surgeons with a special skill in this field.

If phlebography has shown that extensive valveless deep veins are present and causing venous ulceration, it is sometimes possible to reroute these by implanting them into a neighbouring major vein that is valved, for example transposing a superficial femoral vein into a well-valved profunda femoris vein (Fig. 5.3(b)). Transplanting valves from the brachial vein or the long saphenous vein of the opposite limb is a theoretical possibility, but is seldom a convincing form of treatment in practice (Fig. 5.3(c)).

Conservative management

Usually a policy of conservative management will have to be followed. This will be by strong elastic support to compress the angiomatous lesions and to prevent progressive enlargement; special fitting of a full thigh-length stocking with waist attachment may be required. In addition it is essential that a policy of elevation at every spare moment is followed in order to reduce venous hypertension and keep ulceration at bay.

Usually the limb is good in other respects and serves the patient well, so that amputation must not be an option. With good conservative management a useful limb can be maintained indefinitely in a satisfactory state.

Box 8.3   Principles in treatment of congenital venous lesions

Localized angiomas
Sclerotherapy May be well worth giving this a trial in stages.
Laser and high-intensity light treatment May be well worth giving this a trial.
Surgical excision This is practical if the lesion is relatively small and overlying skin is not involved. These lesions are ill-defined and cross anatomical boundaries so that considerable skill may be required. If the skin is involved, this will not tolerate undermining and a plastic procedure will be needed to provide new skin coverage (pedicle flap graft or free microvascular grafting). Control of haemorrhage from the fringe of remaining angioma may be a problem. In favourable lesions excision may be carried out in several stages.
Anomalous veins Study them carefully by phlebography to understand their distribution and the status of the normal anatomical major veins which may be hypoplastic and unable to carry the load if the anomalous vessels are taken away. Even so, elimination of the abnormal veins may bring little benefit and it is often best to settle for elastic support

Diffuse cavernous angiomatosis and Klippel–Trenaunay syndrome
Problems and solutions are as follows
Appearance

- Application of cosmetic pastes.
- Covering with elastic stocking.
- Sclerotherapy should be given a trial and may prove helpful in lesser examples.
- Laser or high-intensity light therapy by appropriate specialist. This can be very effective if the lesion is not too massive.

Venous insufficiency due to valveless veins and consequent ulceration

- Full evaluation of status of normal major veins and of the abnormal veins by phlebography.
- Consider *valve transplantation* to valveless channels or *transposition of valveless major veins into well-valved veins* nearby (these operations are described in Chapter 5).
- Follow a policy of elastic support and elevation overnight and, whenever possible, by day.

Overlengthening of affected limb
Consult orthopaedic surgeon who may:

- Elevate shoe on normal side. This is necessary to prevent progressive damage to lumbar spine caused by tilting of the pelvis.
- Carry out epiphysiodesis to limit further bone growth in the affected limb.
- Wait until bone growth has ceased and then carry out a subtrochanteric bone-shortening procedure if the vascular state allows this and it is considered desirable.

General comment
With angiodysplasia and venous anomalies, including Klippel–Trenaunay syndrome, *do not consider amputation as an option*. These limbs can usually be kept in good condition and serve a useful function throughout life. In most cases elastic stocking support and coverage is the best policy. If ulceration from venous insufficiency threatens, elevate at night and whenever possible by day. As with chronic venous insufficiency from other causes, treat an active ulcer by a period of high elevation and then ambulation in a paste bandage (see Chapter 6 and Fig. 6.5). These patients are among the most difficult to manage well and there should be no hesitation in obtaining the advice of an experienced specialist in this field.

Congenital multiple arteriovenous fistulas in a limb (Parkes–Weber syndrome)

Congenital arteriovenous fistulas may be localized to, for example, part of the foot or leg (Figs 8.2(i) and 8.2(j) or multiple fistulas may extend over the whole limb and perhaps even the adjoining pelvis (Fig. 8.2(k)). There is a corresponding overgrowth of neighbouring bone, with enlargement of the bony structure of the foot if localized there, or, if the entire limb is involved, 5 cm or more increase in its length.

The communications between artery and vein are through sponge-like vascular formations, each supplied by a single large artery which breaks into multiple branches connecting with a leash of enlarged veins running from it (Fig. 8.2(l)). An obvious pulsatile swelling may be present with discoloration of the overlying skin and large veins radiating from it; with a stethoscope, a machinery pumping bruit can be heard extensively over the limb. Massive arteriovenous shunting may cause an increased pulse rate which drops back to normal when the main artery to the limb is temporarily occluded (Branham's sign). The constant struggle to maintain blood pressure and the premature return of a large volume of blood may cause considerable cardiac enlargement with eventual heart failure. Brown pigmentation and ulceration of the skin in the distal limb is often present owing to the sustained venous hypertension characteristic of this condition.

Box 8.4 Arteriovenous fistulas (Parkes-Weber syndrome)

An arteriovenous fistula created by trauma is usually a single point of communication but the congenital lesion consists of numerous apertures based on feeding arteries. They may be localized to one area or be multiple and widespread throughout the whole limb.

Main features of multiple arteriovenous fistulas

Made up of units consisting of:

- an enlarged feeding artery
- capillary bed replaced by a widely open vascular spongework which, in effect, gives multiple direct communications between artery and vein, without the normal resistance offered by capillaries
- enlarged veins leading away to join the normal route of venous return.

These units may be single or multiple and extensive over the limb.

Haemodynamic effects

The feeding artery and the main artery from which this arises become greatly enlarged (a recognized effect caused by wide excursion in pulse pressures owing to lack of peripheral resistance).

The venous pressure in the neighbouring veins is raised to near arterial levels and is pulsatile. This local venous hypertension causes the typical manifestations of venotension, skin pigmentation, and ulceration. The combined heavy wastage of arterial pressure through the arteriovenous shunts and a high venous pressure makes the pressure gradient across normal capillaries precariously low, so that treatment by arterial occlusion may cause an abrupt switch to ischaemia.

With extensive lesions, the lack of peripheral resistance in the arterial system and the rapid return of a significant proportion of cardiac output through the fistulas become so great that the heart has to respond by increasing its output, its rate is increased, and progressive cardiac hypertrophy develops. Eventually, cardiac failure may occur early in adult life.

Clinical features

These are present at birth but tend to become more obvious as the child grows. A small lesion may be no more than a raised pulsatile swelling a few centimetres across, but an extensive lesion may involve the whole limb and beyond into the trunk.

Locally, or distally in whole-limb involvement, there is skin pigmentation and often ulceration due to venous hypertension. The veins are prominent compared with the normal side and warm to touch.

Depending on the position and extent of the lesions, overgrowth of bone gives visible enlargement of the foot or lengthening of the limb, perhaps by up to 5 cm, with corresponding tilting of the pelvis. If not corrected, this asymmetry causes osteo-arthritis of the lumbar spine prematurely in the adult.

An obvious machinery murmur is present over the fistulas, and the main artery supplying the area emits a distinctive humming bruit arising from its large calibre and the high velocity of flow.

The heart may show clinically detectable enlargement and a tachycardia which immediately slows if the main artery (here the femoral artery) is temporarily occluded by finger pressure (Branham's sign).

Investigations

Doppler flowmetry to veins locally detects strong pulsatile flow and high velocity.

Ultrasonography will show pulsatile flow in the veins leading away, and abnormal enlargement of arteries. Fistulous areas of confused high velocity flow may be seen.

Arteriography will show enlarged arteries leading to diffusely filling areas of fistulas and rapid transit into the veins.

Chest *radiography* may show cardiac hypertrophy.

Complications

- Progressive enlargement
- Haemorrhage from ulcer
- Cardiac failure

Diagnosis

The diagnosis is usually evident on clinical grounds and by the finding that Doppler flowmetry shows strong pulsation within the superficial veins. Arteriography with serial pictures will confirm the diagnosis and will often outline individual areas of fistulous communication and the arteries feeding them.

Treatment of congenital arteriovenous fistulas

Very localized lesions can be surgically excised after careful evaluation by arteriography. However, even comparatively small lesions may be better treated by transluminal embolization as described below. Amputation of a limb must not be resorted to except *in extremis*; it may not solve the problem which can continue in the stump.

Active treatment by transluminal occlusion

This requires expert planning and should be performed by an experienced vascular radiologist. A special indication for this is in cardiac failure when it is considered essential to reduce the arteriovenous shunting. The basis is occlusion of the feeding artery by transluminal introduction of an occlusive device, such as the Gianturco coil, under radiological control (Fig. 8.2(m)). This is far better than attempted surgical ligation. However, it is possible to cut off too much arterial supply and abruptly reduce arterial pressure below that of the abnormally high venous pressure so that capillary flow ceases, resulting in extensive ischaemic changes.

Conservative treatment

In most patients conservative treatment will be the mainstay of treatment. Very strong elastic containment and elevation of the limb at every available moment will be essential. If ulceration or haemorrhage occur, inelastic containment by paste bandage, maintained for many weeks, can be most valuable.

Many young patients reach adult life without mishap and continue successfully, even through pregnancy (Fig. 8.2(k)), using the methods outlined above. It is wrong to counsel anxious parents at an early age that the limb should be amputated either at that time or later, but rather to emphasize that every effort will be made to extend the useful state of the limb indefinitely.

Box 8.5   Treatment for congenital arteriovenous fistulas

Small lesions can excised but it is better to occlude the feeding artery by transluminal occlusion, for example, using a Gianturco coil introduced by a catheter controlled by radiographic or ultrasound imaging.

In more extensive or widespread lesions surgical removal is not feasible. Amputation must not be considered except as a last resort, as these limbs can usually be controlled for many years with good function; moreover amputation can offer considerable danger if the fistulous process extends above the level of intended amputation, as is often the case.

Policy of containment

This aims to restrain the excessive blood flow by external compression by the strongest elastic support that the patient can tolerate. This will control progressive enlargement and give some protection to the heart by reducing the massive arteriovenous shunt. This does appear to be of real value, and every encouragement should be given for the young patient to continue with this permanently. A policy of elevation to reduce venous hypertension whenever possible, and certainly overnight, must be maintained to help protect the skin from deterioration and ulceration.

In times of crisis, for instance when an ulcer is active or when haemorrhage occurs, firm compression with paste bandage plus elastic compression should be used, combined with high elevation (with movement) to minimize the venous pressure until the crisis has passed.

Reduction of arterial inflow

This is best achieved by arterial catheterization to occlude (by a Gianturco coil or similar device) carefully selected feeding arteries. This can improve troublesome areas and reduce the cardiac burden. However, there are limits to this procedure, and if a distal main artery becomes occluded it is possible for arterial pressure beyond this to be reduced below that required for perfusion of normal tissues. The high venous pressure now actually exceeds the reduced arterial perfusion pressure so that capillary flow ceases and there is an abrupt change to ischaemia and the threat of gangrene, despite a massive but useless arteriovenous flow nearby. For this reason, it is wisest to arrange this form of treatment cautiously in stages, each treating a limited area. If ischaemia does occur, the limb must be placed horizontally and compression bandaging abandoned; spontaneous improvement is possible. The perfusion of normal tissue in this sort of limb is precarious, and the response to interference with its blood supply is not easy to predict and may be unexpectedly adverse. The golden rule is only to attempt elimination of feeder arteries to grossly abnormal tissue, i.e. where the fistulas lie. The arterial supply to normal tissue (even if shared with fistulas, as is the case with a main artery) must never be interfered with. These feeder arteries are distinctive and readily identified radiographically or by ultrasonography.

Orthopaedic correction for lengthened limb

If detectable lengthening of the limb is present, orthopaedic advice should be sought to correct this by raising the opposite shoe. This will require adjusting as the child grows, but should give protection against eventual harm to the lumbar spine. Surgical epiphysiodesis or bone-shortening operations may not be feasible in these limbs.

Comment

Fortunately these cases are rare, but much can be done to help the preserve a useful limb and protect them from its dangers.

9 Ulcers of the leg

Chronic ulceration of the leg often causes considerable disability and is a common problem with significant economic consequences for the individual and for society. In European countries nearly 80 per cent of these ulcers arise from one or other of the venous disorders described above, but in the remainder there are many other causes; in these, treatment suitable for venous ulceration may be in direct conflict with that actually required, and in the case of ischaemic ulceration may jeopardize the limb. Because of the prevalence of venous ulcer, it is all too easy to assume that this is the diagnosis and to give wholly inappropriate treatment. It is important to identify the underlying cause accurately in each case so that treatment can be correctly based on this. The diagnosis of 'leg ulcer' is totally inadequate and must always be qualified by a statement of the cause, backed by full evidence for this diagnosis. This requires an understanding of the range of leg ulcers that occur and the disease processes underlying them (Fig. 9.1). The description that follows is appropriate for European countries but it must be remembered that the prevalence of leg ulcers has considerable variation geographically and within ethnic groups. Fortunately, venous ulceration has distinctive features that usually allow positive identification; thus the recognition and treatment of venous ulcers will be considered first. The term 'leg' is used here to describe the portion of the lower limb beneath the knee.

Venous ulceration

For the reasons described earlier, patients with venous disorders are liable, in varying degrees, to develop venous hypertension. If this is sufficiently severe, it causes excess capillary exudation and formation of a fibrin barrier around capillaries, with diminished nutritional exchange between capillary blood and the subcutaneous tissues and skin. An important phenomenon involved in this, which has recently been recognized, is the deposition of leucocytes in capillaries affected by venous hypertension (white cell trapping). Endothelial cells, activated by hypoxia, cause leucocytes to become adherent and release injurious products which damage the endothelium with consequent migration of leucocytes into surrounding tissue to cause further harm there. It is as if the leucocytes with their defensive and scavenging properties, which are so valuable in an inflammatory reaction, are mistakenly attacking impaired capillary walls and neighbouring tissue. The destructive effect is enhanced by obstruction to capillary flow by the adherent layer of leucocytes and by thrombus resulting from the activation of platelets. The precise sequence has yet to be established, but 'leucocyte trapping' seems to play an essential part in the changes leading to venous ulceration. Oedema, induration, and fibrosis, accompanied by pigmentation of the skin, develop progressively and, without treatment, culminate in tissue death and ulceration (Figs 4.17(b), 4.18, 4.28, 5.3(a), and 9.2(b)–9.3(e)) (see also Venous ulceration in Part III). The same characteristic changes also develop distal to arteriovenous fistula (see Chapter 8) owing to the common denominator in all these conditions—venous hypertension. A summary of the main features of typical venous ulcer is given below and in Fig. 9.2(a).

Position

The ulcer occurs at a position where venous pressure is sustained at a high level and upon which unnaturally high peaks of pressure may be superimposed. Usually this is in the lower leg; occasionally it is on the upper aspect of the foot but never on its underside. Although the most common site is just above the medial malleolus, ulcer may occur almost anywhere on the leg according to the pattern of venous failure.

Age and distribution

No age of adult life is immune, but the occurrence of venous ulcer increases with age probably due to progressive deterioration in the musculovenous pumping mechanisms with advancing years. Up to 1 per cent of the adult population may be affected by venous ulceration at some stage in their lives, with women affected slightly more frequently than men.

Manifestations

Ulceration is preceded by venotensive changes of local oedema, induration (lipodermatosclerosis), and brown pigmentation of the skin caused by extravasated haemosiderin. These changes are always found in the vicinity of a venous ulcer, and if surrounding skin pigmentation is not present in a white skin the diagnosis is in doubt. However, haemosiderin is of a similar colour to the melanin in a black skin which may be increased locally around any long-standing skin lesion, and, since the two pigments cannot be easily distinguished, increased pigmentation is not a reliable guide to venotension in black patients. Moreover, melanin may be reduced in various circumstances, such as use of steroid cream, so that lack of surrounding pigmentation cannot be used to exclude a venous ulcer. Nevertheless, all the other evidence of venous insufficiency will be present and recognition of the cause should not be difficult.

Other forms of ulceration do not show these changes, although they may be mimicked to some extent by a surrounding cellulitis. Fluid exudate is usual and, depending on prevailing bacteria and the

LEG ULCERS

Four out of five leg ulcers are venous in origin

BUT

One in five has another cause

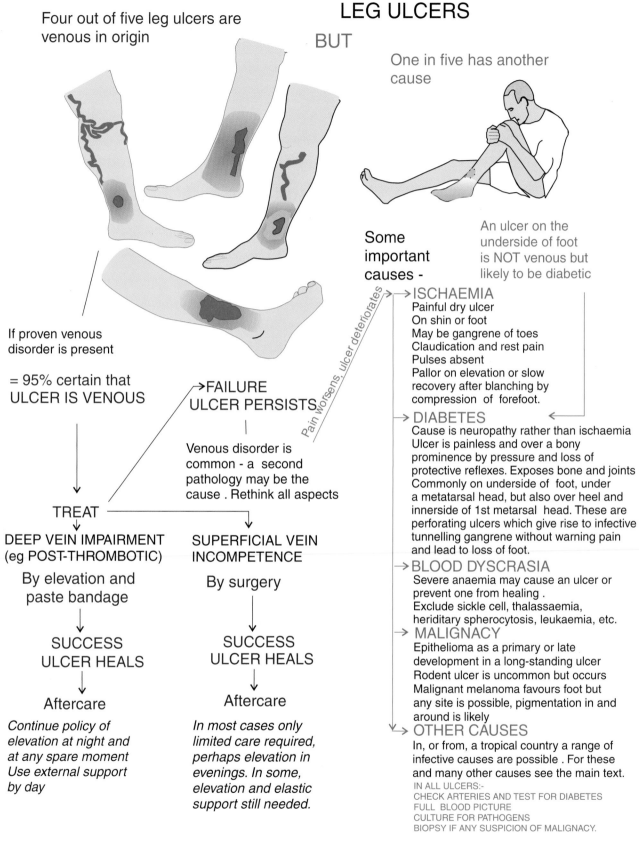

If proven venous disorder is present

= 95% certain that ULCER IS VENOUS

→FAILURE ULCER PERSISTS

Venous disorder is common - a second pathology may be the cause . Rethink all aspects

TREAT

DEEP VEIN IMPAIRMENT (eg POST-THROMBOTIC)

By elevation and paste bandage

↓

SUCCESS ULCER HEALS

↓

Aftercare

Continue policy of elevation at night and at any spare moment Use external support by day

SUPERFICIAL VEIN INCOMPETENCE

By surgery

↓

SUCCESS ULCER HEALS

↓

Aftercare

In most cases only limited care required, perhaps elevation in evenings. In some, elevation and elastic support still needed.

Some important causes -

An ulcer on the underside of foot is NOT venous but likely to be diabetic

Pain worsens, ulcer deteriorates

→ISCHAEMIA
Painful dry ulcer
On shin or foot
May be gangrene of toes
Claudication and rest pain
Pulses absent
Pallor on elevation or slow recovery after blanching by compression of forefoot.

→ DIABETES
Cause is neuropathy rather than ischaemia
Ulcer is painless and over a bony prominence by pressure and loss of protective reflexes. Exposes bone and joints
Commonly on underside of foot, under a metatarsal head, but also over heel and innerside of 1st metarsal head. These are perforating ulcers which give rise to infective tunnelling gangrene without warning pain and lead to loss of foot.

→BLOOD DYSCRASIA
Severe anaemia may cause an ulcer or prevent one from healing .
Exclude sickle cell, thalassaemia, heriditary spherocytosis, leukaemia, etc.

→ MALIGNACY
Epithelioma as a primary or late development in a long-standing ulcer
Rodent ulcer is uncommon but occurs
Malignant melanoma favours foot but any site is possible, pigmentation in and around is likely

→ OTHER CAUSES
In, or from, a tropical country a range of infective causes are possible . For these and many other causes see the main text.
IN ALL ULCERS:-
CHECK ARTERIES AND TEST FOR DIABETES
FULL BLOOD PICTURE
CULTURE FOR PATHOGENS
BIOPSY IF ANY SUSPICION OF MALIGNACY.

Fig. 9.1 Diagnostic approach to an ulcer on the leg.

VENOUS ULCER

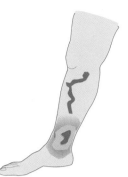

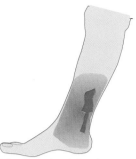

SUPERFICIAL VEIN INCOMPETENCE
Usually varicosities seen
Here a surrounding severe allergic
reaction to antibiotic is depicted

POST-THROMBOTIC SYNDROME
History of deep vein thrombosis
or major fracture to lower limbs

Surrounding skin is pigmented brown with underlying induration
Atrophie blanche or scarring from old ulceraton may be present
Variable amount of swelling

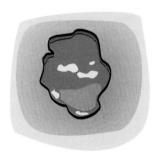

ACTIVE ULCER.
ABRUPT IRREGULAR OUTLINE
WITH RAGGED SKIN EDGE
BASE CONTAINS PUS AND
SLOUGH
Take culture and remove slough;
use hydrocolloid dressing or
similar; avoid allergens.

Always check arterial supply.
TREATMENT
If cause is superficial vein incompetence, treat this
surgically and follow with ambulation and elastic support.
Ulcer should heal but may always require some care by a
gravity counteraction policy (see below).

If it is post-thrombotic, start conservative treatment by spell
of high elevation with external support to leg but allow brief
walks and other activity to preserve muscles and joints.

As ulcer heals apply paste bandage and increase
ambulation but always returning to high elevation.

When fully healed allow increasing time up and about with
external support by stocking or bandage. Patient must learn
to live permanently within a gravity counteraction policy or
ulcer will return.

Gravity counteraction policy
Avoid prolonged standing.
Put leg in high elevation whenever possible, certainly
overnight.
When up and about some form of external support should
be used.
Patient must learn type of external support that suits best.

ULCER IN HEALING PHASE
SMOOTH OUTLINE WITH SHALLOW
SLOPING EDGE. A GREY FILM OF
EPITHELIUM GROWING FROM EDGE
IS CLEARLY VISIBLE.

Fig. 9.2 Leg ulcers.
(a) Main features of venous ulcers.

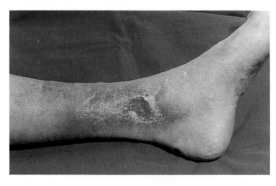

(b) Venous ulcer due to superficial vein incompetence. Commencing venous ulceration. This patient had long neglected her varicose veins and ignored an increasing area of pigmented skin above the medial malleolus. She sought advice only when the shallow ulcer shown here had been present for several weeks. It soon healed with a programme of elevation and use of elastic support. She declined surgical treatment but had learnt how to prevent the ulcer from recurring.

Fig. 9.2 (continued).

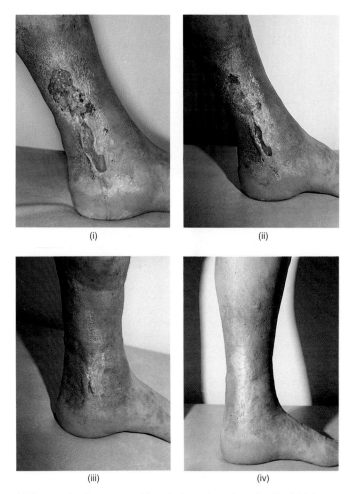

(i)

(ii)

(iii)

(iv)

(d) Venous ulcer in severe post-thrombotic syndrome (see also Fig. 6.3 (g)). This patient was unable to work because of a large painful ulcer. The swelling, induration, and pigmentation surrounding the ulcer are typical of venous hypertension, in this case caused by incurable deep vein impairment so that only conservative treatment was feasible. Infection with *Staphylococcus aureus* was present and treated initially by systemic antibiotic. (i)–(iv) These pictures were taken over 4 months to show the gradual but impressive improvement in response to high elevation with active exercise, and eventual mobilization in inelastic (paste bandage) support; later, a knee-length one-way-stretch stocking was substituted. Prevention of recurrence in these circumstances can only succeed with sustained conscientious effort by the patient. When seen 2 years later, this patient was at work, with the limb in good condition.

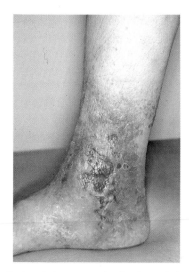

(c) Venous ulceration in valveless states. An ulcer in need of urgent treatment in an elderly patient. The extensive pigmentation and eczema shown here were due to a combination of superficial and deep vein insufficiency (valveless syndrome). The main ulcer is surrounded by satellite ulcers which will coalesce if treatment is not soon started. With a policy of elevation (arterial pulses were present) the ulcer healed. Stripping of the long saphenous vein was carried out subsequently to remove this factor, and the patient was urged to maintain a policy of elevation whenever possible and elastic support.

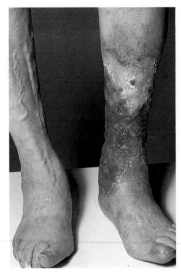

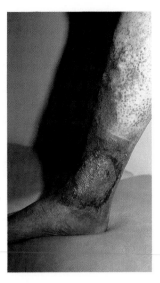

Fig. 9.2   (continued).

(e) Severe ulceration in iliofemoral post-thrombotic syndrome. This picture shows the ulcer illustrated in Fig. 6.4 (d) in more detail. Widespread atrophie blanche is present and indicates impoverished capillary beds. In an ulcer of this size severe anaemia may retard healing, and the possibility of malignant change must not be overlooked. The proliferative appearance suggests that ischaemia is unlikely to be a factor, but this should be verified and, as usual, metabolic factors such as diabetes must be excluded. Skin grafting with conservative treatment to counteract venous hypertension may heal the ulcer but, constant vigilance will be needed thereafter to prevent recurrence.

(f) Medical application to an ulcer may impede healing; for example strong antiseptics may prevent healing and many antibiotics may aggravate surrounding skin by sensitivity reactions. In this patient an exudative eczema in an area of venotensive change rapidly deteriorated when fusidic acid cream was used giving the appearances shown. Antibiotic preparations are particularly likely to cause reaction and should not be used without good reason.

presence of necrotic tissue, it may become purulent, possibly with an offensive odour. The ulcer causes variable discomfort and usually only harmless commensual organisms are found on bacterial culture; however, if it is infected by pathogens, such as *Staphylococcus aureus*, beta-haemolytic streptococci, or anaerobic organisms, invasion of surrounding tissues may cause considerable pain. Pain is also characteristic of an ischaemic ulcer, and the importance of distinguishing this from a venous ulcer is discussed below.

Eczema

This commonly occurs in the pigmented skin of venous disorders, overlying varicosities or alongside venous ulceration. The skin is thickened and lichenified by repeated rubbing in response to itching. A general sensitization may develop, giving rise to patches elsewhere. Its presence in the skin around an ulcer is an added difficulty as increased skin damage and infection are produced by scratching. Another problem is that many ointments applied to give relief may contain allergens that cause a sharp exudative reaction, and great care should be taken to avoid this. A further pitfall is the use of corticosteroids which, although beneficial to the eczema (provided that a sensitizing agent is not included), will prevent healing of the ulcer itself. Care must be taken to apply any corticosteroid sparingly to the skin only, clear of the ulcer.

Diagnosis

Diagnosis is confirmed by the presence of substantial to severe accompanying venous disorder which is readily demonstrated by the usual clinical tests and by the special tests, including Doppler flowmetry, plethysmography, phlebography, or ultrasonography, showing the characteristic abnormalities found in chronic venous insufficiency. Skin in the vicinity will show capillary stasis with laser Doppler rheography and a diminished oxygen tension.

Treatment

This will depend on the type of venous disorder causing ulceration. In superficial vein incompetence, surgery will have a major role by removing the pathway of incompetence, but in most other cases reliance must be placed on conservative treatment by elevation and external support, as discussed earlier. Counteracting venous hypertension is the most important measure in the healing of a venous ulcer, and the most effective way of achieving this is by elevation of the limb (Figs 4.21(g), 4.21(h), 6.5(a), and 9.2(d)). Local applications to the ulcer itself are probably far less important. Strong antiseptics may actually be damaging, and the ulcer is best cleansed by normal saline and covered with an inert non-adherent moisture-preserving material such as a hydrocolloid gel. Steroid applications should be avoided since they may actually delay epithelialization and cause deterioration in the ulcer. Antibiotic preparations should not be used unless there is good reason, for fear of setting up a sensitization reaction in the surrounding skin which is particularly vulnerable to antibiotics (Fig. 9.2(f)) and other materials commonly used in ointments and dressings. If pathogenic organisms have been demonstrated, any necrotic tissue should be excised, and an appropriate antibiotic given systemically for a few days. It must be emphasized that local treatment to the ulcer will not be effective unless venous hypertension is controlled by elevation for a good proportion of the day and all through the night. A sophisticated alternative to high elevation, particularly if oedema is troublesome, is the use of a pneumatic compression device acting sequentially upwards by multiple chambers enclosing the limb. These machines, which are often used in the control of lymphoedema, are widely marketed and can prove very successful in the healing and subsequent prevention of recurrence of ulceration in chronic venous insufficiency.

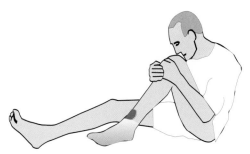

ISCHAEMIC ULCER

The typical posture of rest pain - or patient
may hang leg over edge of bed

Age: usually over 50 but no age immune.

Features: painful dry ulcer on shin or foot, often over a bony prominence such as malleoli or interphalangeal joints.
No surrounding pigmentation of skin. Usually has intermittent claudication and often nocturnal rest pain.
Often no swelling, but may be present due to hanging foot out of bed to relieve rest pain.

Ulcer: There is insufficient arterial supply to develop inflammatory reaction and ulcer is unable to react to
pathogens; little or no pus but destruction of tissue may be massive exposing necrotic muscles, tendons, and bones.
Pain usually severe and prolonged. May be gangrene on toes. (Venous ulcer shows none of these features)

Diagnosis: Absent pulses confirmed by Doppler index below 30%. Pallor of toes and forefoot on elevation, slow
recovery of colour when horizontal again; rubor develops by gravitational refilling with oxygenated blood on
dependency but slowly changes to a puce colour by stasis.

Treatment: Nurse with bed tilted to give slight foot-down position to let gravity assist arterial blood to reach the
forefoot but encourage patient to move foot frequently to promote venous return. Expose foot to room temperature;
use cage to protect from weight of bedclothes. Keep patient's body warm to create a 'physiological sympathectomy'.
Short walks are permitted.
If arterial reconstruction or balloon angioplasty is not possible, amputation may be the only way to relieve rest pain;
sympathectomy may at best give marginal benefit. Vasodilators are ineffective.

Clinical assessment of arterial supply. Signs of critical ischaemia.
Is arterial pressure sufficient to overcome gradient to forefoot?

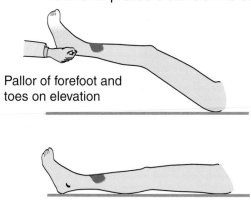

Pallor of forefoot and
toes on elevation

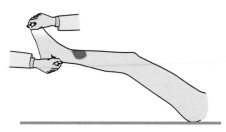

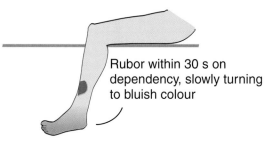

Colour takes 30 s + to return when flat again

Blanching by compression with hand
either persists or colour takes 30 s +
before returning, if foot kept in elevation

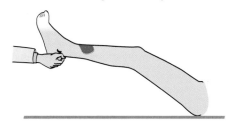

Rubor within 30 s on
dependency, slowly turning
to bluish colour

Fig. 9.2 (continued).

(g) Main features of ischaemic ulcers.

Most venous ulcers will heal under the regimen just outlined, and often it may be combined with limited ambulation if external support with a paste bandage is used. If the ulcer is particularly large, the process can be speeded up surgically by removing excess granulation tissue and applying some form of split skin graft. This should only be done when the ulcer has clearly reached a healing phase with sloping edges and a thin grey line of epithelial ingrowth. In cases where surgical control of venous hypertension is not possible, the ulcer will soon recur unless the patient has been instructed in an appropriate way of life which will include elevation of the limb whenever possible and the use of external support (Figs 4.21 and 6.5). If a large ulcer proves intractable or recurs repeatedly, a plastic procedure in which the ulcer is excised and skin cover is provided by a pedicle graft, or by a myocutaneous free graft vascularized by microvascular surgery, may give a fresh start but will require prolonged care to prevent eventual recurrence. In these circumstances it is imperative to make sure beforehand that ischaemia or malignancy is not the real cause for the ulcer's unsatisfactory response to treatment. The possible role of ligation of perforating veins is discussed earlier.

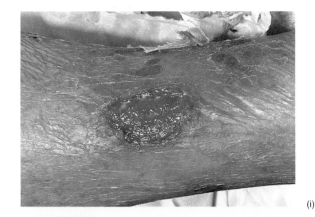

(i)

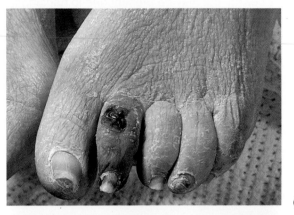

(ii)

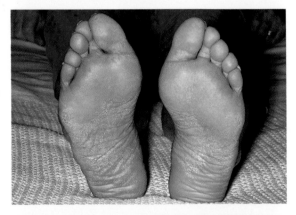

(iiia)

Fig. 9.2   (continued).

(h) Ischaemic ulceration. (i) An ischaemic ulcer is not surrounded by typical venotensive change and will be dry with sparse granulation tissue. The illustration shows an ischaemic ulcer on the shin of an elderly person.
(ii) Gangrene of the toes is a common accompaniment of ischaemic ulceration. In this illustration, the wrinkled skin on the forefoot is due to recent subsidence of dependency oedema caused by the previous habit of hanging the leg out of bed to relieve rest pain. This is on the same limb as that illustrated in (i).
(iii) Critically ischaemic foot: (*a*) colour is present in both feet when horizontal; (*b*) after elevation for 30 s the right forefoot and toes show obvious blanching because arterial perfusion pressure is insufficient to overcome the gradient.

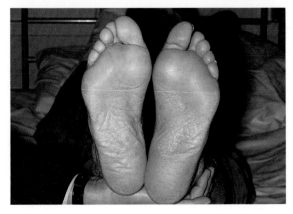

(iv*b*)

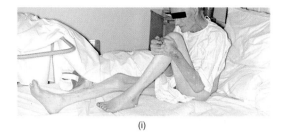

(i)

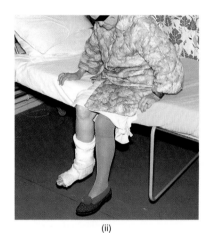

(ii)

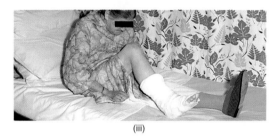

(iii)

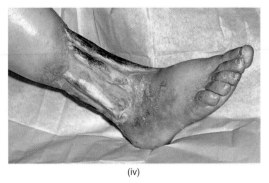

(iv)

Fig. 9.2 (continued).

(i) Characteristic postures of patients with ischaemic rest pain. (i) The typical 'knee-up' position of a patient with severe rest pain. This posture, or hanging the leg over the side of bed, brings a small measure of relief by using gravity to help arterial circulation at knee level down to the foot. (ii), (iii) This elderly patient endured severe ischaemic rest pain for 3 months, sitting endlessly over the edge of the bed or in a 'knee-up' position. (iv) The massive ischaemic ulcer under the bandages of the last patient. Essentially, it is a dry ulcer without granulation tissue or pus (there is not sufficient circulation to give inflammatory reaction) and with necrotic tendons exposed. A venous ulcer does not expose deeper tissues in this fashion. Amputation was necessary here, but arterial reconstruction to the left side succeeded in saving this limb when severe ischaemic rest pain developed a few months later.

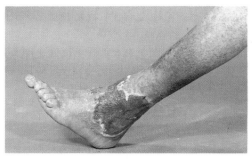

(j) Combination of chronic venous insufficiency and ischaemia. Illustrated here is massive ulceration in the left limb of a 65-year-old man. Originally, both lower limbs were similarly affected and it was found that gross long saphenous incompetence was present together with bilateral occlusion of the superficial femoral arteries. This provided an opportunity to cure the venous incompetence by removing the long saphenous veins and using them as femoropopliteal grafts to restore arterial supply. One limb responded dramatically with healing of the ulcer; the other limb, shown in the illustration, failed to do so and amputation was eventually resorted to, even though the arterial reconstruction remained open; it is possible that widespread occlusion of tibial and peroneal arteries caused this failure. Two years later the right limb remained in good condition with the patient using it actively.

Box 9.1
Factors causing or aggravating leg ulcers

General factors

- Anaemia and blood dyscrasias.
- Malnutrition: deficiency of vitamins, protein and/or minerals. This can arise in the elderly or in countries with widespread poverty.
- Abnormal metabolic states, such as diabetes, renal disease, or liver disease.
- Systemic, autoimmune, and microvascular diseases (e.g. vasculitis in rheumatoid arthritis).
- Poor health or generalized illness.
- Specific illness (e.g. syphilis, tuberculosis, AIDS).

Local factors that must be reversed or removed for healing to occur

- Venotension (including arteriovenous fistula)
- Ischaemia
- Oedema
- Malignancy
- Pathogenic bacteria or parasites
- Allergy to dressings or medical applications, particularly those containing antibiotics, antiseptics, and preservatives (see Box 9.6). This is a common pitfall.
- Continuing or repeated trauma (including self-inflicted trauma from malingering or hysteria).

Some initiating factors

- Physical trauma.
- Burns
- Chemical (to surface or by injection) or radiation damage
- Insect bite (necrotoxins or implantation of infestation.

DIABETIC ULCER (Diabetes mellitus)

Age: All ages but frequency increases with age.
Features: Painless, perforating ulcer exposing a
bony prominence: diabetes +ve.

Essential cause is **diabetic neuropathy** with
arterial supply usually good and not a factor.
Loss of protective reflexes causes skin over
bony prominences to break down to expose
underlying bone and joint.

Diagnostic features: Urine sugar +ve and
blood glucose raised. Position of ulcers over
prominent bones and joints; edges have
sharp punched-out appearance. Evidence of
peripheral neuropathy; ankle jerks and
sensation in toes and forefoot diminished or
absent. No surrounding pigmentation. Warm
foot with good blood supply - ankle pulses
often present or detected by Doppler
flowmeter.

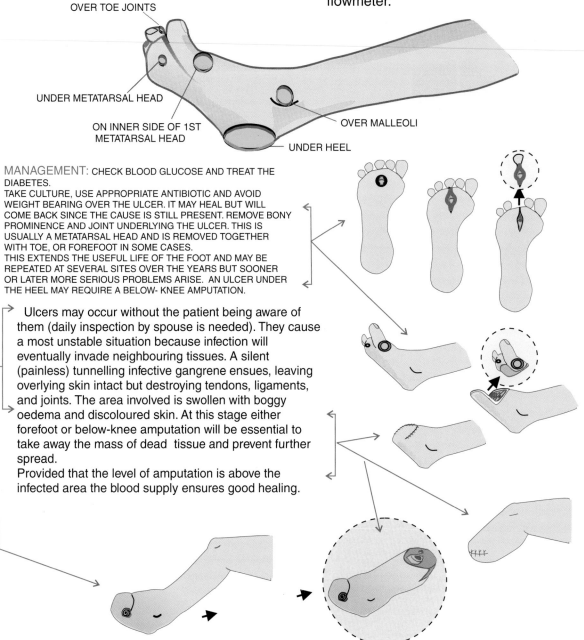

OVER TOE JOINTS

UNDER METATARSAL HEAD

ON INNER SIDE OF 1ST
METATARSAL HEAD

OVER MALLEOLI

UNDER HEEL

MANAGEMENT: CHECK BLOOD GLUCOSE AND TREAT THE
DIABETES.
TAKE CULTURE, USE APPROPRIATE ANTIBIOTIC AND AVOID
WEIGHT BEARING OVER THE ULCER. IT MAY HEAL BUT WILL
COME BACK SINCE THE CAUSE IS STILL PRESENT. REMOVE BONY
PROMINENCE AND JOINT UNDERLYING THE ULCER. THIS IS
USUALLY A METATARSAL HEAD AND IS REMOVED TOGETHER
WITH TOE, OR FOREFOOT IN SOME CASES.
THIS EXTENDS THE USEFUL LIFE OF THE FOOT AND MAY BE
REPEATED AT SEVERAL SITES OVER THE YEARS BUT SOONER
OR LATER MORE SERIOUS PROBLEMS ARISE. AN ULCER UNDER
THE HEEL MAY REQUIRE A BELOW- KNEE AMPUTATION.

Ulcers may occur without the patient being aware of
them (daily inspection by spouse is needed). They cause
a most unstable situation because infection will
eventually invade neighbouring tissues. A silent
(painless) tunnelling infective gangrene ensues, leaving
overlying skin intact but destroying tendons, ligaments,
and joints. The area involved is swollen with boggy
oedema and discoloured skin. At this stage either
forefoot or below-knee amputation will be essential to
take away the mass of dead tissue and prevent further
spread.
Provided that the level of amputation is above the
infected area the blood supply ensures good healing.

Fig. 9.2   (continued).

(k) Main features of diabetic ulcers.

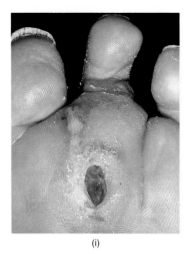

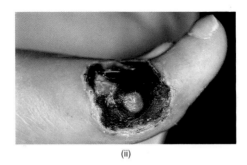

(i)   (ii)

(l) Diabetic ulcer and complications. (i) Typical neuropathic diabetic ulcers occur over bony prominences, as in this example over the head of the second metatarsal bone. Healing this ulcer might be possible but it will keep recurring unless the metatarsal head is removed. (ii) A similar ulcer over the head of the first metatarsal bone and opening into the joint. Stability was restored by removing the distal part of the first metatarsal and the great toe. The blood supply was ample to give good healing.

Fig. 9.2   (continued).

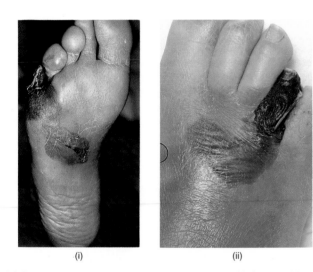

(i)   (ii)

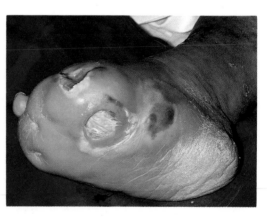

(n) The ultimate fate of a diabetic neuropathic foot. Over the course of many years the foot has been rescued from neuropathic ulcers by removing the heads of various metatarsal bones. In the illustration, further ulceration has occurred over the stumps of remaining metatarsals and has allowed infection to enter. This has tunnelled painlessly through the foot and into the lower leg, and was ignored by the patient as it spread slowly over the preceding weeks. The foot could not be saved but a below-knee amputation healed well.

(m) Consequence of an open lesion in a diabetic neuropathic foot: a painless tunnelling gangrene that is likely to be ignored until it is too late to save the foot. (i) A lesion of the little toe has allowed infection to spread painlessly and insidiously into the deep compartments of the foot over the course of some weeks. The plantar tendons were found to be necrotic and surrounded by pus. In this patient there was inadequate healthy skin to permit a forefoot amputation. (ii) A similar lesion on the dorsum of the foot, again painless and very destructive in the deeper layers.

MALIGNANT ULCER

Venous, ischaemic, and diabetic ulcers all represent a loss of substance, notably the skin.
A malignant ulcer essentially generates substance, with ulceration caused by necrosis within this. The growing outer edge reflects this proliferation by being raised. Within this lies the hollow of an ulcer caused by necrosis. Varicose veins and other venous disorders are very common on the legs, and a separate pathology is easily mistaken as venous, especially if it is malignancy complicating a long-standing venous ulcer. There should never be an automatic assumption that an ulcer is venous.

SQUAMOUS CARCINOMA (epithelioma) is the most likely form to be seen on the leg. The irregular firm, raised everted edge is characteristic. It may occur in any position and its size varies from early small to very large late. The latter may be due to malignant change in a long standing venous ulcer (Marjolin's ulcer). It is important not to miss this since it is actively malignant both locally and by metastasis to lymph nodes and by bloodstream. Biopsy if the raised edge of an ulcer causes any doubt. .

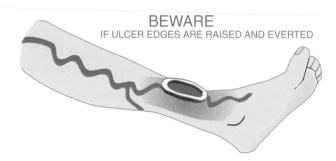

BEWARE
IF ULCER EDGES ARE RAISED AND EVERTED

BASAL CELL CARCINOMA (rodent ulcer). This is uncommon on the leg but amongst obvious varicose veins may be mistaken. Its edge is beaded and only slightly raised with some puckering of neighbouring skin. Within lies an ulcer with a characteristic scab which is shed at intervals. It is a low-grade malignancy and seldom metastasizes to lymph nodes or elsewhere, but can be destructive if neglected too long. If suspected, it is easy to excise at same time as any operation on the veins..

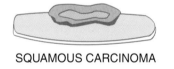

SQUAMOUS CARCINOMA

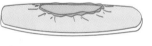

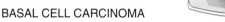

BASAL CELL CARCINOMA

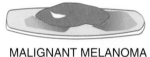

MALIGNANT MELANOMA

MALIGNANT MELANOMA. This is not often an ulcerative lesion but it is pigmented (melanin), although, of course, this has no relationship to venous pigmentation (haemosiderin). Malignant melanoma may arise from a pre-existing benign mole or as a completely fresh growth in an adult. Various types are described, giving a variety of shape (flattened or raised) and manifestation, such as colour which may be brown through to blue-black and may be variegated or even have nonpigmented areas. Some danger signals to look out for, whether in an existing mole or in a new development, are: Increase in size, including height and prominence; change in shape or colour; itching, exudate, crusting, or bleeding; ulceration. The edge has a reddened inflamed appearance. Size above 8 mm in a new lesion.
The pigmentation is in the lesion but invasion of surrounding skin can discolour this and might be misleading. Ulceration, if present, is clearly a lesser feature. Predominantly it is a pigmented lesion, slightly or substantially raised, possibly with a halo of colour by invasion of adjacent skin. It bears no real resemblance to a venous ulcer which essentially is an ulcer without any raising of its edges and there is no pigment within its substance but brown discoloration and induration diffusely for some distance around. A venous ulcer may be covered with a black crust, but this is clearly dead tissue or congealed discharge, and not malignant tissue.

Fig. 9.2   (continued).

(o) Main features of malignant ulcers.

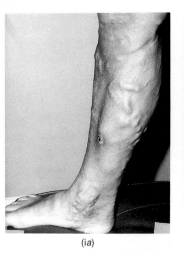

(i*a*)

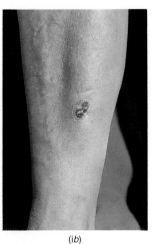

(i*b*)

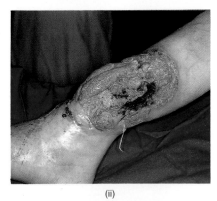

(ii)

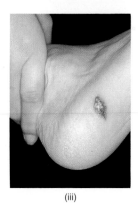

(iii)

Fig. 9.2   (continued).

(p) Malignant ulcers on leg and foot. (i) Basal cell carcinoma. (*a*) This small ulcer with surrounding pigmentation appeared over massive varicose veins due to long saphenous incompetence. There was some surrounding pigmentation and it was assumed to be venous. (*b*) Surgery to the veins gave a good result but the ulcer persisted, although pigmentation around it had gone. Its appearance 1 year later is shown and suggests a rodent ulcer. On excision, a basal cell carcinoma was confirmed. (ii) Squamous carcinoma—Marjolin's ulcer. In this patient, an ulcer had been present for many years, and was assumed to be venous. At the stage shown here, the first attendance at hospital, a massive proliferative ulcer was present, involving underlying muscle and causing pathological fracture of the bone, and immediately recognizable as malignant. Biopsy confirmed a squamous carcinoma and amputation was the only feasible treatment. (iii) Malignant melanoma. The foot and toes are common sites for malignant melanoma and an example is shown here.

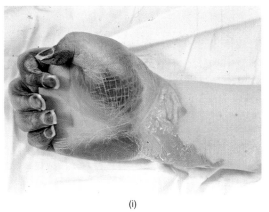 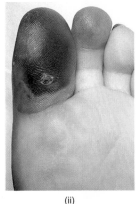 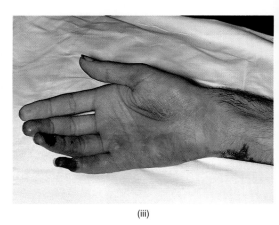

(i)   (ii)   (iii)

Fig. 9.2   (continued).

(q) Lesions caused by intra-arterial injection. (i) Gangrene of a child's hand seen in the early days of intravenous barbiturate anaesthesia; in this case it was undoubtedly intra-arterial, a danger against which all anaesthetists take strict precautions. (ii) Gangrene of the great toe following injection of a commonly used venous sclerosant (sodium tetradecyl sulphate) in the treatment of a plantar wart. The dosage was very small but sufficient to cause this damage by entering the artery supplying the wart. (iii) Ischaemic damage to tissues of wrist and hand, with gangrene in three fingers. This occurred in a drug addict and was caused by a misplaced self-injection of a barbiturate into the ulnar artery.

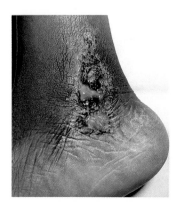 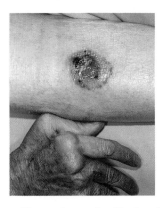

(r) Ulceration at the ankle in sickle cell anaemia. Note the non-specific increase in melanin pigmentation around the ulcer which may be confused with the discoloration by haemosiderin around a venous ulcer. Other blood dyscrasias may cause ulceration, and severe anaemia from any cause will prevent healing.

(s) Ulceration from vasculitis, seen here on the shin of a patient with rheumatoid arthritis.
((r) and (s) by courtesy of Dr Terence Ryan.)

Other causes of leg ulcer

Ischaemic ulcer (arterial insufficiency)

This state is comparatively common and its management conflicts directly with that of venous ulcer, so that distinguishing one from the other is of crucial importance. The ischaemia is usually due to atherosclerosis, so that the older patient is most commonly affected, but it can be encountered in young adults. It may arise in a patient with preexisting varicose veins or other venous disorder so that it is assumed that this is the cause – a bad error that must be avoided.

Main features

The ulcer is usually painful and situated on the toes, foot, or leg; it is particularly likely to occur over bony prominences, such as toe joints, the malleoli, or the shin, where the impoverished skin is easily damaged by external pressure against the unyielding bone.

The ulcer is 'dry', with no exudate or pus because the circulation is insufficient to support inflammatory reaction (Figs 9.2(g), 9.2(h), and 9.2(i) (iii)); this may lead to gross underestimation of the true state when a pathogen, such as *Staphylococcus aureus* or a beta haemolytic streptococcus, is present and has invaded surrounding skin which, although dying, is unable to show any response except a greyish-blue disoloration. There will usually be a story of intermittent claudication, numbness of the toes and forefoot on walking, and a typical nocturnal ischaemic rest pain, which is relieved by sitting in the knee-up position or hanging the foot out of bed (Fig. 9.2(i)), and made worse by elevation. The ankle pulses will be greatly reduced or missing, and this is confirmed by Doppler flowmetry. Sensation may be reduced, and the toes and forefoot show pallor on elevation (Fig. 9.2(h) (iii)) with considerable delay in return of colour when the leg is placed horizontally again. Brown pigmentation of the surrounding skin, typical of venous ulceration, will not be present.

Box 9.3
Venous leg ulcer

Characteristics

A venous ulcer only develops when venous hypertension is well established, and this is readily demonstrated by clinical features and special investigations. It will fall into one of three categories.

- Due to superficial vein incompetence: the ulcer will respond well to conservative treatment but surgery can usually provide a lasting cure.
- Due to deep vein impairment (various forms are described in Chapters 5–8). Surgery is seldom likely to bring benefit and conservative treatment will be required.
- Due to a combination of both: surgery may have a useful role but conservative treatment is likely to be the mainstay of management.

Clinical features and special investigations

- May occur in young adult and onwards but the frequency rises with age.
- Patient complains of discomfort or actual pain (this suggests infection with a pathogen), discharge of exudate or pus, and, in some cases, unpleasant odour.
- History of previous deep vein thrombosis, or major fractures in the lower limbs or pelvis indicate that deep vein impairment (post-thrombotic syndrome) is likely.
- Enlarged or varicose veins usually visible on the leg. Oedema may be present.
- Position of the ulcer is usually in the gaiter area, but may be above this and on any aspect of the leg or the upper surface of the foot. An ulcer on the underside of foot is *not* venous but likely to be diabetic.
- Surrounding skin will show brown pigmentation and underlying in duration (liposclerosis).

Ethnic skin colouring and venous pigmentation

Haemosiderin and melanin are entirely different materials but share a similar colour. Brown pigmentation in venous hypertension (haemosiderin) is a valuable sign in the white skin but may be obscured by the melanin pigment in black skin.

Venous pigment in a black skin can usually be recognized as increased darkening if the background colour is not too intense. However, this tends to be non-specific, as the black skin may react to any local disease by becoming darker so that a non-venous ulcer may show this feature. Depigmentation can occur from a variety of circumstances, including any long-standing skin condition. Nevertheless, venous pigmentation will be detectable in most black skins and at least suffice to indicate this possibility, which can be confirmed easily by the other signs of venous disorder and by the special investigations. Eczema is a common accompaniment.

Evidence of venous disorder is obtained as follows

- Selective Trendelenburg test (if positive, indicates superficial vein incompetence).
- Doppler flowmetry to superficial veins to distinguish type of venous disorder (see Chapter 3).
- Plethysmography: when venous hypertension is sufficiently severe to cause an ulcer, photoplethysmography or a similar method will clearly show this by inadequate response to exercise and a short recovery time afterwards. It may also be possible to return this temporarily to normal by occlusion of incompetent superficial veins if the fault lies there. This is perhaps plethymography's most effective role (see Chapter 3).
- Ultrasonography (see Chapter 3) to display superficial and deep veins.
- Functional phlebography to display superficial and deep veins, but only use in special circumstances (see Chapter 3).

Note. Venous disorder is sufficiently common for a second unrelated pathology causing ulceration to be an occasional possibility.

Additional investigations

In all ulcers:

- Check arterial supply (See Ischaemic ulcer)
- Exclude diabetes by urine and/or blood sugar.
- Exclude anaemia and the blood dyscrasias by full haematology
- Culture for pathogens (particularly *Staphylococcus aureus*, beta haemolytic streptococci and anaerobic organisms). Harmless commensals are always present
- Consider biopsy to ulcer edge if there is any suspicion of malignancy.
- If any doubt, blood chemistry or other blood tests relevant to circumstances should be obtained (e.g. antinuclear and rheumatic factors).

Continued

Box 9.3 *Continued*
Venous leg ulcer

Management
Decide on category of disorder. *Is arterial supply good? If not, the treatment given below can be harmful.*

- If superficial incompetence, carry out surgery as soon as the ulcer has entered the healing phase; it is not necessary to wait for full healing. Until then treat by elevation and/or ambulant elastic compression.
- If deep vein impairment (typically post-thrombotic syndrome), commence treatment by a spell of elevation and external support (see Chapter 6). When the ulcer shows a healing response, increasing ambulation in a paste bandage (inelastic external support) may be commenced until the ulcer is healed. Follow this by maintenance care to prevent recurrence of the ulcer (elevation at any spare moment by day, and certainly in the evening and overnight, with continued use of external support).

Gravity counteraction policy
Venous pressure in the lower limb arises from the hydrostatic pressure created by gravity in the upright position. Normally, muscle pumping action is constantly reducing this, but in deep vein impairment (typically post-thrombotic syndrome) this is irreparably reduced. This harmful state can be mitigated by the policy of counteracting the effect of gravity summarized below.

- Avoid prolonged standing, but when doing so move frequently to use remaining pump action. Sitting substantially reduces venous tension at ankle.
- Elevate the limbs above heart level whenever possible, and certainly in the evenings and in bed overnight. This reduces the venous hydrostatic pressure to zero. The greater the proportion of time spent in elevation, the greater is the benefit.
- Use external support when up and about. Depending on the stage of ulcer healing, response to treatment and severity of venous hypertension, this may be:
    inelastic containment (paste bandage)
    elastic stocking
    elastic bandage, either geometric stretch pattern or short-stretch type.

It is quite possible for venous ulceration to be accompanied by ischaemia, with each condition aggravating the ill effects of the other (Fig. 9.2(j)). Treatment of ischaemic ulceration is summarized in Fig. 9.2(g), but it must be emphasized that elevation of an ischaemic limb or use of a compression bandage can only reduce further its depleted arterial supply which has barely sufficient pressure to overcome the gradient to the forefoot. Treating an ischaemic ulcer as a venous ulcer is a serious error. Pain in a leg ulcer, particularly if it is made worse by elevation, should always suggest that ischaemia is present and the adequacy of arterial supply should be assessed. If there is any doubt, the limb should not be raised above the horizontal.

Diabetic neuropathic ulceration

The most common cause of neuropathic ulceration is diabetes, but other neurological conditions, including spina bifida, tables dorsalis, syringomyelia, spinal cord or nerve injury, and even leprosy, should not be overlooked. The cause for ulceration here is loss of protective reflexes due to neuropathy. This leads to the skin in the foot being given prolonged compression by body weight against bony prominences, such as the underside of a metatarsal head (Fig. 9.2(l)), the calcaneum, or the malleoli, without the patient's being aware that damage is occurring. The arterial supply may be good and ischaemia is not usually a factor.

Diagnostic features

The ulcer is characteristically punched out and situated over a bony prominence. Evidence of the accompanying neuropathy may be provided by absent ankle jerks and diminished sensation in the toes and foot. In diabetes the diagnosis is easily confirmed by raised fasting levels of blood glucose.

These ulcers eventually allow entry of infection to surrounding tissues and set up a smouldering cellulitis that painlessly destroys the interior of the foot by necrosis of ligaments, tendons, and muscles (Figs 9.2(m) and 9.2(n)). A diabetic ulcer is an unstable state which may eventually cause loss of a foot in this fashion and it should not be allowed to continue unhealed. Healing is achieved by control of the diabetes and protection of the ulcer from external pressure, or by surgery to remove the underlying bony prominence, or, if need be, by forefoot amputation (Fig. 9.2(k)).

Of course, diabetes may coexist with true venous ulceration and should always be excluded as a factor in leg ulcers.

Neoplastic ulcers

A primary neoplastic ulcer of the skin, such as malignant melanoma or epithelioma, is always possible. Basal cell carcinoma (rodent ulcer) is uncommon on the lower limb but can occur in an area of venotensive change (Fig. 9.2(p) (i)). Malignant change in a long-standing venous ulcer is a well-known possibility (Marjolin's ulcer), but even so there may be a long delay before this change is recognized (Fig. 9.2(p) (ii)). The foot and toes are a relatively common site for malignant melanoma which may ulcerate (Figs 9.2(o) and 9.2(p) (iii)). Always look for enlarged lymph glands in the groin.

Tropical ulcers

Tropical ulcers, including cutaneous leishmaniasis and fungus infections, may be brought into temperate countries by travellers from abroad.

Box 9.4
Local treatment of venous ulcer

Avoid

- Simple gauze which sticks tenaciously to ulcer is painful to remove, may damage new epithelium and allows drying.
- Tulle gras has same problem of sticking and may contain antibiotic or antiseptics likely to cause a damaging allergic reaction.
- Any creams or ointments containing allergens. Some notable allergens are lanolin, antibiotics (particularly sodium fucidate, neomycin, and soframycin), antiseptics, preservatives, and certain rubbers. If in doubt, test for sensitivity to the material by patch tests to the skin of the back.
- Corticosterioids will delay healing and should not be used on the ulcer itself, but they can be valuable when used sparingly on surrounding skin to control eczema. Non-sticking dressings of rayon or polyester (e.g. NA knitted viscose gauze or Melolin perforated film on an absorbent backing) are acceptable if used with a non-allergenic cream, but allow undue drying when used on their own.

Use

- A dressing that provides a protective cover, preserves moisture, and absorbs exudate and pus, but does not stick so that frequent change for cleansing is possible without pain. Examples are hydrocolloid (Granuloflex) and hydrogel (Geliperm) (see Box 9.6).

Note: Strict sterility goes without saying and proprietary materials in packs ensure this.

Additional measures
- Skin grafting
- Pedicle graft
- Myocutaneous free graft by microvascular surgery.
- Power-operated pneumatic sequential compression. (see below and Appendix)

When should skin grafting be considered?
There must be a good arterial supply to the limb. The intended advantage of skin grafting is to hasten the process of complete epithelial covering. However, if venotension is well controlled, natural epithelial ingrowth soon achieves this. Nevertheless, the larger the ulcer the more tempting it is to gain time by grafting.

An ulcer caused by superficial vein incompetence should heal within a few weeks if the cause is dealt with surgically. This should be done when the ulcer has responded to elevation by commencing epithelial ingrowth. The patient then follows an ambulant postoperative policy of external support and elevation whenever possible until epithelial ingrowth is complete. Skin grafting will offer little advantage here. However, many of these patients have developed ulceration because they have a relatively weak musculovenous pump that is easily overwhelmed. These patients will be prone to a recurrence if they do not take reasonable care (avoiding prolonged standing, using gravity counteraction measures whenever possible, and perhaps using medium elastic support). Skin grafting will not protect them from this vulnerability and they will need careful instruction and regular follow-up.

With a long-established ulcer from deep vein impairment, where the cause cannot be removed, ulcer healing may take many weeks and skin grafting may save time. However, grafts will not take unless the ulcer is in a healing phase (with epithelial ingrowth signifying that venotension is being satisfactorily counteracted and an adequate arterial supply is present) and is maintained there. Whether healed with or without skin grafting, the ulcer will soon reappear if the gravity counteraction policy is not conscientiously followed. A skin graft does not confer an improved robustness but only the possibility of earlier coverage in a large ulcer.

If skin grafting is to be used
The first requirement is a clean ulcer in a healing phase as shown by epithelial ingrowth (which signifies that it is now graft receptive and free from pathogens), otherwise the graft will fail. There is no need to excise the ulcer. Scrape away proliferative granulation tissue to give a clean bed and apply the skin graft. This may be split-skin grafts as a mesh (best) or as stamps. Pinch grafts also work well but leave an unsightly donor area. No stitches should be used and a light compression pad and bandage are sufficient.

The whole procedure need take only a short time and can be done under local or general anaesthetic. The policy of elevation and external support must continue until full healing is secured and, in modified form, indefinitely afterwards. The grafted area is equally vulnerable to breakdown as an area healed by natural epithelial ingrowth; the key is long term control of venotension by gravity counteraction measures and this requires instruction by the surgeon and self-discipline by the patient.

In some circumstances with a very large slow healing ulcer a myocutaneous free graft by microvascular surgery may be considered in consultation with a plastic surgeon. However, although this may be successful at first, it soon breaks down because of the persisting venous hypertension which the valves in the graft are unable to combat. For this reason it offers little advantage over healing by epithelial ingrowth or simple skin grafting. Whatever form of skin coverage is achieved, the patient will always be prone to recurrence if gravity counteraction measures are not maintained.

Free myocutaneous or pedicle grafts are essentially methods to bring in new tissue to fill in deficiency and give good-quality skin coverage. They are only suitable when there is a satisfactory vascular background without active venous hypertension. These methods may have a helpful role in some congenital venous lesions, such as covering a knee joint after removing a cavernous angioma, but this is territory only for the expert!

Continued

Box 9.4 *Continued*
Local treatment of venous ulcer

Power operated pneumatic sequential compression
Several types of electrically powered pneumatic devices giving repeated ripples of compression up the limb are available (see Appendix). The limb is enclosed in a garment which is divided into a number of compartments that are inflated in sequence to create a wave of compression travelling from the foot upwards with a strong massaging effect. They are designed for shared use by day-patients in a hospital clinic or, in a smaller version, for use in the patient's home. They are undoubtedly very effective in severe oedema, and they can also be real value in a post-thrombotic limb with considerable oedema and intractable ulceration. At home, these devices have the advantage that they can be used overnight as well for spells during the day. They should certainly be considered in a long-standing problem which stubbornly refuses to improve with the usual methods described above. However, the patient must not cease to follow a gravity counteraction policy and should be as physically active as the circumstances allow.

Box 9.5
Bacteriology in leg ulcers

Granulation tissue is usually effective in resisting pathogens, and this is so with most venous ulcers, but it is always colonized by a wide range of harmless commensals which require no treatment and can almost be regarded as a favourable sign. However, harmful pathogens can become established and may account for deterioration and pain in an ulcer, with an active cellulitis by invasion of surrounding tissues. Such organisms contain necrotoxins which destroy skin (particularly skin grafts) and thrive in the ensuing slough which the body defences cannot penetrate. There is no great need to take cultures from a clean ulcer that is responding to treatment *but if there is pus, debris, or slough, or evidence of surrounding cellulitis causing pain, then a culture becomes imperative*. However, this needs to be directed to identifying the most damaging organisms, which may not be picked up by a routine swab. The most harmful organism is *the beta haemolytic streptococcus (Lancefield type A)* and the microbiology laboratory should be consulted upon the best means for detecting this, together with *Staphylococcus aureus*.

The following pathogens are likely to be found in an ulcer with significant infection, either alone or in combination with one or more of the others (I.V. Schraibman, Phlebology, **2**, 265–7 (1987)).

Gram negative
- Mixed coliforms
- Pseudomonas
- Proteus
- Bacteroides

Gram
- Beta haemolytic streptococcus, Lancefield type A, B, C, G
- Staphylococcus aureus

In 35 per cent of clinically infected ulcers beta haemolytic streptococcus was found to be present, but Staphylococcus aureus less frequently so. Other authorities have found a predominance of Staphylococcus aureus, but the difference may be due to the effort made to isolate the streptococcus in Schraibman's series. It should be noted that both these organisms can be found in ulcers that are doing well clinically so that the findings must be interpreted in the light of the clinical state. The exotoxins of the streptococcus are a formidable array of necrotoxins and spreading factors so that its potential for damage is great.

Treating the ulcer that is clinically infected

- Take swabs in conjunction with advice from the bacteriology laboratory.
- Carry out surgical debridement of the wound to take away all dead substance.
- Give appropriate antibiotic systematically (local application may cause skin sensitization, which is a considerable added difficulty).
- Cleanse the ulcer and the surrounding skin daily with saline.
- Use a non-allergenic absorbent moisture-preserving dressing such as hydrocolloid.
- Skin grafting should not be employed until the ulcer is free from pathogens.

Box 9.6
Skin sensitization: common allergens

Many applications to ulcers can trigger sensitization reactions in neighbouring skin.
Common allergens are listed below.

- Ointment bases: lanolin and wood alcohol.
- Preservatives in base: parabens, propylene glycol, chloracresol.
- Fragrances included in base.
- Antibacterial agents: sodium fucidate, gentamycin sulphate, neomycin, soframycin, and quioline mix are amongst those most likely to be at fault.
- Materials added to bandages: ester gum resin, dyes, some rubber constituents.
- Household medical applications: some anaesthetic creams, antihistamine creams, some commonly used antiseptics.

This list can only indicate some common possibilities, but is a reminder of how ubiquitous allergens can be in materials used on ulcers. The index of suspicion for this possibility must be high when unexpected skin reactions occur and, in this event, all applications likely to be at fault should be changed. The skin in venotensive areas has a heightened sensitivity to allergens, and the reaction can quickly become more severe if the offender is not withdrawn. Patch testing on the patient's arm or back for sensitivity to a series of likely allergens is easy to do and will identify the material(s) to be avoided.

Box 9.7
Pharmacology to assist ulcer healing

The effects of pharmaceutical products are insignificant compared with the gravity counteraction measures described above, but they may be able to enhance such treatment and also play a role in preventing recurrence.

Fibrinolysis
Stanozolol (Stromba), a fibrinolytic agent, has been tested with the intention of reducing the pericapillary cuff of fibrin believed to play a part in hindering nutritional exchange to the skin and its consequent breakdown into an ulcer. Several years of trial have shown only marginal benefit, at best, and it has not been generally accepted for this purpose.

Improving flow within capillaries
Pentoxifyline (Trental) improves the deformability of red cells and in this way promotes capillary flow. It also can diminish white cell trapping, which is believed to play an important part in delaying capillary flow and causing an undesirable increase in capillary permeability. Theoretically, improving these aspects should have a favourable influence in a venous ulcer by improving skin nutrition and reducing filtration of fluid and protein into the extracellular space. Again, trials over several years have not yet shown convincing benefits to the patient.

Reducing capillary permeability
Hydroxyethylrutosides (Paroven and variants of this) in the laboratory reduce capillary permeability and for many years have been used to diminish discomfort and mild swelling in varicose veins. These products have also been tested carefully to see if they can improve healing and help prevent recurrence of venous ulcers. There has been much debate, but universal agreement upon their benefits has not been achieved.

Specific infection

Ulceration, including that due to tuberculosis and syphilis, may be caused either as part of a systemic illness or as a localized infection. The possibility of lesions due to acquired immune deficiency syndrome (AIDS) should not be overlooked.

Blood dyscrasias

Any severe anaemia, sickle cell anaemia, thalassaemia, hereditary spherocytosis, polycythaemia vera, or leukaemia can provide obscure forms of chronic leg ulceration (Fig. 9.2(r)). It is wise to carry out a routine blood examination at an early stage in the management of chronic leg ulcer

Nutritional and metabolic disturbances

Vitamin and nutritional deficiencies, uraemia, and other metabolic disorders may cause or aggravate chronic ulceration.

Skin sensitivity or allergy

Skin sensitivity or allergy to materials at work, or applied medicinally or for cosmetic reasons, can either cause or aggravate ulceration. It is commonplace for leg ulcers to be exacerbated by inappropriate ointments, particularly antibiotics, cortisone, and antiseptics (Fig. 9.2(f)). A wide range of drugs taken internally may cause skin reactions and eventually ulceration, but these lesions are likely to be widespread and not confined to a limb.

Trauma

Trauma as a single episode commonly sets off an ulcer in the presence of venous stasis, ischaemia, and in many of the generalized states referred to in this section. The skin of patients on corticosteroids becomes fragile and particularly vulnerable to minor trauma.

Necrosis by injection of chemical, insect bite, or radiation

Misplaced injections during sclerotherapy may cause skin necrosis and prolonged ulceration. Many chemicals used medically or industrially can have the same effect. Inadvertent intra-arterial injection is particularly dangerous, and many pharmaceuticals, including sclerosants and barbiturates, can cause extensive gangrene in the extremity; this may occur in medical procedures or by self-injection in drug addiction (Fig. 9.2(q)). High-pressure injection of grease used in servicing automobiles can cause widespread destruction of subcutaneous tissue and skin. Insect bites may inject necrotoxins that produce unpleasant prolonged ulceration. Insect bites may also implant parasitic or protozoal organisms which cause chronic lesions, but these are uncommon in temperate climates.

Box 9.8
Chronic leg ulcers in the tropics

This book is written mainly from the perspective of countries in temperate regions, but an additional range of infective ulcers are seen in the tropics, many of them commonplace. International travel is now so widespread that these conditions must not be overlooked because even the holiday traveller to exotic places may bring home an ulcer not usually seen outside the tropics. The account here cannot be complete and is only intended to be a reminder of this important group of leg ulcers.

The term **tropical ulcer** describes an ulcer frequently seen on the lower leg and foot in Africa (Naga sore), South Asia, and tropical America. It is probably the result of infection introduced by insect bite or trauma, against a background of nutritional deficiency. The principle organisms are *Fusobacterium ulcerans* and *Borrelia vincenti* acting synergistically, but other bacteria such as Proteus and Pseudomonas are often present as well. It develops over some weeks to give an extensive area of necrotic skin with a foul-smelling discharge; after this initial acute stage it becomes chronic as a large painful ulcer that will not heal spontaneously and persists indefinitely unless it is treated. Its situation and appearance on the lower leg might suggest a venous ulcer but will lack any of the other features of venous hypertension. Diagnosis is by bacteriology, microscopy, and exclusion of the many other conditions listed below. Eventually, after some years, it is prone to malignant change as squamous cell carcinoma; this is often preceded by loss of melanin pigment in overlying skin at the ulcer edge and biopsy should be taken from here.

Many other infective ulcers occur in the tropics and subtropics, including yaws, leprosy, tuberculosis, syphilis, AIDS, amoebiasis, and a variety of fungus infections; these must all be distinguished from the non-infective conditions which are the main topic of this chapter. Cutaneous leishmaniasis is a protozoal infection which is acquired through the sandfly bite or by direct contact. It is known by various names, such as oriental sore or Aleppo boil, according to the country of origin, and is caused by the same organism as kala-azar which occurs widely in North Africa, the Middle and Far East, and South America. These ulcers can have some similarity to venous ulceration but will not, of course, have any of the essential features of venous insufficiency; a positive diagnosis can be made by microscopy of smears, biopsy, serology, or positive leishmanin skin test. This condition is seen from time to time in travellers returning from subtropical regions.

Repeated trauma

Recurring trauma, either caused at work or self-inflicted in psychiatric disorders or malingering (dermatitis artefacta), can be an occasional cause of ulceration. Injury to the skin may occur from radiation or chemicals, possibly without the patient realizing it.

Rheumatoid arthritis: pyoderma gangrenosum

Patients with rheumatoid arthritis may develop intractable ulceration on the legs or feet caused by vasculitis, which is sometimes mistaken for venous ulceration (Fig. 9.2(s)). In common with other arthropathies, rheumatoid arthritis can also cause pyoderma gangrenosum, with extensive necrosis of the skin creating a severe ulcerative lesion on the leg. This can also be a complication of other conditions, including ulcerative colitis, Crohn's disease, acute leukaemia, and polycythaemia.

Systemic, autoimmune, and microvascular disease

Disorders such as systemic lupus erythematosus and polyarteritis can form lesions on the legs; these resemble the eczematous changes seen in venous disorder and eventually ulcerate. This can be very misleading when it occurs over incidental varicose veins.

Conclusion

The list of causes of leg ulceration given above is by no means complete but serves to illustrate the need to be constantly aware that one chronic leg ulcer in five will not be venous in origin and will call for a special skill in diagnosis.

Bibliography to Part I

General

The following authoritative works give detailed accounts of the venous disorders and their treatment, together with comprehensive references to relevant publications.

Altenkamper, H. and Eldenburg, M. (1994). *A colour atlas of venous disease*. Manson, London.

Belcaro, G., Nicolaides, A.N., and Veller, M. (1995). *Venous disorders*. Saunders, London.

Bergan, J.J. and Kistner, R.L. (1992). *Atlas of venous surgery*. Saunders, Philadelphia, PA.

Bergan, J.J. and Yao, J.S.T. (1985). *Surgery of the veins*. Grune and Stratton, New York.

Bergan, J.J. and Yao, J.S.T. (1991). *Venous disorders*. Saunders, Philadelphia, PA.

Browse, N.L., Burnand, K.G., and Lea Thomas, M. (1988). *Diseases of the veins: pathology, diagnosis and treatment*. Arnold, London.

Coleridge Smith, P.D. (ed.) (1992). The management of patients with venous disease. *Phlebology*, 7 (Supplement 1).

Dodd, H. and Cockett, F.B. (1976). *The pathology and surgery of the veins of the lower limbs*. Churchill Livingstone, Edinburgh.

Gardner, A.M.N. and Fox, R.H. (1989). *The return of blood to the heart: venous pumps in health and disease*. Libbey, London.

Lea Thomas, M. (1982). *Phlebography of the lower limb*. Churchill Livingstone, Edinburgh.

May, R. (1979). *Surgery of the veins and the pelvis*. Saunders, Philadelphia, PA; Thieme, Stuttgart.

Negus, D. (1991). *Leg ulcers*. Butterworth-Heinemann, Oxford.

Negus, D. and Jantet, G. (ed.) (1986). *Phlebology '85*, pp. 65–7. Libbey, London.

Negus, D., Jantet, G., and Coleridge Smith, P. (ed.) (1995). *Phlebology '95*. Springer-Verlag, London. (published in two volumes as Supplement 1 to *Phlebology*).

Nicolaides, A.N. and Sumner, D.S. (1991). *Investigation of patients with deep vein thrombosis and chronic venous insufficiency*. Med-Orion, London.

Nicolaides, A., Christopoulos, D., and Vasdekis, S. (1989). Progress in the investigation of chronic venous insufficiency. *Ann. Vasc. Surg.*, 3, 278–92.

Ruckley, C.V. (1988). *A colour atlas of surgical management of venous disease*. Wolfe Medical, London.

Tibbs, D.J. (1992). *Varicose veins and related disorders*. Butterworth-Heinemann, Oxford.

Some historical or notable papers and publications

Bjordal, R. (1970), Simultaneous pressure and flow recordings in varicose veins of the lower extremity. *Acta Chir. Scand.*, 136, 309.

Bjordal, R.I. Haemodynamic studies of varicose veins and the postthrombotic syndrome. In: *The treatment of venous disorders* (ed. J.T. Hobbs), pp. 37–53. MTP, Lancaster.

Browse, N.I., Burnand, K.G. and Lea Thomas, M. (1988) *Diseases of the veins: pathology, diagnosis and treatment*. Arnold, London; (Chapter 1 gives a valuable summary of major contributions to the understanding of venous problems made over the centuries).

Cockett, F.B. (1956). Diagnosis and surgery of high-pressure leaks in the leg. *Br. Med. J.*, ii, 1399–13.

Cockett, F.B. and Elgan Jones, D.E. (1953). The ankle blow-out syndrome. *Lancet*, 17–23.

Fegan, W.G. (1960). Continuous uninterrupted compression technique of injecting varicose veins. *Proc. R. Soc. Med.*, 53, 837–40.

Fegan, W.G. (1967). *Varicose veins*. Heinemann, London.

Fegan, W.G. and Kline, A.L. (1972). The cause of varicosity in superficial veins of the lower limb. *Br. J. Surg*, 59, 798–801.

Harvey, W. (1628). *Exercitatio anatomica de motu cordis et sanguini animalibus*. Fitzer, Frankfurt.

Holman, E. (1954). The obscure physiology of poststenotic dilatation: its relation to the development of aneurysms. *J. Thorac. Surg.*, 28, 109.

Keller, W.I. (1905). A new method of extirpating the internal saphenous and similar veins in varicose conditions: a preliminary report. *NY Med. J.*, 82, 385–9.

Linton, R.R. (1938). The communicating veins of the lower leg and the operative technic for their ligation. *Ann. Surg.*, 107, 582–93.

Loftgren, K.A. (1958). An evaluation of stripping versus ligation for varicose veins. *AMA Arch. Surg.*, 76, 310–16.

McPheeters, H.O. (1929). Varicose veins—the circulation and direction of the venous flow. *Surg. Gynecol. Obstet.*, 44, 29–33.

Mayo, C.H. (1906). Treatment of varicose veins. *Surg. Gynecol. Obstet.*, 2, 385–8.

Myers, T.T. (1957). Results and technique of stripping operation for varicose veins. *J. Am. Med. Assoc.*, 163, 87–92.

Pegum, J.M. and Fegan, W.G. (1967). Physiology of venous return from the foot. *Cardiovasc. Res.*, 1, 249.

Todd, A.S. (1959). The histological localisation of fibrinogen activator. *J. Pathol. Bacteriol.*, 78, 281.

Trendelenburg, F. (1891). Uber die Unterbindung der Vena saphena magna bei Unterschenkelvaricen. *Beitr. Klin. Chir.*, 7, 195–210.

Virchow, R. (1846). *Beitr. Exp. Path. Physiol.*, 21.

Classification by chapter and topic

These publications are not referred to in the text but their relevance is clear from the titles of each publication. Some are included to help in the evaluation of alternative viewpoints not expressed in the text.

Chapter 1 Normal anatomy and physiology

Butterworth, D.M., Rose, S.S., Clark, P., *et al.* (1992). Light microscopy, immunohistochemistry and electron microscopy of the valves of the lower limb veins and jugular veins. *Phlebology*, 7, 27–30.

Cockett, F.B. (1991). Venous valves: history up to the present day. *Phlebology*, 6, 63–73.

Davies, M.G., Fulton, G.J., and Hagen, P.O. (1995). Clinical biology of nitric oxide. *Br. J. Surg.*, 82, 1598–1610.

Dodd, H. and Cockett, F.B. (1976). *The pathology and surgery of the veins of the lower limbs.* Churchill Livingstone, Edinburgh.

di Giacomini, G. (1893). *Accad. Med. Torini*, 14.

Gardner, A.M.N. and Fox, R.H. (1989). *The return of blood to the heart: venous pumps in health and disease.* Libbey, London.

Hamblin, T.J. (1990). Endothelins. *Br. Med. J.*, 301, 568.

Komori, K., Okadome, K., and Sugimachi, K. (1991). Endothelium-derived relaxing factor and vein grafts. *Br. J. Surg.*, 78, 1027–30.

McMullen, E.T. (1995). Anatomy of a physiological discovery; William Harvey and the circulation of the blood. *J. R. Soc. Med.*, 88, 491–8.

May, R. (1979). *Surgery of the veins and the pelvis.* Saunders, Philadelphia, PA; Thieme, Stuttgart.

Ortega, F., Samiento, L., Mompeo, B., *et al.* (1994). Morphological study of the valvular distribution in the long saphenous vein. *Phlebology*, 9, 59–62.

Payne, S.K., Sayers, R.D., Watt, P.A.C., *et al.* (1993). Endothelium-derived relaxing factor release from normal and varicose human saphenous veins. *Phlebology*, 8, 107–10.

Pegum, J.M. and Fegan, W.G. (1967). Physiology of venous return from the foot. *Cardiovasc. Res.*, 1, 249.

Sharpey-Schafer, E.P. (1961). Venous tone. *Br. Med. J.*, 2, 1589–95.

Todd, A.S. (1959). The histological localisation of fibrinogen activator. *J. Pathol. Bacteriol.*, 78, 281.

Chapter 2 Disordered venous function

Allen, A.J., Wright, D.I.I., McCollum, C.N., and Tooke, J.E. (1988). Impaired postural vasoconstriction: a contributory cause of oedema in patients with chronic venous insufficiency. *Phlebology*, 3, 163–8.

Baglin, T. (1996). Disseminated intravascular coagulation: diagnosis and treatment. *Br. Med. J.*, 312, 683–7.

Bradbury, A.W., Murie, J.A., and Ruckley, C.V. (1993). Role of the leucocyte in the pathogenesis of vascular disease. *Br. J. Surg.*, 80, 1503–12.

Cockett, F.B. (1991). Venous valves: history up to the present day. *Phlebology*, 6, 63–73.

Committee of American Venous Forum (Chairman, A.N Nicolaides) (1995). Classification and grading of chronic venous disease in the lower limbs: a consensus statement. *Phlebology*, 10, 42–5.

Holman, E. (1954). The obscure physiology of poststenotic dilatation: its relation to the development of aneurysms. *J. Thorac. Surg.*, 28, 109.

Leu, H.J. (1993). Morphological findings in chronic venous insufficiency. *Phlebology*, 8, 48–9.

Mani, R., White, J.E., Barrett, D.F., and Weaver, P.W. (1989). Tissue oxygenation, venous ulcers and fibrin cuffs. *J. R. Soc. Med.*, 82, 345–6.

Michel, C.C. (1990). Oxygen diffusion in oedematous tissue and through pericapillary cuffs. *Phlebology*, 5, 223–30.

Powell, J.T. and Higman, D.J. (1994). Smoking, nitric oxide and the endothelium. *Br. J. Surg.*, 81, 785–7.

Scott, H.J., Cheatle, T.R., McMullin, G.M., *et al.* (1990). Reappraisal of the oxygenation of blood in varicose veins. *Br. J. Surg.*, 77, 934–6.

Stibe, E., Cheatle, T.R., Coleridge Smith, P.D., and Scurr, J.H. (1990). Liposclerotic skin: a diffusion block or a perfusion problem. *Phlebology*, 5, 231–6.

Strandness, D.E. (1978). Applied venous physiology in normal subjects and venous insufficiency. In: *Venous problems*, pp. 24–45. Year Book, Chicago, IL.

Sumner, D.S. (1985). Applied physiology in venous problems. In: *Surgery of the veins* (ed. J.J. Bergan and J.S. Yao), pp. 3–23. Grune and Stratton, New York.

Thulesius, O. (1993). Vein wall characteristics and valvular function in chronic venous insufficiency. *Phlebology*, 8, 94–8.

Chapter 3 Clinical examination and special investigations

General

Abramowitz, H.B., Queral, L.A., Flinn, W.R., *et al.* (1979). The use of photoplethysmography in the assessment of venous insufficiency: a comparison to venous pressure measurements. *Surgery*, 86, 434–41.

Akesson, H., Brudin, L., Jensen, R., *et al.* (1989). Physiological evaluation of venous obstruction in the post-thrombotic leg. *Phlebology*, 4, 3–14.

Avruscio, G.P., Battocchio, F., De Santis, L., *et al.* (1995). Echo color flow in varicose veins: its usefulness. In: *Phlebology '95* (ed. D. Negus, G. Jantet, and P. Coleridge Smith). *Phlebology*, **Suppl. 1**, 241–2.

Bergan, J.J. and Yao, J.S.T. (1991). *Venous disorders.* Saunders, Philadelphia, PA.

Cheatle, T.R., McMullin, G.M., Farrah, J., *et al.* (1990). Three tests of microcirculatory function in the evaluation of treatment. *Phlebology*, 5, 165–72.

Cheatle, T.R., Shami, S.K., Stibe, E., *et al.* (1991). Vasomotion in venous disease. *J.R. Soc. Med.*, 84, 261–3.

Cheatle, T.R., Perrin, M., Hiltbrand, B., *et al.* (1994). Investigation of popliteal fossa venous reflux. *Phlebology*, 9, 25–7.

Christopoulos, D.G., Nicoliades, A.N., Szendro, G., *et al.* (1987). Air-plethysmography and the effect of elastic compression on venous haemodynamics. *J. Vasc. Surg.*, 5, 148–59.

Christopoulos, D., Nicolaides, A.N., and Szendro, G. (1988). Venous reflux: quantification and correlation with the clinical severity of chronic venous disease. *Br. J. Surg.*, 75, 352–6.

Coleridge Smith, P.D. (1990). Noninvasive venous investigation. *Vasc. Med. Rev.*, 1, 139–66.

DePalma, R.G., Hart, M.T., Zanin, L., and Massarin, E.H. (1993). Physical examination, Doppler ultrasound and colour flow duplex scanning: guides to therapy for primary varicose veins. *Phlebology*, 8, 7–11.

Fernandes, E., Fernandes, J., Horner, J., *et al.* (1979). Ambulatory calf volume plethysmography in the assessment of venous insufficiency. *Br. J. Surg.*, 66, 327–30.

Hurlow, R.A. and Strachan, C.J.L. (1978). The clinical scope and potential of isotope angiology. *Br. J. Surg.*, 65, 688–91.

Iafrati, M.D., O'Donnell, T.F. Jr, Kunkemueller, A., *et al.* (1994). Clinical examination, duplex ultrasound and plethysmography for varicose veins. *Phlebology*, 9, 114–18.

Irvine, A.T. and Lea Thomas, M. (1991). Colour-coded duplex sonography in the diagnosis of deep vein thrombosis: a comparison with phlebography. *Phlebology*, **6**, 103–9.

Jackson, J.R. and Mathews, J.A. (1977). A gravimetric plethysmograph and its evaluation in clinical use. *Br. J. Surg.*, **64**, 876–82.

Jensen, C., Lomholdt Knudsen, L., and Hegedus, V. (1983) The role of contact thermography in the diagnosis of deep venous thrombosis. *Eur. J. Radiol.*, **3**, 99–102.

Kalodiki, E., Calahoras, L., and Nicolaides, A.N. (1993). Make it easy: duplex examination of the venous system. *Phlebology*, **8**, 17–21.

Klein Rouweler, B.J.F., Brakkee, A.J.M., and Kuiper, J.P. (1989). Plethysmographic measurement of venous resistance and venous capacity in the human leg. Parts I, II. *Phlebology*, **4**, 241–57.

Klein Rouweler, B.J.F., Kuiper, J.P., and Brakkee, A.J.M. (1990). Plethysmographic measurement of venous flow resistance and venous capacity in humans with deep venous thrombosis. *Phlebology*, **5**, 21–9 (and the two succeeding papers by same authors).

Labropoulos, N., Volteas, M., Leon, S.K., *et al.* (1995). Air plethysmography in the detection of suspected acute deep vein thrombosis. *Phlebology*, **10**, 28–31.

Lancaster, J., Lucarotti, M., and Leaper, D.J. (1987). Laser Doppler velocimetry. *J.R. Soc. Med.*, **80**, 729–30.

Lancaster, J., Lucarotti, M., Mitchell, A., and Leaper, D. (1988). Laser Doppler flowmetric and waveform changes in patients with venous reflux. *Phlebology*, **3**, 69–72.

Lea Thomas, M. (1982). *Phlebography of the lower limb*. Churchill Livingstone, New York.

Lees, T.A. and Holdsworth, J.D. (1995). Assessment and treatment of varicose veins in the Northern Region. *Phlebology*, **10**, 56–61.

McIrvine, A.J., Corbett, C.R.R., Aston, N.O., *et al.* (1984). The demonstration of saphenofemoral incompetence; Doppler ultrasound compared with standard clinical tests. *Br. J. Surg.*, **71**, 809–10.

McMullin, G.M., Scott, H.J., Coleridge Smith, P.D., and Scurr, J.H. (1989). A comparison of photoplethysmography, Doppler ultrasound and duplex scanning in the assessment of venous insufficiency. *Phlebology*, **4**, 75–82.

McMullin, G.M., Coleridge Smith, P.D., and Scurr, J.H. (1991). A study of tourniquets in the investigation of venous insufficiency. *Phlebology*, **6**, 133–9.

Milliken, J.C., Dinn, E., O'Connor, R., and Greene, D. (1986). A simple Doppler technique for the rapid diagnosis of significant sapheno-femoral reflux. *Phlebology*, **1**, 125–8.

Mitchell, D.C., Grasty, M.S., Stebbings, W.S.L., *et al.* (1991). Comparison of duplex ultrasonography and venography in the diagnosis of deep venous thrombosis. *Br. J. Surg.*, **78**, 611–13.

Mosquera, D.A., Manns, R.A., and Duffield, G.M. (1995). Phlebography in the management of recurrent varicose veins. *Phlebology*, **10**, 19–22.

Nicolaides, A.N. and Miles C. (1987). Photoplethysmography in the assessment of venous insufficiency. *J. Vasc. Surg.*, **5**, 405–12.

Nicolaides, A.N. and Sumner, D.S. (1991). *Investigation of patients with deep vein thrombosis and chronic venous insufficiency*. Med-Orion, London.

Nicolaides, A., Christopoulos, D., and Vasdekis, S. (1989) Progrés dans l'exploration de l'insuffisance veineuse chronique. *Ann. Chir. Vasc.*, **3**, 278–92.

Norgren, L., Thulesius, O., Gjores, J.E., and Soderlundh, S. (1974). Foot volumetry and simultaneous venous pressure measurements for evaluation of venous insufficiency. *VASA*, **3**, 140–7.

Nuzzaci, G., Mangoni, N., Tonarelli, A.P., *et al.* (1986). Our experience on light reflection rheography (LRR): a new non-invasive method for the lower limbs venous examination. *Phlebology*, **1**, 231–42.

Ohgi, S., Tanaka, K., Araki, T., *et al.* (1990). Quantitative evaluation of calf muscle pump function after deep vein thrombosis by non-invasive venous tests. *Phlebology*, **5**, 51–9.

Payne, S.P.K., Thrush, A.J., London, N.J.M., *et al.* (1993). Venous assessment using air plethysmography: a comparison with clinical examination, ambulatory venous pressure measurement and duplex scanning. *Br. J. Surg.*, **80**, 967–70.

Pochaczevsky, R., Pillari, G., and Feldman, F. (1982). Liquid crystal contact thermography of deep venous thrombosis. *Am. J. Radiol.*, **138**, 717–23.

Porter, J.M., Swain, I.D., and Shakespeare, P.G. (1985). Measurement of limb flow by electrical impedance plethysmography. *Ann. R. Coll. Surg. Eng.*, **67**, 169–72.

Richardson, G.D. and Beckwith, T. (1990). Duplex scanning of recurrent varicose veins. *Phlebology*, **5**, 281–4.

Richardson, G.D., Beckwith, T.C., and Sheldon, M. (1991). Ultrasound windows to abdominal and pelvic veins. *Phlebology*, **6**, 111–25.

Rosfors, S. (1992). A methodological study of venous valvular insufficiency and musculovenous pump function in the lower leg. *Phlebology*, **7**, 12–19.

Sarin, S., Sommerville, K., Farrah, J., *et al.* (1994). Duplex ultrasonography for assessment of venous valvular function of the lower limb. *Br. J. Surg.*, **81**, 1591–5.

Schindler, J.M., Kaiser, M., Gerber, A., *et al.* (1990). Colour coded duplex sonography in suspected deep vein thrombosis of the leg. *Br. Med. J.*, **301**, 1369–70.

Schmid-Schonbein, G.W. (1995). Activated leuckocytes and endothelium in chronic venous insufficiency. In: *Phlebology '95* (ed. D. Negus, G. Jantet, and P. Coleridge Smith). *Phlebology*, **Suppl. 1**, 90–2.

Schraibman, I.G., Mott, D., Naylor, G.P., and Charlesworth, D. (1975). Comparison of impedance and strain gauge plethysmography in the measurement of blood flow in the lower limb. *Br. J. Surg.*, **62**, 909–12.

Scott, H.J., Coleridge Smith, P.D., McMullin, G.M., and Scurr, J.H. (1990). Venous disease: investigation and treatment, fact or fiction? *Ann. R. Coll. Surg. Engl.*, **72**, 188–92.

Strandness, D.E., Schultz, R.D., Sumner, D.S., and Rushmer, R.F. (1967). Ultrasonic flow detection. *Am. J. Surg.*, **113**, 311–20.

Struckmann, J.R. (1987). Ambulatory strain gauge plethysmography: correlation to symptoms and skin changes in patients with venous insufficiency. *Phlebology*, **2**, 75–80.

Struckmann, J., Stranfe-Vognsen, H.H., Andersen, J., and Hauch, O. (1986). Venous muscle pump function in patients with primary lymphoedema: assessment by ambulatory strain gauge plethysmography. *Br. J. Surg.*, **73**, 886–7.

Tibbs, D.J. (1992). *Varicose veins and related disorders*. Butterworth-Heinemann, Oxford.

Tibbs, D.J. and Fletcher, E.W.L. (1983). Direction of flow in the superficial veins as a guide to venous disorders in the lower limbs. *Surgery*, **93**, 758–67.

Valentin, L.I., Valentin, W.H., Mercado, S., and Rosado, C.J. (1993). Venous reflux localization: comparative study of venography and duplex scanning. *Phlebology*, **8**, 124.

van den Broek, T.A.A., Rauwerda, J.A., Kuijper, C.F., *et al.* (1989). Comparison of strain gauge and photocell venous function testing with invasive pressure measurements. A prospective study in deep vein insufficiency. *Phlebology*, **4**, 223–30.

Vasdekis, S.N., Clarke, G.H., Hobbs, J.T., and Nicoliades, A.N. (1989). Evaluation of non-invasive and invasive methods in the assessment of short saphenous vein termination. *Br. J. Surg.*, **76**, 929–32.

Vasdekis, S.N., Clarke, H.G., and Nicolaides, A.N. (1989). Quantification of venous reflux by means of duplex scanning. *J. Vasc. Surg.*, **10**, 670–7.

Whitehead, S., Lemenson, G., and Browse, N.L. (1983). The assessment of calf pump function by isotope plethysmography. *Br. J. Surg.*, **70**, 675–9.

Ziegenbein, R.W., Myers, K.A., Matthews, P.G., and Zeng, G.H. (1994). Duplex ultrasound scanning for chronic venous disease: techniques for examination of the crucial veins. *Phlebology*, **9**, 108–13.

Phlebography — media

Grainger, R.G. and Dawson, P. (1990). Low osmolar contrast media: an appraisal. *Clin. Radiol.*, **42**, 1–5.

Katayama, H. (1987). Clinical survey on adverse reactions of iodinated contrast media. In: *Advance and future trends of contrast media (Proc. Int. Symp. on Contrast Media, Tokyo)*, Nos. 6, 7.

Palmer, F.J. (1988). The RACR Survey of intravenous contrast media reactions, final reports. *Australas. Radiol.*, **32**, 426–8.

Thornbury, J.R. and Fischer, H.W. (1989). Issues in uroradiology. *Curr. Imaging*, **1**, 3–9.

Phlebography

Ackroyd, J.S., Lea Thomas, M., and Browse, N.L. (1986). Deep vein reflux: an assessment by descending phlebography. *Br. J. Surg.*, **73**, 31–3.

Corbett, C.R., McIrvine, A.J., Aston, N.O., *et al.* (1984). The use of varicography to identify the sources of incompetence in recurrent varicose veins. *Ann. R. Coll. Surg. Engl.*, **66**, 412–15.

Corcos, L., Peruzzi, G., Romeo, V., and Fiori, C. (1987). Intraoperative phlebography of the short saphenous vein. *Phlebology*, **2**, 241–8.

Craig, J.O.M.C. (1977). Investigation of the leg veins by venography. In: *The treatment of venous disorders* (ed. J.T. Hobbs), pp. 83–95. MTP, Lancaster.

Dow, J.D. (1951). Venography of the leg with particular reference to acute deep thrombophlebitis and to gravitational ulceration. *J. Fac. Radiol. London*, **2**, 180–205.

Ferreira, J.A., Villamil, E.J.F., and Ciruzzi, A.O. (1951). Dynamic phlebography. *Angiology*, **2**, 350–73.

Fletcher, E.W.L. and Tibbs, D.J. (1986). Functional phlebography in chronic venous disorders of the lower limbs. In: *Phlebology '85*. (ed. D. Negus and G. Jantet), pp. 51–4. Libbey, London.

Gardner, A.M.N. and Fox, R.H. (1989). *The return of blood to the heart: venous pumps in health and disease*. Libbey, London.

Grainger, R.G. (1984). Low osmolar contrast media. *Br. Med. J.*, **289**, 144–5.

Hughes, D.G., Dixon, P.M., and Fletcher, E.W.L. (1987). Augmentation of upper limb venography with digital subtraction. *Phlebology*, **2**, 125–7.

Lea Thomas, M. (1982). *Phlebography of the lower limb*. Churchill Livingstone, London.

Lea Thomas, M. and Mahraj, R.P.M. (1988). A comparison of varicography and descending phlebography in clinically suspected recurrent groin and upper thigh varicose veins. *Phlebology*, **3**, 155–62.

Neiman, H.L. (1985). Venography in acute and chronic venous disease. In: *Surgery of the veins*. (ed. J.J. Bergan and J.S.T. Yao), pp. 73–87. Grune and Stratton, London.

Perrin, M., Bolot, J.E., Genevois, A., and Hiltbrand, B. (1988). Dynamic popliteal phlebography. *Phlebology*, **3**, 227–35.

Tibbs, D.J. (1992). *Varicose veins and related disorders*. Butterworth-Heinemann, Oxford.

Vandendriessche, M. (1989). Association between gastrocnemial vein insufficiency and varicose veins (with invited comment by A.N. Nicolaides, D., Christopoulos, and S. Vasdelis). *Phlebology*, **4**, 171–84.

Chapter 4 Clinical patterns of venous disorder I. Superficial vein incompetance

General

Andrew, V.O., Wu, Y., and Mansfield, A. (1979). The fibrinolytic activity of the vein following venous stasis. *Br. J. Surg.*, **66**, 637–9.

Austrell, C., Nilson, L., and Norgren, L. (1993). Maternal and fetal haemodynamics during late pregnancy: effect of compression hosiery treatment. *Phlebology*, **8**, 155–7.

Bfergqvist, D. and Jaroszewski, H. (1986). Deep vein thrombosis in patients with superficial thrombophlebitis of the leg. *Br. Med. J.*, **292**, 658–9.

Bjordal, R. (1970). Simultaneous pressure and flow recordings in varicose veins of the lower extremity. *Acta Chir. Scand.*, **136**, 309.

Bjordal, R.I. (1977). Haemodynamic studies of varicose veins and the post-thrombotic syndrome. In: *The treatment of venous disorders* (ed. J.T. Hobbs), pp. 37–53. MTP, Hancaster.

Bjordal, R.I. (1986). The clinical role of dilated perforating veins in varicose disease. In: *Phlebology' 85* (ed. D. Nogus and G. Jantet), pp. 42–4. Libbey, London.

Blackett, R.L. and Heard, G.E. (1988). Pulsatile varicose veins. *Br. J. Surg.*, **75**, 866–8.

Burnand, K.G., Whimster, I.W., Clemenson, G., *et al.* (1981). The relationship between the number of capillaries in the skin of the venous ulcer bearing area of the lower leg and the fall in foot vein pressure during exercise. *Br. J. Surg.*, **68**, 297–300.

Burnand, K.G., Whimster, I., Naidoo, A., *et al.* (1982). Pericapillary fibrin in the ulcer bearing skin of the lower leg. The cause of lipodermatosclerosis and venous ulceration. *Br. Med. J.*, **285**, 1071–2.

Callam, M.J., Harper, D.R., Dale, J.J., and Ruckley, C.V. (1987). Arterial disease in chronic leg ulceration: an underestimated hazard. *Br. Med. J.*, **294**, 929–31.

Callam, M.J., Ruckley, C.V., Dale, J.J., and Harper, D.R. (1987). Hazards of compression treatment of the leg from Scottish surgeons. *Br. Med. J.*, **295**, 1382.

Campbell, B. (1996). Thrombitis, phlebitis, and varicose veins. *Br. Med. J.*, **312**, 198.

Campbell, W.B. (1990). Varicose veins. *Br. Med. J.*, **300**, 763–4.

Campbell, W.B. and Ridler, B.M.F. (1995). Varicose vein surgery and deep vein thrombosis. *Br. J. Surg.*, **82**, 1494–7.

Chiedozi, L.C. and Aghahowa, J.A. (1988). Mondor's disease associated with breast cancer. *Surgery*, **103**, 438–9.

Christopoulos, D. and Nicolaides, A.N. (1991). The long-term effect of elastic compression on the venous haemodynamics of the leg. *Phlebology*, **6**, 85–93.

Coleridge Smith, P.D. (1995). Recurrence at the sapheno-femoral junction. *Phlebology*, **10**, 13.

Corcos, L., Peruzzi, G., and Romeo, V. (1987). Intraoperative phlebography of the short saphenous vein. *Phlebology*, **2**, 241–8.

Daseler, E.H., Anson, B.J., Reimann, A.F., and Beaton, L.E. (1946). The saphenous tributaries and related structures in relation to the technique of high ligation. *Surg. Gynecol. Obstet.*, **82**, 53–63.

Davy, A. and Ouvry, P. (1986). Possible explanations for recurrence of varicose veins. *Phlebology*, **1**, 15–21.

Dayantas, J., Liatus, A.C., and Lazarides, M. (1990). Pulsatile varicose veins caused by tricuspid valve regurgitation. *Phlebology*, **5**, 189–91.

Dickson Wright, A. (1931). The treatment of indolent ulcer of the leg. *Lancet*, 457–60.

Dodd, H. and Cockett, F.B. (1976). *The pathology and surgery of the veins of the lower limbs*. Churchill Livingstone, Edinburgh.

Eklof, B. (1988). Modern treatment of varicose veins. *Br. J. Surg.*, **75**, 297–8.

Gardner, A.M.N. and Fox, R.H. (1989). *The return of blood to the heart*. Libbey, London.

Glass, G.M. (1987). Neovascularization in restoration of continuity of the rat femoral vein following surgical interruption. *Phlebology*, **2**, 1–5.

Glass, G.M. (1987). Neovascularization in recurrent of the varicose great saphenous vein following transection. *Phlebology*, **2**, 81–91.

Glass, G.M. (1995). Neovascularization in recurrent sapheno-femoral incompetence of varicose veins: surgical anatomy and morphology. *Phlebology*, **10**, 136–42.

Goren, G. and Yellin, A.E. (1990). Primary varicose veins: topographic and hemodynamic correlations. *J. Cardiovasc. Surg.*, **31**, 672–7.

Guex, J.J., Hiltbrand, B., Bayon, J.M., *et al.* (1995). Anatomical patterns in varicose vein disease: a duplex scanning study. *Phlebology*, **10**, 94–7.

Guillebaud, J. (1985). Surgery and the pill. *Br. Med. J.*, **291**, 498–9.

Henry, M. and Corless, C. (1989). The incidence of varicose veins in Ireland. *Phlebology*, **4**, 133–7.

Hobbs, J.T. (1977). Superficial thrombophlebitis. In: *The treatment of venous disorders* (ed. J.T. Hobbs), pp. 414–27. MTP, Lancaster.

Hobbs, J.T. (1980). Per-operative phlebography to ensure accurate sapheno-popliteal ligation. *Br. Med. J.*, **2**, 1578.

Hobbs, J.T. (1985). A new approach to short saphenous vein varicosities. In: *Surgery of the veins* (ed. J.J. Bergan and J.S.T. Yao), pp. 301–21. New York.

Hobbs, J.T. (1988). The enigma of the gastrocnemius vein. *Phlebology*, **3**, 19–30.

Hubner, H.J. and Schultz-Ehrenburg, U. (1986). Simple and hidden Satypical refluxes of the leg veins. In: *Phlebology '85* (ed. D. Negus and G. Jantet), pp. 58–60. Libbey, London.

Khaira, H.S., Crowson, M.C., and Parnell, A. (1996). Colour flow duplex in the assessment of recurrent varicose veins. *Ann. R. Coll. Surg. Engl.*, **78**, 139–41.

Lorenzi, G., Bavera, P., Cipolat, L., and Carlesi, R. (1986). The prevalence of primary varicose veins among workers of a metal and steel factory. In: *Phlebology '85* (ed. D. Negus and G. Jantet), pp. 18–21. Libbey, London.

Milliken, J.C., Dinn, E., O'Connor, R., and Greene, D. (1986). A simple Doppler technique for the rapid diagnosis of significant sapheno-femoral reflux. *Phlebology*, **1**, 125–8.

Obitsu, Y., Ishimaru, S., Furukawa, F., and Yoshihama, I. (1990). Histopathological studies of the valves of varicose veins. *Phlebology*, **5**, 245–54.

Quaile, A. and Rowland, F.H. (1986). A retrospective study of the epidemiology and treatment of varicose veins. In: *Phlebology '85* (ed. D. Negus and G. Jantet), pp. 33–7. Libbey, London.

Rose, S. (1986). The aetiology of varicose veins. In: *Phlebology '85*, (ed. D. Negus and G. Jantet), pp. 6–8. Libbey, London

Rose, S.S. (1991). Commentary: the aetiology of varicose veins. *Phlebology*, **6**, 215–17.

Sakaguchi, S., Koyano, K., Hishiki, S., and Takihara, M. (1986). A modified stripping operation for varicose veins of the legs based on Doppler flowmetric findings. In: *Phlebology '85* (ed. D. Negus and G. Jantet), pp. 206–8. Libbey, London.

Sethia, K.K. and Darke, S.G. (1984). Long saphenous incompetence as a cause of venous ulceration. *Br. J. Surg.*, **71**, 754–5.

Sheppard, M. (1986). The incidence, diagnosis and management of sapheno-popliteal incompetence. *Phlebology*, **1**, 23–32.

Somjen, G.M., Donlan, J., Hurse, J., *et al.* (1995). Venous reflux at the sapheno-femoral junction. *Phlebology*, **10**, 132–5.

Sutton, R. and Darke, S.G. (1986). Stripping the long saphenous vein: preoperative retrograde saphenography in patients with and without venous ulceration. *Br. J. Surg.*, **73**, 305–7.

Thulesius, O., Al-Dourary, A., Eklof, B., *et al.* Incidence of venous disease in Kuwait (1984). In *Phlebology '85*, (ed. D. Negus and G. Jantet), pp. 38–40. Libbey, London.

Thulesius, O., Gjores, J.E., and Berlin, E. (1986). Valvular function and venous distensibility. In: *Phlebology '85* (ed. D. Negus and G. Jantet), pp. 26–9. Libbey, London.

Tibbs, D.J. (1986). The intriguing problem of varicose veins. *Int. Angiol.*, **4**, 289–95.

Tibbs, D.J. and Flectcher, E.W.L. (1983). Direction of flow in superficial veins as a guide to venous disorders in the lower limbs. *Surgery*, **93**, 758–67.

Tibbs, D.J. (1992). *Varicose veins and related disorders*. Butterworth-Heinemann, Oxford.

Vandenriessche, M. (1989). The association between gastrocnemial vein insufficiency and varicose veins (including 'Invited comment' by A.N. Nicolaides, D. Christopoulos, and S. Vasdekis). *Phlebology*, **4**, 171–84.

Vasdekis, S.N., Clarke, G.H., Hobbs, J.T., and Nicolaides, A.N. (1989). Evaluation of non-invasive and invasive methods in the assessment of short saphenous vein termination. *Br. J. Surg.*, **78**, 929–32.

Widmer, L.K., Mall, Th., and Martin, H. (1977). Epidemiology and sociomedical importance of peripheral venous disease. In: *The treatment of venous disorders* (ed. J.T. Hobbs), pp. 3–12. MTP, Lancaster.

Widmer, L.K., Stahelin, H.B., Nissen, C., and da Silva, A. (1981). *Venen-, Arterien- Krankheiten, koronare Herzkrankheit bei Berufstatigen*. Bern.

Widmer, L.K., Zemp, E., Delley C., and Biland, L. (1986). Varicosity: prevalence and medical importance. In: *Phlebology '85* (ed. D. Negus and G. Jantet), pp. 87–90. Libbey, London.

Wolfe, J.H.N., Morland, M., and Browse, N.L. (1979). The fibrinolytic activity of varicose veins. *Br. J. Surg.*, **66**, 185–7.

Zelikovski, A., Haddad, M., Sahar, G., and Reiss, R. (1986). The role of ambulatory surgery of thrombosed varicose veins. *Phlebology*, **1**, 135–7.

Pelvic congestion syndrome and ovarian vein incompetence

Beard, R.W., Highman, J.W., Pearce, S., and Reginald, P.W. (1984). Diagnosis of pelvic varicosiites in women with chronic pelvic pain. *Lancet*, **ii**, 946–9.

Beard, R.W., Reginald, P.W., and Pearce, S. (1986). Pelvic pain in women. *Br. Med. J.*, **293**, 1160–2.

Dodd, H. and Payling Wright, H. (1959). Vulval varicose veins in pregnancy. *Br. Med. J.*, **1**, 831–32.

Hobbs J.T. (1976). The pelvic congestion syndrome. *Practitioner*, **216**, 529–40.

Lea Thomas, M., Fletcher, E.W.L., Andress, M.R., and Cockett, F.B. (1967). The venous connections of vulval varices. *Clin. Radiol.*, **18**, 313–17.

Lechter, A., Alvarez, A., and Lopez, G. (1987). Pelvic varices and gonadal veins. *Phlebology*, **2**, 181–8.

Lechter, A., Franco, C.A., Bayona, G., *et al.* (1995). Varices of pelvic origin: Reappraisal of a clinical, radiological and surgical condition. In: *Phlebology '95* (ed. D. Negus, G. Jantet, and P. Coleridge Smith). *Phlebology*, **Suppl. 1**, 1039–41.

May, R. (1979). *Surgery of the veins of the leg and pelvis*. Saunders, Philadelphia, PA.

Hereditary and congenital aspects

Belcaro, G.V. (1986). Saphneno-femoral incompetence in young asymptomatic subjects with a family history of varices of the lower limbs. In: *Phlebology '85* (ed. D. Negus and G. Jantet), pp. 30–2. London, Libbey.

Gunderson, J. (1977). Hereditary factors in varicose veins. In: *The treatment of venous disorders* (ed. J.T. Hobbs), pp. 13–17. MTP, Lancaster.

Schulltz-Ehrenburg, U. and Weindorf, N. (1986). Prospective epidemiological study on the development of varicosis in German grammar schools (Bochum study 1). In: *Phlebology '85* (ed. D. Negus and G. Jantet), pp. 22–5. Libbey, London.

Conservative treatment of venous disorders

Anderson, J.H., Geraghty, J.G., Wilson, Y.T., *et al.* (1990). Paroven and graduated compression hosiery for superficial venous insufficiency. *Phlebology*, **5**, 271–6.

Brakkee, A.J. and Kuiper, J.P. (1988). The influence of compressive stockings on the haemodynamics of the lower extremities. *Phlebology*, **3**, 147–53.

Burnand, K.G. and Layer, G.T. (1986). Graduated elastic stockings. *Br. Med. J.*, **293**, 224–5.

Chant, A.D.B., Magnussen, P., and Kershaw, C. (1985). Support hose and varicose veins. *Br. Med. J.*, **290**, 204.

Cheatle, T.R., Scurr, J.H., and Coleridge Smith, P.D. (1991). Drug treatment of chronic venous insufficiency and venous ulceration: a review. *J R. Soc. Med.*, **84**, 354–8.

Christopoulos, D.G., Nicolaides, A.N., Szendro, G., *et al.* (1987). Air-plethysmography and the effect of elastic compression on venous hemodynamics of the leg. *J. Vasc. Surg.*, **5**, 148–59.

Cornwall, J., Dore, C.J., and Lewis, J.D. (1987). Graduated compression and its relationship to venous refilling time. *Br. Med. J.*, **295**, 1087–90.

Dodd, H. and Cockett, F.B. (1976). *The pathology and surgery of the veins of the lower limb.* Churchill Livingstone, Edinburgh.

Drug Tariff (National Health Service England and Wales). (1989). *Graduated compression hosiery*, pp. 79–83a. HMSO, London.

Fegan, W.G. (1967). *Varicose veins.* Heinemann, London.

Fegan, W.G., Beesley, W.H., and Fitzgerald, D.E. (1964). Prophylaxis of superficial and deep venous thrombosis in the lower limbs. *J. Irish Med. Asoc.*, **54**, 110–13.

Fentem, P.H., Goddard, M., and Gooden, B.A. (1976). Support for varicose veins. *Br. Med. J.*, **1**, 254–6.

Gundersen, J. (1992). Bandaging of the lower leg. *Phlebology*, **7**, 150–3.

Horner, J., Lowth, L.C., and Nicolaides, A.N. (1980). A pressure profile for elastic stockings. *Br. Med. J.*, **1**, 818–20.

Jones, N.A.G., Webb, P.J., Rees, R.L., and Kakkar, V.V. (1980). A physiological study of elastic compression stockings in venous disorders of the leg. *Br. J. Surg.*, **67**, 569–72.

Large, J. (1990). The treatment of varicose veins: a personal review. *Phlebology*, **5**, 141–6.

Sigg, K. (1977). Treatment of varicose veins by injection-sclerotherapy: a method practised in Switzerland. In: *The treatment of venous disorders* (ed. J. Hobbs), pp. 113–37. MTP, Lancaster.

Stacey, M.C., Burnand, K.G., Layer, G.T., and Pattison, M. (1988). Calf pump function in patients with healed venous ulcers is not improved by surgery to the communicating veins or by elastic stockings. *Br. J. Surg.*, **75**, 436–9.

Stemmer, R. (1969). Ambulatory elasto-compressive treatment of the lower extremities particularly with elastic stockings. *Kassenarzt*, **9**, 1–8.

Struckman, J. (1986). Compression stockings and their effect on the venous pump—a comparative study. *Phlebology*, **1**, 37–45.

Struckman, J., Christensen, S.J., Lendorf, A., and Mathiesen, F. (1986). Venous muscle pump improvement by low compression elastic stockings. *Phlebology*, **1**, 97–103.

Sclerotherapy

Abramowitz, I. (1973). The treatment of varicose veins in pregnancy by empty vein compression sclerotherapy. *SA Med. J.*, **47**, 607–10.

Conrad, P., Malouf, G.M., and Stacey, M.C. (1994). The Australian polidocanol (Aethoxysklerol) study: results at 1 year. *Phlebology*, **9**, 17–20.

Conrad, P. (1975). Sclerostripping—a 'new' procedure for the treatment of varicose veins. *Med. J. Aust.*, **2**, 42–4.

Consensus Paper. Union Internationale de Phlebologie and Italian Ministry of Health (Initiator G. Buccaglini). (1996). Sclerotherapy of varicose veins of the lower limbs. *Scope*, **3**, 4–17.

Fegan, W.G. (1960). Continuous uninterrupted compression technique of injecting varicose veins. *Proc. R. Soc. Med.*, **53**, 837–40.

Gachet, G. (1995). L'echosclerose des varices. In: *Phlebology '95* (ed. D. Negus, G. Jantet, and P. Coleridge Smith). *Phlebology*, **Suppl. 1**, 527–9.

Goldman, M.P. (1995). Laser and non-coherent pulsed light treatment of leg telangiectasias and venules. *Phlebology '95* (ed. D. Negus, G. Jantet, and P. Coleridge Smith). *Phlebology*, **Suppl. 1**, 504–7.

Goren, G. (1988). Sclerotherapy for truncal varicose veins. The concomitant high ligation and single session perfusion-compression method. Personal communication from Vein Disorders Center, Encino, CA.

Goren, G. (1991). Injection sclerotherapy for varicose veins: history and effectiveness. *Phlebology*, **6**, 7–11.

Grondin, L. and Soriano, J. (1992). Duplex echosclerotherapy: the quest for the safe technique. In: *Phlebologie 1992* (ed. R. Raymond-Martimbeau, R. Prescott, and M. Zummo), pp. 824–5. Libbey Eurotext, Paris.

Hobbs, J.T. (1974). Surgery and sclerotherapy in the treatment of varicose veins. *Arch. Surg.*, **109**, 793–6.

Hobbs, J.T. (1977). The treatment of dilated venules. In: *The treatment of venous disorders* (ed. J.T. Hobbs), pp. 399–413. MTP, Lancaster.

Hobbs, J.T. (1977). A random trial of the treatment of varicose veins by surgery and sclerotherapy. In: *The treatment of venous disorders* (ed. J.T. Hobbs), pp. 195–207. MTP, Lancaster.

Hobbs, J.T. (1978). Compression sclerotherapy of varicose veins. In: *Venous problems* (ed. J.J. Bergan and J.S.T. Yao). Year Book, Chicago, IL.

Hoerdegen, K.M. and Sigg, K. (1988) Injection–compression sclerotherapy of the greater saphenous vein with proximal incompetence (cross insufficiency) as an alternative treatment to surgery. *Phlebology*, **3**, 41–8.

Jakobsen, B.H. (1979). The value of different forms of treatment for varicose veins. *Br. J. Surg.*, **66**, 182–4.

Knight, R.M., Vin, F., and Zygmunt, I.A. (1989). Ultrasonic guidance of injection into the superficial venous system. In: *Phlebologie 1989* (ed. A. Davy and R. Stemmer), pp. 339–41. Libbey Eurotext, Paris.

McDonagh, D.B. (1995). How compression and ambulation robs you of success in the sclerotherapy of large varicose veins. In: *Phlebology '95* (ed. D. Negus, G. Jantet, and P. Coleridge Smith). *Phlebology*, **Suppl. 1**, 591–2.

McFarland, R.J., Scott, H.J., Kay, D.N., and Scott, R.A.P. (1988). High injection sclerotherapy for varicose veins in the presence of femoro-saphenous reflux. *Phlebology* **3**, 49–54.

Marks, C.G. (1974) Localized hirsuties following compression sclerotherapy with sodium tetradecyl sulphate. *Br. J. Surg.*, **61**, 127–8.

Neglen, P., Einarsson, E., and Eklof, B. (1986). High tie with sclerotherapy for saphenous vein insufficiency. *Phlebology*, **1**, 105–11.

Neglen, P., Jonsson, B., Einarsson, E., and Eklof, B. (1986). Socio-economic benefits of ambulatory surgery and compression sclerotherapy for varicose veins. *Phlebology*, **1**, 225–30.

Ouvry, P.A. and Davy, A. (1986). Traitement sclerosant de la saphene extern variqueuse. In: *Phlebology '85* (ed. D. Negus and G. Jantet), pp. 115–18. Libbey, London.

Ouvry, P.A. and Davy, A. (1986). Sclerotherapie apres stripping. In: *Phlebology '85* (ed. D. Negus and G. Jantet), pp. 125–8. Libbey, London.

Schadeck, M. (1987). Doppler and echotomography in sclerosis of the saphenous veins. *Phlebology*, **2**, 221–40.

Schadeck, M. (1993). Echo-sclérose de la grande saphène. *Phlebologie*, **46**, 673–82.

Schadeck, M. (1995). Duplex scanning in the mechanism of sclerotherapy: the initial stage. In: *Phlebology '95* (ed. D. Negus, G. Jantet, and P. Coleridge Smith). *Phlebology*, **Suppl. 1**, 614.

Schadeck, M. and Allaert, F.A. (1991). Echotomographie de la sclérose. *Phlebologie*, **4**, (1), 111–30.

Schadeck, M. and Allaert, F.A. (1995). Post sclerosis recurrences of the great saphenous vein. In: *Phlebology '95*, (ed. D. Negus, G. Jantet, and P. Coleridge Smith). *Phlebology*, **Suppl. 1**, 614.

Shouler, P.J. and Runchman, P.C. (1989). Varicose veins: optimum compression after surgery and sclerotherapy. *Ann. R. Coll. Surg. Engl.*, **71**, 402–4.

Stother, I.G., Bryson, A., and Alexander, S. (1974). The treatment of varicose veins by compression sclerotherapy. *Br. J. Surg.*, **61**, 387–90.

Tennant, W.G. and Ruckley, C.V. (1996). Medicolegal action following treatment for varicose veins. *Br. J. Surg.*, **83**, 291–2.

Tournay, R. (1990). How should resistant varicose veins be sclerosed? *Phlebology*, **5**, 151–5.

Villavicencio, J.L., Collins, G.J., Youkey, J.R., *et al.* (1985). Nonsurgical management of lower extremity venous problems. In: *Surgery of the veins* (ed. J.J. Bergan and J.S.T. Yao), pp. 323–45. Grune and Stratton, New York.

Various authors (1977). Techniques of sclerotherapy. In: *The treatment of venous disorders* (ed. J. Hobbs). MTP Lancaster.

Wallois, P. (1980). Indications et techniques de la sclerose des varices. *Bull. Actual. Ther.*, **25**, 2485–95.

Compression bandaging in sclerotherapy

Batch, A.J.G., Wickremesinghe, S.S., Gannon, M.E., and Dormandy, J.A. (1980). Randomised trial of bandaging after sclerotherapy for varicose veins. *Br. Med. J.*, **281**, 423.

Fraser, I.A., Perry, E.P., Hatton, M., and Watkin, D.F.L. (1985). Prolonged bandaging is not required following sclerotherapy of varicose veins. *Br. J. Surg.*, **72**, 488–90.

Raj, T.B., Goddard, M.D., and Makin, G.S. (1980). How long do compression bandages maintain their pressure during ambulatory treatment of varicose veins? *Br. J. Surg.*, **67**, 122–4.

Reddy, P., Wickers, J., Terry, T., *et al.* What is the correct period of bandaging following sclerotherapy? *Phlebology*, **1**, 217–20.

Scurr, J.H., Coleridge-Smith, P., and Cutting, P. (1985). Varicose veins: optimum compression following sclerotherapy. *Ann R. Coll. Surg. Engl.*, **67**, 109–11.

Complications of sclerotherapy and surgery: medicolegal aspects

Callum, M.J., Ruckley, C.V., Dale, J.J. and Harper, D.R. (1987). Hazards of compression treatment of the leg: an estimate from Scottish surgeons. *Br. Med. J.*, **295**, 1382.

Cockett, F.B. (1986). Arterial complications during surgery and sclerotherapy of varioce veins. *Phlebology*, **1**, 3–6.

Conrad, P. (1987). Injection of varicose veins and spider veins. *Aus. Fam. Physician*, **16**, 451–4.

Eklof, B. (1988). Modern treatment of varicose veins. *Br. J. Surg.*, **75**, 297–8.

Fegan, W.G. and Pegum, J.M. (1974). Accidental intra-arterial injection during sclerotherapy of varicose veins. *Br. J. Surg.*, **61**, 124–6.

Fletcher, I.R. and Healy, T.E. (1983). The arterial tourniquet. *Ann. R. Coll. Surg. Engl.*, **65**, 409–17.

Hadfield, G. (1971). Thromboembolism in patients under injection treatment. In: *Stoke Mandeville Symposium. The treatment of varicose veins by injection and compression*, p. 52. Pharmaceutical Research, London.

Hoyte, P. (1987). Hazards of injections. *J. Med. Defence Union*, **Summer**, 9.

Keddie, N.C. (1987). Medico-legal problems from the treatment of varicose veins. *J. Med. Defence Union*, **Winter**, 8–9.

MacGowan, W.A.L. (1985). Sclerotherapy—prevention of accidents: a review. *J. R. Soc. Med.*, **78**, 136–7.

MacGowan, W.A.L., Holland, P.D.J., Browne, H.I., and Byrnes, D. (1972). The local effects of intra-arterial injections of sodium tetradecyl sulphate (STD) 3 per cent: an experimental study. *Br. J. Surg.*, **59**, 101–4.

Oesch, A., Mahler, F., and Stirnemann, P. (1986). Acute ischaemia of the foot following sclerotherapy. In: *Phlebology '85* (ed. D. Negus and G. Jantet), pp. 122–4. Libbey, London.

Tennant, W.G. and Ruckley, C.V. Medicolegal action following treatment for varicose veins. *Br. J. Surg.*, **83**, 291–2.

Thompson, Hon. Mr. Justice. (1975). Transcript of Proceedings. Judgement (revised). Queen's Bench Division, 15 July 1975, 74/NJ/3104.

The contraceptive pill

Aitenhead, A.R. (1990). Prudence with the pill. *J. Med. Defence Union*, **6**, 62–4.

Guillebaud, J. (1985). Surgery and the pill. *Br. Med. J.*, **291**, 498–9.

Robinson, G.E., Burren, T., Mackie, I.J., *et al.* (1991). Changes in haemostasis after stopping the combined contraceptive pill: implications for major surgery. *Br. Med. J.*, **302**, 269–71.

Vessey, M.P., Doo, R., and Fairbairn, A.S. (1970). Post-operative thromboembolism and the use of oral contraceptives. *Br. Med. J.*, **iii**, 123–6.

Surgery

Babcock, W.W. (1907). A new operation for the extirpation of varicose veins of the leg. *NY Med. J.*, **86**, 153–6.

Bishop, C.C.R. and Jarrett, P.E.M. (1986). Outpatient varicose vein surgery under local anaesthesia. *Br. J. Surg.*, **73**, 821–2.

Clinton, O. and Negus, D. (1990). Suitability for day-care varicose vein surgery. *Phlebology*, **5**, 277–9.

Conrad, P. (1992). Groin-to-knee downward stripping of the long saphenous vein. *Phlebology*, **7**, 20–2.

Corcos, L., Peruzzi, G.P., Romeo, V., and Procacci, T. (1989). Preliminary results of external valvuloplasty in saphenofemoral junction insufficiency. *Phlebology*, **4**, 197–202.

Dodd, H. (1964). The diagnosis and ligation of incompetent perforating veins. *Ann. R. Coll. Surg. Engl.*, **34**, 186–96.

Dodd, H. and Cockett, F.B. (1976). *The pathology and surgery of the veins of the of the lower limb*, p. 106. Churchill Livingstone, Edinburgh.

Dunn, J.M., Cosford, E.J., Kernick, V.F.M., and Campbell, W.B. (1995). Surgical treatment for venous ulcers: is it worthwhile? *Ann. R. Coll. Surg. Engl.*, **77**, 421–4.

Fullarton, G.M. and Calvert, M.H. (1987). Intraluminal long saphenous vein stripping: a technique minimizing perivenous tissue trauma. *Br. J. Surg.*, **74**, 255.

Gaylis, H. (1968). Subcutaneous implantation of varicose veins for future arterial grafting. *Surgery*, **63**, 591–3.

Gilliland, E.L., Gerber, C.J., and Lewis, J.D. (1987). Short saphenous vein surgery, pre-operative Doppler ultrasound marking compared with on-table venography and operative findings. *Phlebology*, **2**, 109–14.

Goren, G. and Yellin, A.E. (1991). Ambulatory stab evulsion phlebectomy for truncal varicose veins. *Am. J. Surg.*, **162**, 166–74.

Groen, G. and Yellin, A.E. (1995). Minimally invasive surgery for primary varicose veins: limited invaginated axial stripping and tributary (hook) stab avulsion. *Ann. Vasc, Surg.*, **9**, 401–14.

Hobbs, J.T. (1980). Pre-operative venography to ensure accurate sapheno-popliteal ligation. *Br. Med. J.*, **ii**, 1578.

Juhan, C., Haupert, S., Miltgen, G., *et al.* Recurrent varicose veins. *Phlebology*, **5**, 201–11.

Li, A.K.C. (1975). A technique for re-exploration of the saphenofemoral junction for recurrent varicose veins. *Br. J. Surg.*, **62**, 745–6.

Loftgren, K.A. (1978). Management of varicose veins: Mayo Clinic experience. In: *Venous problems* (ed. J.J. Bergan and J.S.T. Yao), Year Book, Chicago, IL.

Nabatoff, R.A. (1953) A complete stripping operation of varicose veins under local anaesthesia. *NY J. Med.*, **53**, 1445.

McMullin, G.M., Coleridge Smith, P.D., and Scurr, J.H. (1991) Objective assessment of high ligation without stripping the long saphenous vein. *Br. J. Surg.*, **78**, 1139–42.

Martin, A.G., Wainwright, A.M., and Lear, P.A. (1995). Crochet hooks in varicose vein surgery. *Ann. R. Coll. Surg. Engl.*, **77**, 460–1.

Oesch, A. (1993). 'Pin-stripping': a novel method of atraumatic stripping. *Phlebology*, **8**, 171–3.

Sarin, S., Scurr, J.H., and Coleridge Smith, P.D. (1992). Assessment of stripping the long saphenous vein in the treatment of primary varicose veins. *Br. J. Surg.*, **79**, 889–93.

Sheppard, M. (1978). A procedure for the prevention of recurrent saphenofemoral incompetence. *Aust. NZ J. Surg.*, **48**, 322–6.

Sheppard, M. (1986). The incidence and management of saphenopopliteal incompetence. *Phlebology*, **1**, 23–32.

Staelens, I, and van der Stricht, J. (1992). Complication rate of long stripping of the greater saphenous vein. *Phlebology*, **7**, 67–70.

Taylor, E.W., Fielding, J.W., Keighley, M.R., and Alexander-Williams, J. (1981). Long saphenous vein stripping under local anaesthesia. *Ann. R. Coll. Surg. Engl.*, **63**, 206–7.

Travers, J.P., Berridge, D.C., and Makin, G.S. (1990). Surgical enhancement of skin oxygenation in patients with venous lipodermatosclerosis. *Phlebology*, **5**, 129–33.

van der Stricht, J. (1963). Saphenectomie par invagination sur fil. *Presse Med.*, **71**, 1081–2.

Zamboni, P. and Liboni, A. (1991). External valvuloplasty of the sapheno-femoral junction using perforated prosthesis. *Phlebology*, **6**, 141–7.

Chapter 5 Clinical patterns of venous disorder II. Valve deficiency and weak vein walls

General

Almgren, B. (1990). Non-thrombotic deep venous incompetence with special reference to anatomic, haemodynamic and therapeutic aspects. *Phlebology*, **5**, 255–70.

Browse, N.L., Clemenson, G., and Lea Thomas, M. (1980). Is the postphlebitic leg always postphlebitic? Relation between phlebographic appearances of deep vein thrombosis and late sequelae. *Br. Med. J.*, **281**, 1167–70.

Guamera, G., Furgiuele, S., Di Paola, F.M., and Camilli, S. (1995). Recurrent varicose veins and primary deep venous insufficiency: relationship and therapeutic implications. *Phlebology*, **10**, 98–102.

Kistner, R.L. (1980). Primary venous valve incompetence of the leg. *Am. J. Surg.*, **140**, 218–24.

Kistner, R.L. (1985). Venous valve surgery. In: *Surgery of the veins* (ed. J.J. Bergan and J.S.T. Yao), pp. 205–17. Grune and Stratton, New York.

Ludbrook, J. (1966). *Aspects of venous function in the lower limbs.* Thomas, Springfield, IL.

Perrin, M. (1995). Surgical technique of vlavuloplasty in the deep vein. In: *Phlebology '95* (ed. D. Negus, G. Jantet, and P. Coleridge Smith). *Phlebology*, **Suppl. 1**, 971.

Rose, S. (1986). The aetiology of varicose veins. In: *Phlebology '85* (ed. D. Nogus and G. Jantet), pp. 6–9. Libbey, London.

Rose S. (1986). The aetiology of varicose veins. In: *Progressi in flebologia* (ed. M. Tesi *et al.*), pp. 47–8. Minerva Medica, Turin.

Taheri, S.A., Heffner, R., Meenaghan, M.A., *et al.* (1985). Technique and results of venous valve transplantation. In: *Surgery of the veins* (ed. J.J. Bergan and J.S.T. Yao), pp. 219–31. Grune and Stratton, London.

Hereditary and congenital aspects

Lodin, A., Lindvall, N., and Gentele, H. (1958–9). Congenital absence of venous valves as a cause of leg ulcers. *Acta Chir. Scand.*, **116**, 256–61.

El-Gohary, M.A. (1984). Boyhood varicocele: an overlooked disorder. *Ann. R. Coll. Surg. Engl.*, **66**, 36–8.

Friedman, W.I., Taylor, L.M., and Porter, J.M. (1988). Congenital venous valvular aplasia of the lower extremities. *Surgery*, **103**, 24–7.

Kistner, R.L. (1980). Primary venous valve incompetence of the leg. *Am. J. Surg.*, **140**, 218–24.

Lodin, A. and Lindvall, N. (1961). Congenital absence of valves in the deep veins of the leg. A factor in venous insufficiency. *Acta. Derm. Venereol. (Stockholm)*, **41** (Suppl. 45), 7–91.

Partsch, B., Mayer, W., and Partsch, H. (1992). Improvement in ambulatory venous hupertension by narrowing of the femoral vein in congential absence of venous valves. *Phlebology*, **7**, 101–4.

Plate, G., Brudin, L., Eklof, B., *et al.* (1986). Physiological and therapeutic aspects of congenital vein valve aplasia of the lower limb. In: *Phlebogy '85* (ed. D. Negus and G. Jantet). Libbey, London.

Rabe, E. (1987). Acute and chronic venous insufficiency in infancy and childhood. *Phlebology*, **2**, 249–55.

Chapter 6 Clinical patterns of venous disorder III. Deep vein impairment (post-thrombotic syndrome)

General

Adamson, A.S., Littlewood, T.J., Poston, G.J., *et al.* (1988). Malignancy presenting as peripheral venous gangrene. *J.R. Soc. Med.*, **81**, 609–10.

Baumgartner, I., Franzeck, U.K., and Bollinger, A. (1992). Venous claudication evaluated by ambulatory plethysmography. *Phlebology*, **7**, 2–6.

Belcaro, G.V. and Nicolaides, A.N. (1994). Effects of intermittent sequential compression in venous hypertensive microangiopathy. *Phlebology*, **9**, 99–103.

Cheatle, T.R. and Perrin, M. (1993). Primary venous aneurysms of the popliteal fossa. *Phlebology*, **8**, 82–5.

Cheatle, T.R., McMullin, G.M., and Scurr, J.H. (1991). Deep vein reflux is reduced by compression of the foot venous plexus. *Phlebology*, **6**, 75–7.

Chilton, C.P. and Darke, S.G. (1980). External iliac venous compression by a giant iliopsoas rheumatoid bursa. *Br. J. Surg.*, **67**, 641.

Christopoulos, D., Nicoliades, A.N., Belcaro, G., and Duffy, P. (1990). The effect of elastic compression on calf muscle pump function. *Phlebology*, **5**, 13–19.

Cockett, F.B. (1991). Venous valves: history up to the present day. *Phlebology*, **6**, 63–73.

Gajraj, H. and Browse, N.L. (1991). Fibrinolytic activity and calf pump failure. *Br. J. Surg.*, **78**, 1009–12.

Hobbs, J.T. (1988). The enigma of the gastrocnemius vein. *Phlebology*, **3**, 19–30.

Hudson, I. and Sadow, G.J. (1990). An unusual cause of femoral vein obstruction. *J.R. Soc. Med.*, **83**, 331–2.

Hughes, G.R. and Pridie, R.B. (1970). Acute synovial rupture of the knee—a differential diagnosis from deep vein thrombosis. *Proc. R. Soc. Med.*, **63**, 587–90.

Kistner, R.L. (1980). Primary venous valve incompetence of the leg. *Am. J. Surg.*, **140**, 218–24.

Lea Thomas, M. (1982). *Phlebography of the lower limb*. Churchill Livingstone, Edinburgh.

Lea Thomas, M. and Solis, G. (1992). The phlebographic distribution of deep venous thrombosis in the calf and its relevance to duplex ultrasound. *Phlebology*, **7**, 64–6.

Mestres, C.A., Ninot, S., Guerola, M., *et al.* (1987). Spontaneous iliacocaval arteriovenous fistula: the case for differential diagnosis. *Br. J. Surg.*, **74**, 1178–9.

Nicolaides, A.N., Zukowski, A., and Kyprianou, P. (1985). Venous pressure measurements in venous problems. In: *Surgery of the veins* (ed. J.J. Bergan and J.S.T. Yao), pp. 111–19. Grune and Stratton, New York.

Shull, K.C., Nicolaides, A.N., Fernandes, F., *et al.* (1979). Significance of popliteal reflux in relation to ambulatory venous pressure and ulceration. *Arch. Surg.*, **114**, 1304–6.

Tibbs, D.J. and Fletcher, E.W.L. (1983). Direction of flow in superficial veins as a guide to venous disorders inlowerlimbs. *Surgery*, **93**, 758–67.

Tibbs, D.J. and Fletcher, E.W.L. (1986). Further experience with directional Doppler flowmeter applied to superficial veins in the diagnosis of venous disorders of the lower limbs. In: *Progress in flebologia* (ed. M. Tesi), pp. 90–6. Minerva Medica, Turin.

Watts, R.A. and Bretland, P.M. (1990). Necrotizing fasciitis mimicking a ruptured popliteal cyst. *J. R. Soc. Med.*, **83**, 52–3.

Welch, G.H., Reid, D.B., Pollock, J.G. (1990). Infected false aneurysms in the groin of intravenous drug abusers. *Br. J. Surg.*, **77**, 330–3.

Pharmaceuticals

Coleridge Smith, P.D. (1994). Pharmacological treatment for venous disease. *Phlebology*, **9**, 47.

Monreal, M., Callejas, J.M., Martorell, A., *et al.* (1994). A prospective study of the long-term efficacy of two different venoactive drugs in patients with post-thrombotic syndrome, *Phlebology*, **9**, 37–40.

Post-thrombotic syndrome and liposclerosis

Bauer, G.A. (1942). Roentgenological and clinical study of the sequelae of thrombosis. *Acta Chir. Scand.*, **74**, 1.

Bjordal, R.I. (1977). Haemodynamic studies of varicose veins and the post-thrombotic syndrome. In: *The treatment of venous disorders* (ed. J.T. Hobbs), pp. 37–55. MTP, Lancaster.

Bollinger, A. and Jager, K. (1986). Intermittent venous claudication evaluated by strain-gauge plethsmography during treadmill exercise. In: *Phlebology '85* (ed. D. Negus and G. Jantet), pp. 571–3. Libbey, London.

Browse, N. (1985). The pathogenesis of venous ulceration. In: *Surgery of the veins* (ed. J.J. Bergan and J.S.T. Yao), (ed. 25–31. Grune and Stratton, New York.

Browse, N. and Burnand, K. (1978). The postphlebitic syndrome: a new look. In: *Venous problems* (ed. J.J. Bergan and J.S.T. Yao), pp. 395–405. Year Book, Chicago, IL.

Burnand, K., Clemenson, G., Morland, M., *et al.* Venous lipodermatosclerosis: treatment by fibrinolytic enhancement and elastic compression. *Br. Med. J.*, **280**, 7–11.

Burnand, K.G., Whimster, I., Naidoo, A., and Browse, N.L. (1982). Pericapillary fibrin in the ulcer bearing skin of the lower leg. The cause of lipodermatosclerosis and venous ulceration. *Br. Med. J.*, **285**, 1071–2.

Callam, M.J., Harper, D.R., Dale, J.J., and Ruckley, C.V. (1987). Chronic ulcer of the leg: clinical history. *Br. Med. J.*, **294**, 1389–91.

Cockett, F.B. and Lea Thomas, M. (1965). The iliac compression syndrome. *Br. J. Surg.*, **52**, 816.

Cockett, B., Lea Thomas, M., and Negus, D. (1967). Iliac vein compression—its relation to iliofemoral thrombosis and the post-thrombotic syndrome. *Br. Med. J.*, **2**, 14.

Coleridge Smith, P.D., Thomas, P., Scurr, J.H., and Dormandy, J.A. (1988). Causes of venous ulceration: a new hypothesis. *Br. Med. J.*, **296**, 1726–7.

Dodd, H. and Cockett, FB. (1976). The pathology and surgery of the veins of the lower limb. Churchill Livingstone, Edinburgh.

Hobbs, J.T. (1977). The post-thrombotic syndrome. In: *The treatment of venous disorders* (ed. J.T. Hobbs), pp. 253–71. MTP, Lancaster.

Homans, J. (1917). The aetiology and treatment of varicose ulcer of the leg. *Surg. Gynec. Obstet.*, **24**, 300.

Jones, W.M., Taylor, I., and Stoddard, C.J. (1973). Common iliac vein compression syndrome occurring in siblings. *Br. J. Surg.*, **60**, 663–4.

Lagerstedt, C., Olsson, C.G., Fagher, L., *et al.* (1993). Recurrence and late sequelae after first-time deep vein thrombosis: relationship to initial signs. *Phlebology*, **8**, 62–7.

Lawrence, D. and Kakkar, V.V. (1980). Post-phlebitic syndrome–a functional assessment. *Br. J. Surg.*, **67**, 686–9.

Lea Thomas, M., Fletcher, E.W.L., Cockett, F.B., and Negus, D. (1967). Venous collaterals in external and common iliac vein obstruction. *Clin. Radiol.*, **18**, 403–11.

May, R. and Thurner, J. (1957). The cause of the predominantly sinistral occurrence of thrombosis of the pelvic veins. *Angiology*, **8**, 419.

Mudge, M. and Hughes, L.E. (1975). The long term sequelae of deep vein thrombosis. *Br. J. Surg.* **65**, 692–4.

Negus, D. (1970). The post-thrombotic syndrome. *Ann. R. Coll. Surg. Engl.*, **47**, 92–105.

Negus, D. and Cockett, F.B. (1967). Femoral vein pressures in post phlebitic iliac vein obstruction. *Br. J. Surg.*, **54**, 522.

Saarinen, J., Sisto, T., Laurikka, J., *et al.* (1995). Late sequelae of acute deep venous thrombosis: evaluation five and ten years after. *Phlebology*, **10**, 106–9.

Stacey, M.C., Burnand, K.G., Pattison, M., *et al.* (1987). Changes in the apparently normal limb in unilateral venous ulceration. *Br. J. Surg.*, **74**, 936–8.

Stacey, M.C., Burnand, K.G., Lea Thomas, M., and Pattison, M. (1991). Influence of phlebographic abnormalities on the natural history of venous ulceration. *Br. J. Surg.*, **78**, 868–71.

Taheri, S.A., Nowakowski, P., Prendergast, D., *et al.* (1987). Iliocaval compression syndrome. *Phlebology*, **2**, 173–9.

Thomas, P.R.S., Nash, G.B., and Dormandy, J.A. (1988). White cell accumulation in dependent legs of patients with venous hypertension: a possible mechanism for trophic changes in the skin. *Br. Med. J.*, **296**, 1693–5.

Tierney, S., Burke, P., Fitzgerald, P., *et al.* (1993). Ankle fracture associated with prolonged venous dysfunction. *Br. J. Surg.*, **80**, 36–8.

Tronnier, M., Schmeller, W., and Wolff, H.H. (1994). Morphological changes in lipodermatosclerosis and venous ulcers: light microscopy, immunohistochemistry and electron microscopy. *Phlebology*, **9**, 48–54.

Widmer, L.K., Zemp, E., Widmer, M.Th., and Voelin, R. (1986). Thromboembolic recurrence and post-thrombotic syndrome after deep vein thrombosis. In: *Phlebology '85* (ed. D. Negus and G. Jantet), pp. 556–9. Libbey, London.

Wolfe, J.H.N. (1987). Postphlebitic syndrome after fractures of the leg. *Brit. Med. J.*, **295**, 1364–5.

Woodyer, A.B., Walker, R.T., and Dormandy, J.A. (1986). Venous claudication. In: *Phlebology '85* (ed. D. Negus and G. Jantet), pp. 524–7. Libbey, London.

Wright, C.B., Hobson, R.W., Swan, K.G., and Rich, N.M. (1978). The pathophysiology of extremity venous occlusion. In: *Venous problems* (J.J. Bergan and J.S.T. Yao), pp. 451–67. Year Book, Chicago, IL.

Conservative treatment

Villavicencio, J.J., Collins, G.J., Youkey, J.R., *et al.* (1985). Nonsurgical management of lower extremity venous problems. In: *Surgery of the veins* (ed. J.J. Bergan and J.S.T. Yao), pp. 323–45. Grune and Stratton, New York.

Thrombosis

Ghani, A.R. and Tibbs, D.J. (1962). Role of blood-borne cells in organisation of mural thrombi. *Br. Med. J.*, **1**, 1244–7.

Gillespie, G. (1973). Peripheral gangrene as the presentation of myeloproliferative disorders. *Br. J. Surg.*, **60**, 377–80.

Hill, D.A. (1992). Calf vein thrombosis: diagnosis and treatment. *Phlebology*, **7**, 40–4.

Kakkar, V.V., Howe, G.T., Flanc, C.J., and Clarke, M.B. (1969). Natural history of postoperative deep vein thrombosis. *Lancet*, **ii**, 230.

McCollum, C. (1987). Vena caval filters: keeping big clots down. *Br. Med. J.*, **294**, 1566.

Perkins, J.M.T., Magee, T.R., and Galland, R.B. (1996). Phlegmasia caerulea dolens and venous gangrene. *Br. J. Surg.*, **83**, 19–23.

Rickles, F.R. and Edwards, R.L. (1983). Activation of blood coagulation in cancer: Trousseau's syndrome revisited. *Blood*, **62**, 14–32.

Scott, G.B.D. (1970). Concerning the organization of thrombi. *Ann. R. Coll. Surg. Engl.*, **47**, 335–43.

Vessey, M.P., Doo, R., and Fairbairn, A.S. (1970). Post-operative thromboembolism and the use of oral contraceptives. *Br. Med. J.*, **iii**, 123–6.

Surgery

Aitken, R.J., Matley, P.J., and Immelman, E.J. (1989). Lower limb vein trauma: a long-term clinical and physiological assessment. *Br. J. Surg.* **76**, 585–8.

Campbell, J.B., Glover, J.L., and Herring, B. (1988). The influence of endothelial seeding and platelet inhibition on the patency of ePTFE grafts used to repalce small arteries—an experimental study. *Eur. J. Vasc. Surg.*, **2**, 365–70.

Cheatle, T.R. and Perrin, M. (1993). Surgical options in post-thrombotic syndrome. *Phlebology*, **8**, 50–7.

Clarke, J.M.F. and Marston, A. (1988). Seeding of arterial protheses with living cells. *Eur. J. Vasc. Surg.*, **2**, 353–5.

Dale, W.A. (1985). Synthetic grafts for venous reconstruction. In: *Surgery of the veins* (ed. J.J. Bergan and J.S.T. Yao), pp. 233–9. Grune and Stratton, New York.

Dilley, R.J., McGeachie, J.K., and Prendergast, F.J. (1983). Experimental vein grafts in the rat: re-endothelialization and permeability to albumin. *Br. J. Surg.*, **70**, 7–12.

Eklof, B., Einarsson, E., and Plate, G. (1985). Role of thrombectomy and temporary arteriovenous fistula in acute ilio-femoral venous thrombosis. In: *Surgery of the veins* (ed. J.J. Bergan and J.S.T. Yao), pp. 131–44. Grune and Stratton, New York.

Fox, U., Diamantini, S., and Lucani, G. (1996). Surgery of lymphatics. *Scope*, **3**, 18–21. (This gives a good summary of the various surgical procedures, past and present, used in treating lymphoedema.)

Gardner, A.M.N. (1973). Treatment of combined external iliac artery and vein injury by cross-over femorofemoral arterial and venous grafts with temporary arteriovenous shunt. *Br. J. Surg.*, **60**, 744–5.

Gruss, J.D. (1985). The saphenopopliteal bypass for chonic venous insufficiency (May–Husni operation). In: *Surgery of the veins* (ed. J.J. Bergan and J.S.T. Yao), pp. 255–65. Grune and Stratton, New York.

Gruss, J.D. (1988). Venous reconstruction. Part 1. *Phlebology*, **3**, 7–18.

Gruss, J.D. (1988). Venous reconstruction. Part 2. *Phlebology*, **3**, 75–87.

Halliday, P., Harris, J., and May, J. (1985). Femoro-femoral crossover grafts (Palma operation): a long term follow-up study. In: *Surgery of the veins* (ed. J.J. Bergan and J.S.T. Yao), pp. 241–54. Grune and Stratton, New York.

Hardy, E.G. and Tibbs, D.J. (1960). Acute ischaemia in limb injuries. *Br. Med. J.*, **i**, 1001–5.

Ijima, H., Hirabayashi, K., Sakakibara, Y., *et al.* (1990). Results of femoro-femoral vein bypass grafting with temporary arteriovenous fistula for femoroiliac venous thrombosis: differences between operations in the acute and chronic phases. *Phlebology*, **5**, 237–44.

Kistner, R.L. (1978). Transvenous repair of the incompetent femoral valve. In: *Venous problems* (ed. J.J. Bergan and J.S.T. Yao). Year Book, Chicago, IL.

Kistner, R.L. (1985). Venous valve surgery. In: *Surgery of the veins* (ed. J.J. Bergan and J.S.T. Yao), pp. 205–17. Grune and Stratton, New York.

Krige, J.E.J. and Spence, R.A.J. (1987). Popliteal artery trauma: a high risk injury. *Br. J. Surg.*, **74**, 91–4.

McMullin, G.M., Coleridge Smith, P.D., and Scurr, J.H. (1990). Evaluation of Psathakis' silastic sling procedure for deep vein reflux: a preliminary report. *Phlebology*, **5**, 95–106.

McNeill, A.D. and Sorour, N.N. (1980). Veno-venous internal saphenous crossover graft for phlegmasia caerulea dolens. *Br. J. Surg.*, **67**, 877–8.

May, R. (1979). *Surgery of the veins of the leg and pelvis.* Saunders, Philadelphia, PA; Thieme, Stuttgart.

O'Reilly, M.J.G., Hood, J.M., Livingston, R.H., and Irwin, J.W.S. (1980). Penetrating injuries of the popliteal vein: a report on 34 cases. *Br. J. Surg.*, **67**, 337–40.

Psathakis, D. and Psathakis, N. (1992). Popliteal valvular construction using a silastic sling (Technique II) for deep venous insufficiency of the lower limb. *Phlebology*, **7**, 158–65.

Sawyer, P.N. and Kaplitt, M.J. (1978). *Vascular grafts*. Appleton-Century-Crofts, New York.

Schanzer, H., Skladany, M., and Peirce, E.C., II (1994). The role of external banding valvuloplasty in the surgical management of chronic deep venous disease. *Phlebology*, **9**, 8–12.

Shull, K.C., Nicolaides, A.N., Fernandes, F., *et al.* (1979). Significance of popliteal reflux in relation to ambulatory venous pressure and ulceration. *Arch. Surg.*, **114**, 1304–6.

Smith, S.R.G., Mansfield, A.O. and Bradley, J.P.W. (1988). Remotely inserted venous occlusion catheters for the control of venous haemorrhage. *Ann. R. Coll. Surg. Engl.*, **70**, 161–2.

Sottiurai, V.S. (1991). Incompetent transplanted arm vein valves: surgical correction and result. *Phlebology*, **6**, 41–6.

Taheri, S.A., Heffner, R., Meenaghan, M.A., *et al.* (1985). Technique and results of venous valve transplantation. In: *Surgery of the veins* (ed. J.J. Bergan and J.S.T. Yao), pp. 219–31. Grune and Stratton, New York.

Tibbs, D.J. (1962). Acute ischaemia of the limbs. *Proc. R. Soc. Med.*, 593–6.

Vandendriessche, M. (1989). Association between gastrocnemial vein insufficiency and varicose veins (with an invited comment by A.N. Nicoliades, D. Christopoulos, and S. Vasdelis). *Phlebology*, **4**, 171–84.

Vohra, R., Thomson, G.J.L., Carr, H.M.H., *et al.* (1991). Comparison of different vascular protheses and matrices in relationship to endothelial seeding. *Br. J. Surg.*, **78**, 417–20.

Wilson, N.M., Rutt, D.L., and Browse, N.L. (1991). Repair and replacement of deep vein valves in the treatment of venous insufficiency. *Br. J. Surg.*, **78**, 388–94.

Wilson, N.M., Rutt, D.L., and Browse, N.L. (1991). *In situ* venous valve construction. *Br. J. Surg.*, **78**, 595–600.

Cystic adventitial disease in veins and arteries.

Browse, N.L., Burnand, K.G., and Lea Thomas, M. (1988). Cystic degeneration of the vein wall. In: *Disease of the veins*, pp. 661–3. Arnold, London.

Campbell, W.B. and Millar, A.W. (1985). Cystic adventitial disease of the common femoral artery communicating with the hip joint. *Br. J. Surg.*, **72**, 537.

England, P.C., King, J., Beton, D.C., and Hancock, B.D. (1979). Cystic adventitial disease of the popliteal artery. *J. R. Soc. Med.*, **72**, 283–4.

Flanigan, D.P., Burnham, S.J., Goodreau, J.J., and Bergan, J.J. (1979). Summary of cases of adventitial cystic disease of the popliteal artery. *Ann. Surg.*, **189**, 165–75. (Refers to veins affected in three cases.)

Hall, R.I., Proud, G., Chamberlain, J., and McNeil, I.F. (1985). Cystic adventitial disease of the common femoral and popliteal arteries. *Br. J. Surg.*, **72**, 756–8.

Kiskinis, D. and Raithel, D. (1979). Uncommon causes of intermittent claudication: cystic adventitial disease of the popliteal artery and popliteal entrapment syndrome. *Cardiovasc. Res. Center Bull.*, **17**, 69–74.

Macfarlane, R., Livesey, S.A., Pollard, S., and Dunn, D.C. (1987). Cystic adventitial arterial disease. *Br. J. Surg.*, **74**, 89–90.

Shute, K. and Rothnie, N.G. (1973). The aetiology of cystic arterial disease. *Br. J. Surg.*, **60**, 397–400.

Popliteal vein entrapment

Brightmore, T.G.J., and Smellie, W.A.B. (1971). Popliteal artery entrapment. *Br. J. Surg.*, **58**, 481–4.

Connell, J. (1978). Popliteal vein entrapment. *Br. J. Surg.*, **65**, 351.

Inada, K., Hirose, M., Iwashima, Y., and Matsumoto, K. (1978). Popliteal artery entrapment syndrome: a case report. *Br. J. Surg.*, **65**, 613–15.

Iwai, T., Sato, S., Yamada, T., *et al.* Popliteal vein entrapment caused by the third head of gastrocnemius muscle. *Br. J. Surg.*, **74**, 1006–8.

Chapter 7 Clinical patterns of venous disorder IV. Role of the perforator

Akesson, H., Brudin, L., Cwikiel, W., *et al.* (1990). Does the correction of insufficient superficial and perforating veins improve venous function in patients with deep venous insufficieny? *Phlebology*, **5**, 113–23.

Barker, W.F. (1978). The postphlebitic syndrome: management by surgical means. In: *Venous problems* (ed. J.J. Bergan and J.S.T. Yao), pp. 383–93. Year Book, Chicago, IL.

Bjordal, R.I. (1972). Circulation patterns in incompetent perforating veins in the calf and in the saphenous system in primary varicose veins. *Acta Chir. Scand.*, **138**, 251.

Bjordal, R.I. (1974). Circulation patterns in the saphenous system and the perforating veins of the calf in patients with previous deep vein thrombosis. *VASA* (**Suppl.**), **3**.

Bjordal, R.I. (1977). Haemodynamic studies of varicose veins and the post-thrombotic syndrome. In: *The treatment of venous disorders* (ed. J.T. Hobbs), pp. 37–55. MTP, Lancaster.

Bjordal, R.I. (1981). Circulation patterns in incompetent perforating veins of the calf in venous dysfunction. In: *Perforating veins*, (ed. R. May, P. Partsch, and J. Staubesa), pp. 71–88. Urban & Schwarzenberg, Munich.

Cockett, F.B. (1956). Diagnosis and surgery of high-pressure leaks in the leg. *Br. Med. J.*, **ii**, 1399–13.

Cockett, F.B. and Dodd, H. (1976). *The pathology and surgery of the veins of the lower limb.* Churchill Livingstone, Edinburgh.

Cockett, F.B. and Elgan Jones, D.E. (1953). The ankle blow-out syndrome. *Lancet*, 17–23.

Dodd, H., Calo, A.R., Mistry, M., and Rushford, A. (1957). Ligation of ankle communicating veins in the treatment of the venous-ulcer syndrome of the leg. *Lancet*, 1249.

Gasbarro, V.M.D., Pozza, E.M.D., Viaggi, R.M.D., *et al.* (1995). Video-endoscopic surgical treatment of perforating veins. Phlebology '95 (ed. D. Negus, G. Jantet, and P. Coleridge Smith). *Phlebology*, **Suppl. 1**, 991.

Haeger, K. (1977). Leg ulcers. In: *The treatment of venous disorders* (ed. J.T. Hobbs), pp. 272–91. MTP, Lancaster.

Hobbs, J.T. (1988). The enigma of the gastrocnemius vein. *Phlebology*, **3**, 19–30.

Johnston, T.B. and Whillis, J. (1938). *Gray's Anatomy*, p. 666. Longmans Green, London. (It is stated that valves 'are absent in the very small veins, i.e. less than 2 mm in diameter'. This is a general reference, not specifically related to perforating veins, but does raise the possibility that many lesser perforating veins are valveless and, collectively, a number of these could allow appreciable outward flow in certain conditions in the normal limb.)

Linton, R.R. (1938). The communicating veins of the lower leg and the operative technic for their ligation. *Ann. Surg.*, **107**, 582–93.

Linton, R.R. (1953). The post-thrombotic ulceration of the lower extremity: its etiology and surgical treatment. *Ann. Surg.*, **138**, 415–33.

Lockhart-Mummery, H.E. and Smitham, J.H. (1951). Varicose ulcer. *Br. J. Surg.*, **38**, 284.

McMullin, G.M., Scott, H.J., Coleridge Smith, P.D., and Scurr, J.H. (1990). A reassessment of the role of perforating veins in chronic venous insufficiency. *Phlebology*, **5**, 85–94.

May, R. (1979). *Surgery of the veins of the leg and pelvis.* Saunders, Philadelphia, PA.

May, R., Partsch, P., and Staubesand, J. (ed.). (1981). *Perforating veins.* Urban & Schwarzenberg, Munich.

Negus, D. (1985). Perforating vein interruption in the postphlebitic syndrome. In: *Surgery of the veins.* (ed. J.J. Borgan and J.S.T. Yao), pp. 191–204. Grune and Stratton, New York.

Stacey, M.C., Burnand, K.G., Layer, G.T., and Pattison, M. (1988). Calf pump function in patients with healed venous ulcers is not improved by surgery to the communicating veins or by elastic stockings. *Br. J. Surg.*, **75**, 436–9.

Thomson, H. (1979). The surgical anatomy of the superficial and perforating veins of the lower limb. *Ann. R. Coll. Surg Engl.*, **61**, 198–205.

Vandenriessche, M. (1989). The association between gastrocnemial vein insufficiency and varicose veins, (includes 'Invited comment' by A.N. Nicoliades, D. Christopoulos, and S. Vasdekis). *Phlebology*, **4**, 171–84.

Zukowski, A.J., Nicolaides, A.N., Szendro, G., *et al.* (1991). Haemodynamic significance of incompetent perforating veins. *Br. J. Surg.*, **78**, 625–9.

Chapter 8 Congenital venous disorders
General

Browse, N.L., Whimster, I., Stewart, G., *et al.* (1986). Surgical management of 'lymphangioma circumscriptum'. *Br. J. Surg.*, **73**, 585–8.

Browse, N.L., Burnand, K.G., and Lea Thomas, M. (1988). *Diseases of the veins*. Arnold, London.

Carruth, J.A.S. (1984). Argon laser in the treatment of port wine stain. *J.R. Soc. Med.*, **77**, 722–4.

Dodd, H. and Cockett, F.B. (1976). *The pathology and surgery of the veins of the lower limb*, pp. 160–70. Churchill Livingstone, Edinburgh.

Friedman, E.I., Taylor, L.M., and Porter J.M. (1988) Congenital venous valvular aplasia of the lower extremities. *Surgery*, **103**, 24–6.

Hollier, L.H. (1985). Surgical treatment of congenital venous malformations. In: *Surgery of the veins* (ed. J.J. Bergan and J.S.T. Yao), pp. 275–84. Grune and Stratton, London, 1985.

Kheterpal, S. (1991). Angiodysplasia: a review. *J.R. Soc. Med.*, **84**, 615–18.

Kinmonth, J.B. (1972). *The lymphatics: diseases, investigation and treatment*. Arnold, London.

Kinmonth, J.B., Young, A.E., Edwards, J.M., *et al.* (1976). Mixed vascular deformities of the lower limbs, with particular reference to lymphography and surgical treatment. *Br. J. Surg.*, **63**, 899–906.

Lawler, F. and Charles-Holmes, S. (1988). Uterine haemangioma in Klippel–Trenaunay–Weber syndrome. *J.R. Soc. Med.*, **81**, 665–6.

Lea Thomas, M. (1982). *Phlebography of the lower limb*. Churchill Livingstone, Edinburgh

Lechter, A., Lopez, G., Theuzaba, E., *et al.* Angiomatosis at the saphenofemoral junction. *Phlebology*, **8**, 167–70.

Lodin, A. and Lindvall, N. (1961). Congenital absence of valves in the deep veins of the leg. A factor in venous insufficiency. *Acta Dermatol. Venereol. (Stockholm)*, **41** (Suppl. 45), 7–91.

Malan, J.B. and Puglionsi, A. (1964). Congenital angiodysplasias of the extremities. 1: Generalities and classification, venous dysplasia. *J. Cardiovasc. Surg.*, **5**, 87.

Mulliker, J.B. and Young, A.E. (1986). *Vascular birthmarks: haemangiomas and malformations*. Saunders, Philadelphia, PA.

Partsch, B., Mayer, W., and Partsch, H. (1992). Improvement in ambulatory venous hupertension by narrowing of the femoral vein in congential absence of venous valves. *Phlebology*, **7**, 101–4.

Paes, E. and Volmar, J. (1995). Diagnosis and surgical aspects of congenital venous angiodysplasia in the extemities. *Phlebology*, **10**, 160–4.

Rabe, E. (1987). Acute and chronic venous insufficiency in infancy and childhood. *Phlebology*, **2**, 249–55.

Tibbs, D.J. (1953). Metastasizing haemangiomata. *Br. J. Surg.*, **40**, 465–70.

van der Stricht, J. (1988). Classification of vascular malformations. *Phlebology*, **3**, 203–6.

Young, A.E. (1983). Maldevelopments of the vascular system: clinical conundrums. In: *Development of the vascular system, Ciba Found. Symp. 100*, pp. 222–43. Pitman, London.

Bone overgrowth

Clarke, P.J., Tibbs, D.J., and Kenwright, J. (1986). Bone overgrowth and vascular anomalies in the limbs; combined experience of an orthopaedic centre and a vascular clinic. In: *Phlebology' 85* (ed. D. Negus and G. Jantet), pp. 798–800. Libbey, London.

McCullough, C.J. and Kenwright, J. (1970). The prognosis in congenital lower limb hypertrophy. *Acta Orthop. Scand.*, **50**, 307–13.

Parkes-Weber, F. (1907). Angioma formation in connection with hypertrophy of the limbs and hemihypertrophy. *Br. J. Dermatol.*, **19**, 231.

Parkes-Weber, F. (1918). Haemangiectactic hypertrophy of limbs—congenital phlebarteriectasis and so-called congenital varicose veins. *Br. J. Child. Dis.*, **15**.

Venous dysplasias and Klippel–Trenaunay syndrome

Baskerville, P.A., Ackroyd, J.S., Lea Thomas, M., and Browse, N.L. (1985). The Klippel–Trenaunay syndrome: clinical, radiological and haemodynamic features and management. *Br. J. Surg.*, **72**, 232–6.

Baskerville, P.A., Ackroyd, J.S., and Browse, N.L. (1986). Is the Klippel–Trenaunay syndrome a mesodermal abnormality? In: *Phlebology '85* (ed. D. Negus and G. Jantet), pp. 767–9. Libbey, Paris.

Gloviczki, P., Hollier, L.H., Telander, R.L., *et al.* (1983). Surgical implications of Klippel–Trenaunay syndrome. *Ann. Surg.*, **197**, 353–62.

Gorenstein, A., Katz, S., and Schiller, M. (1988). Congenital angiodysplasia of the superficial venous system of the lower extremities in children. *Ann. Surg.*, **207**, 213–18.

Klippel, M. and Trenaunay, P. (1900). Du noevus osteo-hypertrophique. *Arch. Gen. Med.*, **3**, 641–7.

Lawlor, F. and Charles-Holmes, S. (1988). Uterine haemangioma in Klippel–Treanaunay–Weber syndrome. *J.R. Soc. Med.*, **81**, 665–6.

Lendorf, A., Struckmann, J., Strange-Vognsen, H.H., and Nielsen, S.L. (1988). Congenital angiodysplasia of the lower limb: the Klippel–Trenaunay syndrome and arteriovenous fistulae. *Phlebology*, **3**, 31–9.

Lindenauer, M.S. (1971). Congenital arteriovenous fistula and the Klippel–Trenaunay syndrome. *Ann. Surg.*, **174**, 248–63.

Parkes-Weber, F. (1907). Angioma formation in connection with hypertrophy of the limbs and hemihypertrophy. *Br. J. Dermatol.*, **19**, 231.

Parkes-Weber, F. (1918). Haemangiectactic hypertrophy of limbs—congenital phlebarteriectasis and so-called congenital varicose veins. *Br. J. Child. Dis.*, **15**, 13.

Samuel, M. and Spitz, L. (1995). Klippel–Trenaunay syndrome: clinical features, complications and management in children. *Br. J. Surg.*, **82**, 757–61.

Swinn, M.J. and Hargreaves, D.G. (1996). Consequences of lymphatic malformations in the Klippel–Trenaunay syndrome. *J.R. Soc. Med.*, **89**, 106P–7P.

Taheri, S.A., Williams, J., Bowman, L., and Pisano, S. (1988). Superficial femoral vein transposition in Klippel-Trenaunay syndrome. *Phlebology*, **3**, 123–7.

Congenital arteriovenous fistulas

Askerkhanov, R.P. (1972). Clinical aspects and treatment of arteriovenous fistulae. *Khirurgiya (Mosk.), Eng. Abstr.*, **48**, 98–102.

Braithwaite, F. and Tibbs, D. (1955). A case of localised arteriovenous fistulae. *Br. J. Surg.*, **42**, 442–3.

Branham, H.H. (1890). Aneurysmal varix of the femoral artery and vein following gunshot wound. *Int. J. Surg.*, **3**, 250–1.

Cotton, L.T. and Sykes, B.J. (1969). The treatment of diffuse congenital arterio-venous fistulae of the leg. *Proc. R. Soc. Med.*, **62**, 245–7.

Gomes, M.M.R. and Bernatz, P.E. (1970). Arteriovenous fistulas: a review and ten-year experience at the Mayo Clinic. *Mayo Clin. Proc.*, **45**, 81–102.

Greenhalgh, R.M., Rosengarten, D.S., and Calnan, J.S. (1972). A single congenital arteriovenous fistula of the hand. *Br. J. Surg.*, **59**, 76–8.

Haughton, V.M. (1975). Hemoclip- Gelfoam emboli in the treatment of facial arteriovenous malformations. *Neuroradiology*, **10**, 69–71.

Holman, E. (1923). The physiology of an arteriovenous fistula. *Arch. Surg.*, **7**, 64–82.

Holman, E. (1924). Arteriovenous aneurism. *Ann. Surg.*, **December**, 801–16.

Holman, E. (1937). *Arteriovenous aneurysm*. Macmillan, New York.

Lindenauer, M.S. (1971). Congenital arteriovenous fistula and the Klippel–Trenaunay syndrome. *Ann. Surg.*, **174**, 248–63.

Sako, Y. and Varco, R.L. (1970). Arteriovenous fistula: results of managment of congenital and acquired forms, blood flow measurements, and observations on proximal arterial degeneration. *Surgery*, **67**, 40–61.

Parkes-Weber, F. (1907). Angioma formation in connection with hypertrophy of the limbs and hemihypertrophy. *Br. J. Dermatol.*, **19**, 231.

Parkes-Weber, F. (1918). Haemangiectactic hypertrophy of limbs—congenital phlebarteriectasis and so-called congenital varicose veins. *Br. J. Child. Dis.*, **15**, 13.

Partsch, H., Mostbeck, A., and Wolf, C. (1986). AV shunts in congenital vascular malformations of the limbs. New approaches to diagnosis. In: *Phlebology '85* (ed. D. Negus and G. Jantet), pp. 791–4. Libbey, London.

Riche, M.C., Melki, J.P., Laurian, C., *et al.* (1986). Le role de l'hyperpresson veineuse dans les malformations arterioveineuses des membres. In: *Phlebology '85* (ed. D. Negus and G. Jantet), pp. 801–3. Libbey, London.

Sako, Y. and Varco, R.L. (1970). Arteriovenous fistula: results of management of congenital and acquired forms, blood flow measurements, and observations on proximal arterial degeneration. *Surgery*, **67**, 40–61.

Schwartz, R.S., Osmundson, P.J., and Hollier, L.H. (1986). Treatment and prognosis in congenital arteriovenous malformation of the extremity. *Phlebology*, **1**, 171–80.

Chapter 9 Ulcers of the leg

Venous ulcers

General

Adair, H.M. (1977). Epidermal repair in chronic venous ulcers. *Br. J. Surg.*, **64**, 800–4.

Alexander House Group (1992). Consensus paper on venous leg ulcers. *Phlebology*, **7**, 48–58.

Allen, S. (1991). Venous ulceration in drug abusers: an important physical sign. *Phlebology*, **6**, 47–8.

Blair, S.D. Wright, D.D.I., Backhouse, C.M., *et al.* (1988). Sustained compression and healing of chronic venous ulcers. *Br. Med. J.*, **297**, 1159–61.

Browse, N.L. and Burnand, K.G. (1978). The postphlebitic syndrome: a new look. In: *Venous problems* (ed. J.J. Bergan and J.S.T. Yao), pp. 395–405. Year Book, Chicago, IL.

Buxton, P.K. (1987). Leg ulcers. *Br. Med. J.*, **295**, 1542–5.

Callam, M.J., Ruckley, C.V., Harper, D.R., and Dale, J.J. (1985). Chronic ulceration of the leg: extent of the problem and provision of care. *Br. Med. J.*, **290**, 1855–6.

Callam, M.J., Harper, D.R., Dale, J.J., and Ruckley, C.V. (1987). Chronic ulcer of the leg: clinical history. *Br. Med. J.*, **294**, 1389–91.

Cornwall, J.V., Dore, C.J., and Lewis, J.D. (1986). Leg ulcers: epidemiology and aetiolgy. *Br. J. Surg.*, **73**, 693–6.

Dickson Wright, A. The treatment of varicose ulcer. *Proc. R. Soc. Med.*, **23**, 1032.

Dickson Wright, A. (1931). The treatment of indolent ulcer of the leg. *Lancet*, 457–60.

Franks, P.J., Wright, D., and McCollum, C.N. (1989). Epidemiology of venous disease: a review. *Phlebology*, **4**, 143–51.

Hansson, C. and Holm, J. (1995). Frequency of isolated superficial incompetence in patients with venous ulcers as measured by ambulatory strain-gauge plethysmography. *Phlebology*, **10**, 65–8.

Lees, T.A. and Lambert, D. (1993). Patterns of venous reflux in limbs with skin changes associated with chronic venous insufficiency. *Br. J. Surg.*, **80**, 725–8.

Lockhart-Mummery, H.E. and Smitham, J.H. (1951). Varicose ulcer. *Br. J. Surg.*, **38**, 284–95.

McQueen, A. (1980). The skin. In: *Muir's textbook of pathology* (ed. J.R. Anderson), pp. 1049–85. Arnold, London.

Negus, D. (1991). *Leg ulcers*. Butterworth-Heinemann, Oxford.

Rivlin, S. (1951). *The treatment of varicose veins and their complications*. William Heinemann, London.

Rivlin, S. (1958). Gravitational leg ulcer in the elderly. *Lancet*, **i**, 1363–7.

Ryan, T.J. (1987). *The management of leg ulcers* (2nd edn), p. 101. Oxford University Press, Oxford.

Ryan, T.J. and Wilkinson, D.S. (1986). Diseases of the veins and arteries: leg ulcers. In: *Textbook of dermatology* (ed. F.J.G. Ebling, A. Rook, and D.S. Wilkinson), pp. 1187–1227. Blackwell, Oxford.

Shami, S.K., Chittenden, S.J., Scurr, J.H., and Coleridge Smith, P.D. (1993). Skin blood flow in chronic venous insufficiency. *Phlebology*, **8**, 72–6.

Widmer, L.K., Mall, Th., and Martin, H. (1977). Epidemiology and socio-medical importance of peripheral venous disease. In: *The treatment of venous disorders* (ed. J.T. Hobbs), pp. 3–11. MTP, Lancaster.

Factors in causation

Baker, S.R., Stacey, M.C., Jopp-McKay, A.G., *et al.* (1991). Epidemiology of chronic venous ulcers. *Br. J. Surg.*, **78**, 864–7.

Balaji, P. and Mosley, J.G. Evaluation of vascular and metabolic deficiency in patients with large leg ulcers. *Ann. R. Coll. Surg. Engl.*, **77**, 270–2.

Braasch, D. Red cell deformability and capillary blood flow. *Physiol. Rev.*, **51**, 679.

Browse, N. (1985). The pathogenesis of venous ulceration. In: *Surgery of the veins* (ed. J.J. Borgan and J.S.T. Yao), pp. 25–31. Grune and Stratton, New York.

Burnand, K.G., Whimster, I., Clemenson, G., *et al.* (1981). The relationship between the number of capillaries in the skin of the venous ulcer-bearing area of the lower leg and the fall in foot vein pressure during exercise. *Br. J. Surg.*, **68**, 297–300.

Burnand, K.G., Whimster, I., Naidoo, A., *et al.* Pericapillary fibrin in the ulcer bearing skin of the lower leg. The cause of lipodermatosclerosis and venous ulceration. *Br. Med. J.*, **285**, 1071–72.

Cheatle, T.R., McMullin, G.M., Farrah, J., *et al.* (1990). Skin damage in chronic venous insufficiency: does an oxygen diffusion barrier really exist? *J. R. Soc. Med.*, **83**, 493–4.

Cheatle, T.R., Stibe, E.C.L., Shami, S.K., *et al.* (1991). Vasodilatory capacity of the skin in venous disease and its relationship to transcutaneous oxygen tension. *Br. J. Surg.*, **78**, 607–10.

Coleridge Smith, P.D., Thomas, P., Scurr, J.H., and Dormandy, J.A. (1988). Causes of venous ulceration: a new hypothesis. *Br. Med. J.*, **296**, 1726–7.

Dormandy, J.A. (1979). Clinical importance of blood viscosity. *Viscositas*, **1**, 5.

Duruble, M. and Ouvry, P. (1991). Haemodilution in venous disease. *Phlebology*, **6**, 31–6.

Gilliland, E.L., Dore, C.J., Nathwani, N., and Lewis, J.D. (1988). Bacterial colonisation of leg ulcers and its effect on the sucess rate of skin grafting. *Ann. R. Coll. Surg. Engl.*, **70**, 105–8.

Grimaudo, V., Gueissaz, F., Hauert, J., *et al.* (1989). Necrosis of skin induced by coumarin in a patient deficient in protein S. *Br. Med. J.*, **298**, 233–4.

Owens, C.W.I., Al-Khader, A.A., Jackson, M.J., and Prichard, B.N.C. (1981). A severe 'stasis eczema', associated with low plasma zinc, treated successfully with oral zinc. *Br. J. Dermatol.*, **105**, 461–4.

Pflug, J.J. and Davies, D.M. (1985). Chronic swelling of the leg and stasis ulcer. *Br. Med. J.*, **290**, 1273–6.

Prasad, A., Ali-Khan, A., and Mortimer, P. (1990). Leg ulcers and oedema: a study exploring the prevalence, aetiology, and possible significance of oedema in venous ulcers. *Phlebology*, **5**, 181–7.

Reid, H.L., Dormandy, J.A., Barnes, A.J., *et al.* (1976). Impaired red cell deformability in peripheral vascular disease. *Lancet*, **i**, 666.

Ryan, T.J. and Cherry, G.W. (1985). The assessment of vascular abnormalities of the leg. In: *Recent advances in dermatology* (ed. R.H. Champion), pp. 87–101. Churchill Livingstone, Edinburgh.

Schraibman, I.G. (1987). The bacteriology of leg ulcers. *Phlebology*, **2**, 265–70.

Schraibman, I.G. and Stratton, F.J. (1985). Nutritional status of patients with leg ulcers. *J. R. Soc. Med.*, **78**, 39–42.

Senapati, A. and Thompson, R.P.H. (1985). Zinc deficiency and the prolonged accumulation of zinc in wounds. *Br. J. Surg.*, **72**, 583–4.

Stacey, M.C., Burnand, K.G., Pattison, M., *et al.* (1987). Changes in the apparently normal limb in unilateral venous ulceration. *Br. J. Surg.*, **74**, 936–9.

Stacey, M.C., Burnand, K.G., Layer, G.T., and Pattison, M. (1990). Transcutaneous oxygen tension in assessing the treatment of healed venous ulcers. *Br. J. Surg.*, **77**, 1050–4.

Stewart, J.B., Cherry, C.A., Cherry, G.W., and Ryan, T.J. Lymphatic function in patients with venous leg ulcers. *J. Invest. Dermatol.*, **92**, 523.

Thomas, P.R.S., Nash, G.B., and Dormandy, J.A. (1988). White cell accumulation in dependent legs of patients with venous hypertension: a possible mechanism for trophic changes in the skin. *Br. Med. J.*, **296**, 1693–5.

Vanscheidt, W., Kress, O., Hach-Wunderle, V., *et al.* (1992). Leg ulcer patient: no decreased fibrinolytic response but white cell trapping after venous occlusion of the upper limb. *Phlebology*, **7**, 92–4.

Pharmaceutical

Belcaro, G.V. (1986). Treatment of chronic venous hypertension of the lower lionbs by 0-(b- hydroxyethyl)-rutoside and elastic compression. In: *Phlebology '85* (ed. D. Negus and G. Jantet), pp. 834–6. Libbey, Paris.

Burnand, K., Clemenson, G., Morland, M., *et al.* (1980). Venous lipodermatosclerosis: treatment by fibrinolytic enhancement and elastic compression. *Br. Med. J.*, **1**, 7–11.

Colgan, M., Dormandy, J.A., Jones, P.W., *et al.* (1990). Oxpentifylline treatment of venous ulcers of the leg. *Br. Med. J.*, **300**, 972–4.

de Jongste, A.B., ten Cate, J.W., and Huisman, M.V. (1986). The effectiveness of *O*-(b-hydroxyethyl)-rutosides in the post-thrombotic syndrome. In: *Phlebology '85* (ed. D. Negus and G. Jantet), pp. 837–9. Libbey, London.

Layer, G.T., Powell, S., Pattison, M., and Burnand, K.G. (1986). Early results of a trial of adjuvant fibrinolytic enhancement therapy in the healing of venous ulcers. In: *Phlebology '85* (ed. D. Negus and G. Jantet), pp. 587–90. Libbey, London.

Leach, R.D. (1984). Venous ulceration, fibrinogen and fibrinolysis. *Ann. R. Coll. Surg. Eng.* **66**, 258–63.

Pulvertaft, T.B. (1986). General practice treatment of symptoms of venous insufficiency with oxerutins: results of a 660-patient multicentre study in the UK. In: *Phlebology '85* (D. Negus and G. Jantet), pp. 853–6. Libbey, London.

Weitgasser, H. (1983). The use of pentoxifylline ('Trental' 400) in the treatment of leg ulcers: results of a double-blind trial. *Pharmatherapeutica*, **3**, 143–51.

Which? Consumers' Association. (1985). Does Stanozolol prevent venous ulceration? *Drug Ther. Bull.*, **2**, 91–2.

Relationship to ischaemia

Callam, M.J., Harper, D.R., Dale, J.J., and Ruckley, C.V. (1987). Arterial disease in chronic leg ulceration: an underestimated hazard. *Br. Med. J.*, **294**, 929–31.

Callam, M.J., Ruckley, C.V., Dale, J.J., and Harper, D.R., (1987). Hazards of compression treatment of the leg from Scottish surgeons. *Br. Med. J.*, **295**, 1382.

Kulozik, M., Cherry, G.W., and Ryan, T.J. (1986). The importance of measuring the ankle brachial systolic pressure ratio in the management of leg ulcers. *Br. J. Dermatol.*, **115**, 26.

Moffat, C.J., Oldroyd, M.I., Greenhalgh, R.M., and Franks, P.J. (1994). Palpating ankle pulses is insufficient in detecting arterial insufficiency in patients with leg ulceration. *Phlebology*, **9**, 170–2.

Applications and dressings

Backhouse, C.M., Blair, S.D., Savage, A.P., *et al.* (1987). Controlled trial of occlusive dressings in healing chronic venous ulcers. *Br. J. Surg.*, **74**, 625–7.

Beaconsfield, T., Genbacev, O., and Taylor, R.S. (1991). The treatment of long-standing venous ulcers with an extract of early placenta—a pilot study. *Phlebology*, **6**, 153–8.

Callam, M.J., Harper, D.R., Dale, J.J., *et al.* (1992). Lothian and Forth Valley Leg Ulcer Healing Trial, Part 2: knitted viscose dressing versus a hydrocellular dressing in the treatment of chronic leg ulceration. *Phlebology*, **7**, 142–5.

Cherry, G.W., Ryan, T., and McGibbon, D. (1984). Trial of a new dressing in venous leg ulcers. *Practitioner*, **228**, 1175–8.

Efem, S.E.E. (1988). Clinical observations on the wound healing properties of honey. *Br. J. Surg.*, **75**, 679–81.

Lucarotti, M.E., Morgan, A.P., and Leaper, D.J. (1990). The effect of antiseptics and the moist wound environment on ulcer healing: an experimental and biochemical study. *Phlebology*, **5**, 173–9.

Moffat, C.J., Franks, P.J., Oldroyd, M.I., and Greenhalgh, R.M. (1992). Randomized trial of an occlusive dressing in the treatment of chronic non-healing leg ulcers. *Phlebology*, **7**, 115–97.

Partsch, H. (1991). Treatment of resistant leg ulcers by retrograde intravenous pressure infusions of urokinase. *Phlebology*, **6**, 13–21.

Rasmussen, L.H., Karlsmark, T., Avnstorp, C., *et al.* (1991). Topical human growth hormone treatment of chronic leg ulcers. *Phlebology*, **6**, 23–30.

Ryan, T.J. (1985). An environment for healing—the role of occlusion. *Proc. R. Soc. Med. Int. Congr. Symp. Ser.*, **88**, 1–158.

Ryan, T.J. (1988). Beyond occlusion: wound care. *Proc. R. Soc. Med. Int. Congr. Symp. Ser.*, **136**, 141.

Which? Consumers' Association (1986). Skin sensitisers in topical corticosteroids. *Drug Ther. Bull.*, **24**, 57–9.

Wood, M.K. and Davies, D.M. Use of split-skin grafting in the treatment of chronic leg ulcers. *Ann. R. Coll. Surg. Engl.*, **77**, 222–3.

Zumla, A. and Lulat, A. (1989). Honey—a remedy rediscovered. *J. R. Soc. Med.*, **82**, 384–5.

Ischaemic ulcer

Callam, M.J., Harper, D.R., Dale, J.J., and Ruckley, C.V. (1987). Arterial disease in chronic leg ulceration: an underestimated hazard. *Br. Med. J.*, **294**, 929–31.

Eastcott, H.H.G. (1969). *Arterial surgery*. Pitman Medical, London.

Tibbs, D.J. (1962). Acute ischaemia of the limbs. *Proc. R. Soc. Med.*, 593–6.

Diabetic ulcer

Cook, T.A., Rahim, N., Simpson, H.C.R., and Galland, R.B. (1996). Magnetic resonance imaging in the management of diabetic foot infection. *Br. J. Surg.*, **83**, 245–8.

Irwin, S.T., Gilmore, J., McGrann, S., *et al.* (1988). Blood flow in diabetics with foot lesions due to 'small vessel disease'. *Br. J. Surg.*, **75**, 1201–6.

Warren, A.G. (1989). The surgical conservation of the neuropathic foot. *Ann. R. Coll. Surg.*, **71**, 236–42.

Malignant ulcer

Berth-Jones, J., Graham-Brown, R.A.C., Fletcher, A., *et al.* (1989). Malignant fibrous histiocytoma: a new complication of chronic venous ulceration. *Br. Med. J.*, **298**, 231–2.

Damstra, R.J. and Toonstra, J. (1992). Cutaneous B-cell lymphoma mimicking ulcus cruris venosum. *Phlebology*, **7**, 82–4.

Gajraj, H., Barker, S.G.E., Burnand, K.G., and Browse, N.L. (1987). Lymphangiosarcoma complicating chronic primary lymphoedema. *Br. J. Surg.*, **74**, 1180.

Hassan, S.A., Cheatle, T.R., and Fox, J.A. (1993). Marjolin's ulcer: a report of three cases and review of the literatiure. *Phlebology*, **8**, 34–5.

Hughes, L.E., Horgan, K., Taylor, B.A., and Laidler, P. (1985). Malignant melanoma of the hand and foot: diagnosis and management. *Br. J. Surg.*, **72**, 811–15.

Lagattolla, N.R.F. and Burnand, K.G. (1994). Chronic venous disease may delay the diagnosis of malignant ulceration of the leg. *Phlebology*, **9**, 167–9.

Stringer, M.D., Melcher, D., and Stachan, C.L.J. (1986). The lower limb as a presenting site of malignant lymphoma. *Ann. R. Coll. Surg. Engl.*, **68**, 8–11.

Which? Consumer's Association (1988). Malignant melanoma of the skin. *Drug Ther. Bull.*, **26**, 73–5.

Tropical ulcer

Fahal, A.H. and Hassan, M.A. (1992). Mycetoma. *Br. J. Surg.*, **79**, 1138–41.

Manson-Bahr, P.E.C. and Bell, D.R. (1987). *Manson's Tropical diseases*. Ballière Tindall, London.

Marsden, P.D. (1990). Cutaneous leishmaniasis. *Br. Med. J.*, **300**, 1716–17.

Acknowledgements: Part 1

We are indebted to Butterworth-Heinemann Ltd for permission to use many illustrations from: Tibbs DJ. (1992). *Varicose veins and related disorders*. Butterworth-Heinemann Ltd, Oxford. The numerous functional phlebograms in this book were obtained with much skill and patience by EWL Fletcher, Consultant Vascular Radiologist, John Radcliffe Hospital, Oxford. Most of the artwork was prepared by Sylvia Barker, Gillian Lee, and David Tibbs. In the present book this artwork has been redrawn computer-graphically by the Illustration Department of Oxford University Press and to this has been added a number of fresh computer-graphic illustrations by David Tibbs. The best of the original clinical photographs are by David Floyd, but added to these are many 'snapshots' hurriedly taken as opportunity presented in outpatient clinic, theatre, or ward.

The colour scan duplex ultrasonograms in Parts I & II have been provided by J.H. Scurr, P.D. Coleridge Smith, and John Farrah. Dr Naghmana Riazuddin and Allison Bullivant were photographed whilst ably demonstrating practical aspects of ultrasonographic scanning and microsclerotherapy. Jo Mowinski gave indispensible secretarial support.

Other acknowledgements are made individually in captions to illustrations.

The publishers would like to thank Mr David Tibbs for all his assistance with the illustrative material.

Part II

Acute deep vein thrombosis and pulmonary embolism

Mark G. Davies and David C. Sabiston, Jr

10 Acute deep vein thrombosis and pulmonary embolism

Historical aspects

In the peripheral veins, the danger proceeds chiefly from the small branches. By no means rarely do these become quite filled with masses of coagulum. As long, however, as the thrombus is confined to the branch itself so long as the body is not exposed ... only the greater number of the thrombi in the small branches do not content themselves with advancing up to the level of the main trunk, but pretty constantly new masses of coagulum deposit themselves from the blood upon the end of the thrombus layer after layer, the thrombus is prolonged beyond the mouth of the branch into the trunk in the direction of the current of blood, shoots out in the form of a thick cylinder farther and farther and becomes continually larger and larger. From a lumbar vein, for example a plug may extend into the vena cava as thick as the last phalanx of the thumb. There as the thrombi that constitute the source of real danger, it is in them that ensues the crumbling away which leads to secondary occlusion in remote vessels. (Virchow 1856)

In 1856, Virchow introduced the concept of embolism as a result of his extensive autopsy studies. He observed the frequent clinical association of thrombi in the veins of the leg and pelvis with pulmonary embolism and that these thrombi were the same histological age as those found in the lungs.[1] He further characterized this phenomenon by observing that when thrombi were injected into the femoral veins of animals, they ultimately lodged in the lungs. Virchow concluded that thrombi formed in the systemic veins and that they were caused by one or more of three conditions: reduced blood flow in the systemic veins, injury within the veins, and a state of hypercoagulability. These factors remain important in the pathogenesis of pulmonary embolism and are known as 'Virchow's triad'.

The lesion consists of an induration, which is partial and never occupies a large portion of the lung; its usual size is 1 to 4 cubic inches. The surrounding parenchyma is entirely normal—the swollen part is very dark red. The cut surface shows granularity like the hepatized lung, but otherwise these two conditions are entirely different from each other. One encounters two or three such engorgements in one lung and rather frequently both lungs are similarly affected. (Laennec 1819)

Laennec described pulmonary embolism as 'pulmonary apoplexy' and differentiated the condition from other pulmonary disorders that could cause haemoptysis.[2] Rokitansky confirmed Laennec's findings in 1842 and also introduced the term 'haemorrhagic infarct'.[3] Most consider this condition to be a primary process of the pulmonary vasculature and not a secondary phenomenon. The source of these pulmonary thrombi remained unresolved until Virchow's descriptions of the association between peripheral venous thrombosis and pulmonary embolism in 1847.[1] From his experimental work, Virchow showed that embolism alone did not produce pulmonary infarcts and suspected that bronchial collateral circulation present in the pulmonary system prevented most pulmonary emboli from causing infarction. In 1872, Cohnheim showed that not all patients with pulmonary embolism have concomitant pulmonary infarction and that associated congestive heart failure is an important part of the infarction process.[4] In 1948, Blalock confirmed Virchow's earlier findings on pulmonary collateral circulation with the observation of bright red blood perfusing the pulmonary vessels distal to chronic emboli. Collateral perfusion of the lungs by bronchial vessels was confirmed angiographically by Viamonte in 1964.[5] Trendelenburg performed the first pulmonary embolectomy in 1908, describing emergent thoracotomy and removal of emboli in three patients, all of whom succumbed within 40 h.[6,7] In 1924 Kirschner performed the first pulmonary embolectomy with long-term survival.[8] In 1962 Sharp was the first to perform pulmonary embolectomy with cardiopulmonary bypass.[9] The first ante-mortem diagnosis of chronic pulmonary embolism was made in 1950 by Carroll,[10] and the first successful embolectomy for recurrent pulmonary emboli was described by Allison in 1960.[11] In 1987 Daily and colleagues reported bilateral thromboendarterectomies via median sternotomy and extrapericardial dissection of the pulmonary arteries, and in 1989 they reported a series of 100 consecutive patients treated with cardiopulmonary bypass, deep hypothermia, and intermittent circulatory arrest to facilitate embolectomy.[12]

Epidemiology

Venous thromboembolic disease remains a significant problem affecting 2.5 million people each year in the United States. There are more than a quarter of a million hospital admissions each year in the United States for acute deep vein thrombosis and pulmonary embolism.[13–15] In hospital patients without prophylaxis, it is estimated that the incidence of isolated calf deep vein thrombosis (DVT) and proximal DVT is 25 per cent and 7 per cent respectively.[15,16] When thrombosis is proximal to the calf, there is a 50 per cent likelihood of pulmonary embolism. There are geographical differences in reports on DVT, with up to twice the reported incidence of calf DVT in Europe compared with North America.[16] 'Virchow's triad' remains a reasonable basis on which to base the risk assessments for DVT. Consistently quoted risk factors for DVT and odds ratios for DVT are listed in Tables 10.1 and 10.2.[17,18]

Pulmonary thromboembolic disease is cited as the primary cause of death in 100 000 patients each year and is considered to be a contributing cause of death in another 100 000 patients.[19] Fifty per cent of deaths from pulmonary embolism are in patients with a low life expectancy, whereas the remainder occur in patients with an overall favourable prognosis.[20] Routine autopsies in patients over 40 show that two-thirds have either gross or microscopic evidence of pulmonary emboli. Other autopsy studies consistently demonstrate that approximately 10 per cent of deaths in hospital are due to pulmonary embolism.[13–15] Ninety per cent of clinically important pulmonary embolism result from lower-limb DVT.[21] When no risk factors present, it is unusual for a patient to develop venous thromboembolism.[22] The risk increases in direct proportion to the number of predisposing factors identified (Tables 10.1 and 10.3).[18,22]

Of the approximately 200 000 patients who succumb from pulmonary embolism, approximately 11 per cent die within the first hour. The diagnosis is not made in 70 per cent of the survivors, and the mortality of this group is 30 per cent.[2] The estimated risk of death from a pulmonary embolus after a surgical procedure is 0.11 per cent. There has been a progressive increase in the incidence of death from pulmonary embolism and pulmonary infarction in the United States and Europe. This increase has been attributed to increasing numbers of the elderly, greater incidence and magnitude of operative procedures, increased clinical recognition, and the use of oral contraceptives. Most patients with pulmonary embolism have an active fibrinolytic system which causes rapid resolution of pulmonary emboli. Most pulmonary emboli present as acute clinical problems that resolve with few-long term sequelae. In general, it appears that major pulmonary perfusion defects resolve by 21 days after embolism, but may be delayed by congestive cardiac failure.

Intravascular coagulation

Primary haemostasis is a factor of platelet activation while secondary haemostasis is dependent on the coagulation cascades. The normal role of platelets is the arrest of bleeding (physiological haemostasis), and their pathological role is in the formation of vaso-occlusive thrombi (pathological thrombus). Thrombosis is initiated when alterations in the properties of the vascular endothelium allow platelets to adhere to the endothelial cells or to the subendothelial connective tissue (Fig. 10.1). Initial contact of a platelet under high-flow conditions is mediated by the interaction of platelet glycoprotein Ib (GPIb complex) with von Willibrand's factor (vWF), an adhesive molecule in the subendothelium. Early contact under conditions of low flow can be mediated by other platelet receptors, such as GPIa-IIa complex (VLA-2) and GPIc-IIa complex (VLA-5), and components of the extracellular matrix (collagen and fibronectin). The platelets change shape from smooth discs to spiny spheres and spread out. Spreading of platelets is mediated by vWF and by platelet GP IIb-IIIc interacting with vWF, vibronectin, and fibronectin. Following adhesion, activated platelets undergo the release of prepackaged platelet granule constituents (ADP from dense granules and fibrinogen from the α-granules). Adherence of platelets stimulates enzymes that catalyse the release of arachidonic acid, which in turn is converted by cyclo-oxygenase into thromboxane A_2, increasing phospholipase C activity and

Table 10.1   Risk factors for venous thromboembolism

Age over 40

Male

Obesity

Presence of malignancy

Presence of varicose veins

Prior deep venous thrombosis or pulmonary embolism

Type of procedure

    Orthopaedic

    Neurosurgical

    Urological

    Gynaecological

    Any procedure lasting more than 2 h

Oral contraceptive pill

Pregnancy

Presence of hypercoagulable disorder

Adapted from ref. 18.

Table 10.2   Proximal deep venous thrombosis: correlation factors

Deep venous thrombosis signs or symptoms	1:3
Major abdominal surgery (no prophylaxis)	1:20
Major abdominal surgery (prophylaxis)	1:50
Hospital in patients	1:100
General US population (per year)	1:2000

Adapted from ref. 17.

Table 10.3   The proportion of patients with clinically suspected DVT in whom diagnosis was confirmed by objective testing increases with the number of risk factors

Number of risk factors	Confirmed DVT (%)
0	11
1	24
2	36
3	50
4 or more	100

Adapted from ref. 22.

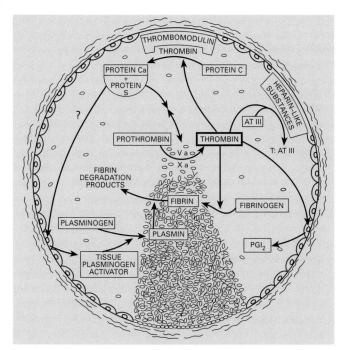

Fig. 10.1 Formation of the haemostatic plug at the site of vascular injury and its control by physiological antithrombotic mechanisms. (Reproduced with permission from J. Loscalzo, M.A., Creager, and V.J. Dzau *Vascular medicine*, Little Brown, Boston, MA.)

further enhancing platelet responsiveness. Release of granules from platelets is partly dependent on *de novo* formation of thromboxane A_2. Platelets release a variety of mediators after activation, including ADP which modifies the platelet surface allowing fibrinogen to attach and link to adjacent platelets. Platelet secretion and degranulation cause adherence of platelets to form a platelet thrombus (a primary haemostatic plug). This thrombotic formation depends on fibrinogen which is derived from plasma and platelet α-granules, interacting with activated platelets via GP IIb-IIIa. Within 45 s of platelet activation, the enzyme thrombin is also formed which allows the local conversion of fibrinogen into fibrin and its adherence to and cross-linking of neighbouring platelets. Thus a platelet fibrin thrombus or a secondary haemostatic plug is formed that is more resistant to the shear stress of blood flow.

The regulation of intravascular coagulation is one of the primary functions of the endothelium.[24] This is achieved by four separate but related mechanisms: (1) participation in and separation of procoagulant pathways, (2) inhibition of procoagulant proteins, (3) regulation of fibrinolysis, and (4) production of thromboregulating compounds.[25] The focal point for the coagulation cascades is the generation of the enzyme thrombin which cleaves fibrinogen to form insoluble fibrin clot. The endothelium participates in this cascade by producing a number of co-factors including high-molecular-weight kininogen (HMWK), factor V, factor VIII, and tissue factor. Tissue factor is a procoagulant enzyme synthesized by the endothelium and is found mainly in the subendothelium. However, basal secretion of tissue factor by the endothelium is low compared with that of the underlying smooth muscle cells and fibroblasts. However, if stimulated or injured, the endothelial cells can increase tissue factor production by a factor of 10–40. The binding of factors VIII and X to the endothelial cell surface lowers the affinity of endothelial cells for factor IX, which allows the binding of factor IX_a and the formation

of IX_a–VIII complexes on the endothelial surface. Once bound to the endothelium, factor IX_a decay is significantly inhibited in the presence of factors VIII and X, thereby providing additional feedback for the perpetuation of cell-bound procoagulant activity. Finally, stimulated endothelial cells can express GMP-140, a surface receptor which preferentially binds platelets. The binding of platelets increases the local availability of platelet activating factor and further accelerates endothelial cell interaction with platelets.

The basic barrier function of the endothelium separates intravascular coagulation factors (factor VII_a) from tissue factor in the subendothelium and also prevents exposure of platelets to the proaggregating constituents of the subendothelium such as collagen and vWF.[26,27] Furthermore, endothelial cells produce and express on their extracellular surfaces small amounts of the proteoglycan heparan sulphate which serves to localize and increase the intrinsic activity of antithrombin III and tissue factor pathway inhibitor (TFPI). Although less than 1 per cent of plasma antithrombin III is bound to the endothelium, this bound pool is at least 1000-fold more reactive than the unbound pool. TFPI is synthesized and released by the endothelium; it complexes with apolipoprotein A-II by a disulphide linkage. This complex is bound to heparan sulphate and other glycosoaminoglycans on the surface of the endothelial cell and acts as a potent inhibitor of factor X_a through its interactions with factor X_a it produces feedback inhibition of the factor VII_a–tissue factor complex.

Endothelial cells inhibit procoagulant proteins with the autoregulatory protein C pathway consisting of three elements: protein C, protein S, and thrombomodulin.[28] After activation by thrombin, protein C_a inactivates factors V_a and VIII_a, and this activity is enhanced by thrombomodulin, an integral membrane glycoprotein on the luminal surface of endothelial cells. The activity of protein C_a is further potentiated by a second endothelial derived peptide, protein S. Protein S promotes the interaction of protein C_a with factors V_a and VIII_a. In addition to its facilitatory effects in the protein C pathway, thrombomodulin removes thrombin from the blood by complexing with the thrombin molecule, facilitating its internalization and subsequent intracellular degradation. As well as its direct effects on activated coagulant factors, protein C_a also increases endothelial cell fibrinolytic activity by complexing with and decreasing the activity of the plasminogen activator inhibitory protein PAI-1 and thereby increasing fibrinolysis. Finally, endothelial cells also secrete protease nexin I, a protease inhibitor that inactivates hrombin and facilitates its degradation by the endothelium.

The endothelium also participates in the regulation of fibrinolysis.[29] For fibrinolysis to occur, plasminogen must be converted to plasmin. Plasminogen (glu-plasminogen) binds to endothelial cells and is converted to a form (lys-plasminogen) which is more efficiently activated. Endothelial cells synthesize the plasminogen activators (PAs) as single-chain proteins, secrete and then bind them to allow their assembly into functional complexes. There are two forms of PA: the urokinase type (uPA) which activates plasminogen in the fluid phase and tissue PA (tPA) which is most active when bound to fibrin. *In vivo*, normal endothelial cells express tPA only. However, if stimulated by a variety of cytokines and circumstances, endothelial cells preferentially synthesize uPA and downregulate tPA synthesis. In addition to these two fibrinolytic enzymes, endothelial cells also secrete two PA inhibitors, PAI-1, and PAI-2. Both are serine protease inhibitors and form equimolar complexes with either active uPA or tPA molecules. PAI-1 requires the presence of vibronectin in the extracellular matrix to maintain its active conformation. It is inactive outside the matrix.

Finally, the endothelium is also a source of thromboregulators which can be defined as physiological substances that modulate the early phases of thrombus formation.[25] Several groups of molecules have been identified as thromboregulators. First, there are the eicosanoids, in particular prostacyclin, which acts as a platelet anti-aggregator, and thromboxane A_2, which acts as a platelet proaggregator. A balance between these two prostanoids helps control platelet reactivity on the surface of the endothelial cells. The second group is endothelium-derived NO which helps to prevent platelet adhesion, activation, and recruitment. The third and final family of thromboregulators is the endothelial surface ectonucleotidases that metabolize ADP to prevent platelet recruitment and form adenosine which can elevate platelet cAMP levels and further inhibit platelet reactivity.

Hypercoaguable states are any events that cause a procoagulant environment and manifest themselves clinically as overt symptoms and sequelae of thromboembolic disease (Table 10.4). Primary disorders involve a specific defect of a haemostatic protein, while secondary disorders result in an indirect effect on the haemostatic pathways.[30–33] All patients with thrombosis at an early age (<45 years), with a positive family history of thrombotic disease, with thrombosis at an unusual site (mesenteric vein, cerebral vein), or with recurrent thromboses without predisposing factors should be screened for hypercoagulability. Many laboratories provide thrombosis panels which are designed to evaluate those proteins which have been clearly identified as inherited thrombotic disorders and usually include functional antithrombin III, functional plasminogen, functional protein C, and functional protein S. Warfarin therapy interferes with measurement of proteins C and S, while heparin therapy lowers antithrombin III levels.

Pathophysiology

Venous stasis is the most important feature predisposing to venous thrombosis. Radio-opaque contrast injected into the deep veins of the leg may take surprisingly long to clear when the postoperative patient remains flat in bed with little movement due to pain. Allison and coworkers showed that, in postoperative patients who are apt to remain still, radio-opaque dye may linger in the calf veins for as long as 25 min after injection.[11] The venous sinuses of the veins are particularly vulnerable to stasis and thrombosis (Fig. 10.2). Propagation of the thrombus may then follow upstream or the process may spread retrograde (Fig. 10.3). Thrombi found in veins when blood flow is reduced are composed predominantly of fibrin and entrapped blood cells with relatively few platelets, and are often termed red thrombi. The friable ends of these thrombi are the source of the material which eventual forms pulmonary emboli. Formation of venous thrombi is typically asymptomatic and may involve the superficial or deep venous systems. Deep venous thrombi can propagate into the superficial system.

Superficial thrombophlebitis is an inflammatory process of the superficial veins of the leg and presents as local pain, erythema, and induration with tenderness along the thrombosed vein. When thrombophlebitis occurs below the knee, management consists of bed rest, leg elevation, and local application of heat to the affected area. The condition is usually self-limiting as obliteration of the affected part of the superficial venous system usually precludes subsequent attacks. The risk of thromboembolism is minimal and anticoagulation is not indicated. When thrombophlebitis extends above the knee, embolization may occur and such patients should be

closely observed for cephalad progression of the thrombus. Anticoagulation is generally indicated.

Pulmonary emboli from recent thrombi are multiple and fragmented, while emboli from older thrombi contain laminated fibrin layers. Emboli that prove fatal are generally 1.5 cm or more in diameter and 50 cm or more in length, and are often fragmented.[34] The right pulmonary artery is more frequently involved than the left, and the lower pulmonary lobes are more often involved than the upper lobes. The majority of pulmonary emboli originate in the iliac and femoral veins, while a minority (about 20 per cent) originate from other sources, including the inferior vena cava and the veins of the arm and neck. The natural history of pulmonary

Table 10.4   Hypercoaguable states

Primary

Antithrombin III deficiency

Heparin co-factor II deficiency

Protein C deficiency

Protein S deficiency

Fibrinolysis deficiencies (dysplasminogenemia, decrease plasminogen activator or increased plasminogen activator inhibitors, dysfibrinogenemia)

Factor VII deficiency

Secondary

Defects of coagulation and fibrinolysis

   Malignancy

   Pregnancy

   Use of oral contraceptive

   Nephrotic syndrome

   Lupus anticoagulant

Defects of platelets

   Myeloproliferative disorders

   Paroxysmal nocturnal hematuria

   Diabetes mellitus

   Hyperlipidemia

   Cushing's syndrome

   Heparin-induced thrombocytopenia

Defects of blood vessels and rheology

   Immobilization

   Postoperative care

   Vasculitis

   Chronic obliterative arterial disease

   Homocystinuria

   Hyperviscosity

   Thrombocytopenic thrombotic purpura

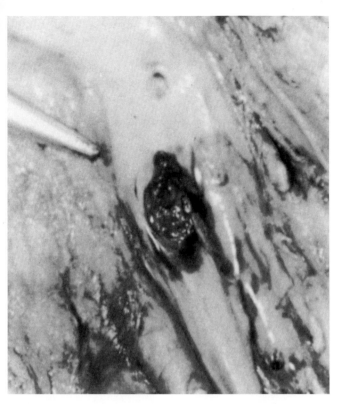

Fig. 10.2   A primary thrombus forming in a valve sinus in the deep femoral vein (from Hume, M., Sevitt, S., and Thomas, D.P., *Venous thrombosis and pulmonary embolism*, Harvard University Press, Cambridge, Ma, 1970. Reproduced with permission from D.C. Sabiston Jr, Pulmonary embolism, *Textbook of surgery* (ed. D.C. Sabiston Jr) (14th edn), Chapter 50, Saunders, Philadelphia, PA, 1991.)

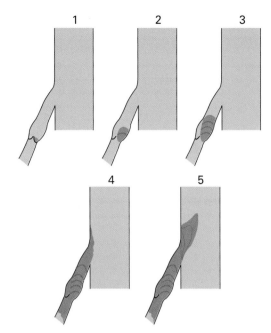

Fig. 10.3   Illustration showing propagation of deep thrombus arising in a valvular pocket with deposition of successive layers and ultimate extension of the non-adherent red thrombus into the lumen of a larger parent vein. (Reproduced with permission from D.C. Sabiston Jr, Pulmonary embolism, *Textbook of Surgery* (ed. D.C. Sabiston Jr) (14th edn), Chapter 50, Saunders, Philadelphia, PA, 1991.)

embolism is spontaneous resolution over time; however, resolution of aged thrombi proceeds more slowly.[35] Pulmonary thromboembolism may be stratified according to its impact on the patient's cardiorespiratory parameters (Table 10.5).

The pulmonary vasculature is a low-vascular-resistance circuit which enables flow in the vascular bed to be increased several-fold with minimal elevation of pulmonary arterial pressure. Occlusion of 30 per cent of the pulmonary vascular tree is usually necessary to elevate the mean pulmonary pressure, while an occlusion of more than 50 per cent is associated with an additional reduction in systemic arterial blood pressure. The degree of pulmonary hypertension is proportional to the degree of angiographic occlusion. When the level of obstruction rises to 75 per cent, the right ventricle must generate a systolic pressure greater than 50 mmHg in order to produce a pulmonary arterial pressure of 40 mmHg, which is the pressure required to preserve pulmonary perfusion. In these conditions, the right ventricle ultimately fails owing to the pressure generation demands. The physiological changes following pulmonary embolism are related to the size of the emboli and can be divided into those that produce microembolism (obstruction of terminal small arteries and arterioles) and those that produce macroembolism (occlusion of the large pulmonary vessels). Experimental emboli formed in the inferior vena cava and embolized to the lungs 2 weeks later cause few changes in central venous, arterial, and cardiac haemodynamic parameters until more than half the pulmonary arterial bed is occluded.[11] In patients with a normal cardiopulmonary reserve, removal of one lung is well tolerated.[36] Similarly, ligation of one pulmonary artery or intraluminal occlusion is also tolerated well and accompanied by few haemodynamic changes.[37] In patients with a reduced cardiopulmonary reserve, unilateral occlusion of the right or left pulmonary artery by a balloon catheter produces a sharp elevation in pulmonary arterial pressure. Similarly, resection of less than one lung may be followed by only minor changes in pulmonary arterial pressure, whereas removal of greater amount of pulmonary tissue produces elevated pulmonary arterial pressure.[36,37] Thus mechanical factors are important determinants of the cardiovascular effects of pulmonary embolism. In contrast, the ventilatory effects associated with pulmonary emboli appear to be due to local neurohumoral mechanisms and feedback loops which produce significant regional bronchoconstriction.[38] Once an embolus lodges in a blood vessel, it interrupts pulmonary blood flow and the ratio of ventilation to perfusion in the affected area increases. The small bronchi in the affected segment respond by constricting to reduce the developing ventilation perfusion mismatch. Experimental studies suggest that both a neural reflex and the local release of vasoactive substances (such as serotonin, prostanoids, and kinins) contribute to the bronchoconstriction, the reduced lung volumes, and the static pulmonary compliance.[39] Arterial emboli produce pulmonary hypertension by mechanical obstruction of main arterial branches, whereas bronchoconstriction and vasoconstriction are produced by arteriolar embolism and are largely mediated by neurohumoral responses. Hypoxia is related to shunting, by overperfusion of the nonembolized lung, a diffusion impairment, and a widened alveolar arterial oxygen gradient. Experimentally, pulmonary emboli induce immediate reduced function of the embolized lung and this pulmonary function returns almost to normal within several weeks as the emboli resolve.

Table 10.5 Stratification of pulmonary thromboembolism

Category	PaO$_2$ (mmHg)	PaCO$_2$ (mmHg)	PA occlusion (%)	HR	CVP	PA (mmHg)	Response
Minor	<80	<35	20–30	Increased	Normal	<20	
Major	<65	<30	30–50	Increased	Elevated	>20	Resuscitation
Massive	<50	<30	>50	Increased	Elevated	>25	Pressor/inotropes
Chronic	<70	30–40	>50	Increased	Elevated	>40	Fixed low CO

PA occlusion, pulmonary artery occlusion; HR, heart rate; CVP, central venous pressure; PA, pulmonary arterial pressure.
Adapted from ref. 97.

Diagnosis

The clinical diagnosis of DVT can be unreliable, as the disease mimics the patterns of many other disorders.[17,40] More than half the patients who present with the classical symptoms of DVT do not have the disease.[17] Clinical suspicion in combination with diagnostic imaging should be used to confirm the diagnosis.[41]. The proportion of patients with clinically suspected DVT, in whom the diagnosis is confirmed by objective testing increases with the number of risk factors identified (Table 10.3). Approximately half the patients with DVT who develop pulmonary embolism have no symptoms of deep venous disease. This causes a delay in the administration of appropriate prophylactic and therapeutic measures. Symptoms of DVT are mild swelling, superficial venous dilatation, and pain in the calf. Examination reveals oedema, tenderness, and an increase in skin temperature. Often a thrombosed vein can be felt at some site from the plantar aspect of the foot to the groin in the affected limb. Homan's sign (tenderness and tightness in the calf with hyperextension of the foot) may be present, but is not necessarily pathognomic of thrombotic disease. Most forms of DVT involve the popliteal vein and its tributaries, but the thrombosis may extend proximally to the femoral and iliac veins. Swelling and pain in the distal thigh are more prominent if femoral vein thrombosis is present, but these signs may be absent. 'Phlegmasia caerulea dolens' occurs when iliofemoral thrombosis is associated with massive swelling of the entire extremity to the inguinal ligament and is characterized by severe pain, tenderness, and cyanosis. Iliofemoral venous thrombosis with altered arterial inflow is known as 'phlegmasia alba dolens'; is characterized by a pale cool extremity with diminished or absent pulses and may threaten viability of the leg. Finally, disease confined to the popliteal vein and its tributaries may be occult or confused with other conditions such as rupture of the gastrocnemius muscle or disorders involving the knee, particularly a ruptured Baker's cyst.

The most specific test for confirmation of the diagnosis of DVT is venography, and it is considered the gold standard by which other modalities are compared. A normal result almost always excludes the presence of venous thrombosis.[42] A positive study is a failure to fill the deep systems with passage of the contrast medium into the superficial system or demonstration of discrete filling defects (Fig. 10.4). Failure to fill the deep system does not provide information concerning the proximal extent of the thrombus. Venography can be complicated by venous thrombosis, extravasation of contrast with subsequent perivasculitis, cellulitis, and ulceration. Venography using radio-isotopes instead of contrast avoids these complications,

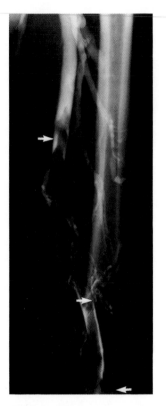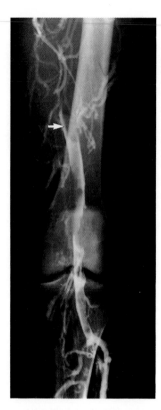

Fig. 10.4 Selected venograms showing intraluminal filling defects within the vascular system are diagnostic of acute thrombosis as outlined by radiographic contrast material (arrows). These are examples of extensive DVT involving the infrapopliteal veins of the calf, the popliteal vein, and the deep venous system of the thigh. The propagating tail of the thrombus is identified in the mid-thigh.

but the disadvantages of the technique include portability, dye loading and ease of repeatability.

Compression ultrasonography (Fig. 10.5) (and see Figure 3.16 and Figure 6.2) is a popular screening method for the non-invasive assessment of blood flow in leg veins and of valve cusp movement.[43] It can also differentiate between acute and chronic venous thrombosis (Table 10.6). All major deep veins of the lower limb can be assessed, but it cannot exclude the presence of thrombi in small veins and is less accurate in demonstrating thrombotic disease of the calf. With experience, ultrasonography is accurate, repeatable,

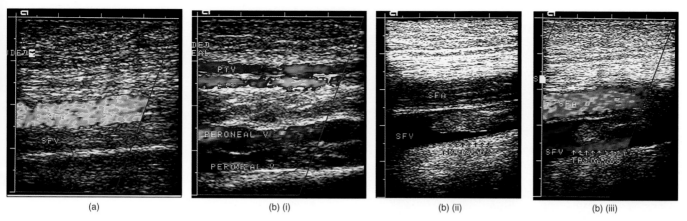

Fig. 10.5 Compression duplex ultrasonography with colour scanning in the diagnosis of DVT. (a) Patient A. The superficial femoral artery is strongly coloured by flow, but although the vein alongside is easily recognized as a dark outline, it was not compressible and did not show any colour flow on release of compression; these features are characteristic of deep vein thrombosis. (b) Patient B. (i) On initial duplex scanning of the calf, one the paired peroneal veins and neighbouring tibial veins showed active colour flow and were compressible. The outline of the other peroneal vein is clearly visible but it was not compressible and there was no colour flow in it, clear evidence that it is filled with thrombus. (ii) On duplex ultrasonography, with the colour scan switched off to give better detail, the superficial femoral vein showed some compressibility, but a large echogenic filling defect within it, seen here, is in keeping with a free-floating thrombus. (iii) With the colour scanning switched on, flow around the filling defect is immediately apparent, confirming the diagnosis. Pulmonary embolus is imminent and urgent treatment is necessary.

and inexpensive.[44] The criteria for a diagnosis on ultrasonography of a DVT and its chronicity are shown in Tables 10.6 and 10.7.

Plethysmography is another non-invasive technique which has a use in DVT evaluation.[45] By measuring changes in the volume of tissue, the oedematous changes associated with thrombosis can be detected. The diagnosis of venous thrombosis depends on the changes in venous capacitance and the rate of emptying after release of the occlusion. Prolongation of the outflow wave suggests major venous thrombosis with a 95 per cent accuracy. It is helpful in demonstrating more proximal thrombotic disease than that occurring in the calf. The advantages of plethysmography are low cost, ease of serial testing, and the ability to detect suprainguinal thrombosis.[46] Plethysmography does not distinguish between intravascular and extravascular compression, and it is also less sensitive for non-obstructing emboli. A normal plethysmographic test is considered reliable, whereas an abnormal test requires cautious interpretation and should suggest further diagnostic imaging.[47]

Intravenous administration of radioactive fibrinogen is another sensitive non-invasive technique that may be used to diagnose DVT.[48] An increase of 20 per cent or more in one area of a limb indicates an underlying thrombus. The modality permits sequential scanning of the extremities over a period of days. This test accurately detects thrombosis in the calf, but high-background radiation from the pelvic bones and urinary tract means that it is not useful in assessing veins in the upper thigh. It has the disadvantage of a minimal delay of 24 h before diagnosis, unsuitability in pregnancy and in the young, viral transmission by the fibrinogen, and invalidation if the targeted limb has had any recent injury, operation, or inflammation.[49] It is seldom used.

Magnetic resonance imaging (MRI) is a reliable method of diagnosing venous thrombosis, particularly in the pelvic veins.[50] It is expensive and time consuming, but does not require venous access or contrast media and can evaluate the entire venous system. Venous thrombi can be visualized using either spin echo or gradient echo MRI techniques. When gradient echo techniques are used, a lower-extremity DVT is diagnosed when a filling defect is seen within a vein or when a low-intensity occlusion of a large vein is imaged (Fig. 10.6). The presence of intraluminal webs or irregular/occluded

Table 10.6 Criteria for ultrasonographic diagnosis of acute versus chronic DVT

	Acute	Chronic
Thrombus	Hypoechoic	Echogenic
Vein lumen	Distended	Narrow irregular
Compressibility	Spongy, partial	Rigid incompressible
Collaterals	Absent	Present

Table 10.7 Criteria for ultrasonographic diagnosis of DVT

The presence of echogenic material within the vein lumen

Non-compressibility of the vein

Venous distension

Free-floating thrombosis

Abnormal spectral waveform

Abnormal colour image

veins in association with collateral veins is suggestive of chronic DVT. MRI and venography have comparable accuracy for diagnosing DVT, but MRI is superior in the ultrasonographically difficult areas (pelvic veins, common femoral veins, and superficial femoral veins in the adductor canal). MRI is recommended if pelvic vein thrombosis is suspected.

The symptoms and signs of pulmonary embolism are similar to those of a number of other cardiopulmonary disorders, so that the diagnosis of pulmonary embolism is often difficult (Table 10.8).[51,52] Dyspnoea, chest pain, haemoptysis, and hypotension are well

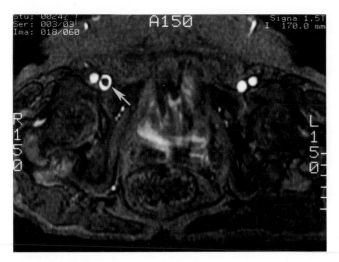

Fig. 10.6 Magnetic resonance image (33/13/60°) showing an intraluminal thrombus (decreased signal) surrounded by flowing blood (high signal) in the right external iliac vein (arrow).

described, but are not specific and are present in only a quarter or less of patients. Many patients have underlying cardiac disease, and dyspnoea and tachypnoea are the most frequent clinical findings. Accentuation of the pulmonary second sound is common. The more classic signs of haemoptysis, pleural friction rub, gallop rhythm, cyanosis, and chest splinting are present in 25 per cent or less of patients.[51,52] Arterial blood gas measurements show a P_aO_2 of less than 60 mmHg in most patients with a widened alveolar arterial oxygen gradient. A reduction in the P_aCO_2 is also helpful in differentiating the diagnosis of major embolism from other causes in the critically ill patient.[51,52]

In acute pulmonary embolism and in the absence of coexisting pulmonary disease, the plain chest radiogram is usually within normal limits (Table 10.9). Diminished pulmonary vascular markings may be presence at the site of the embolus (Westermark's sign) (Fig. 10.7).[53] The electrocardiogram is not specific but changes can be confirmatory. It is probable that more than 10–20 per cent of patients subsequently proven to have a pulmonary embolism show some electrocardiographic changes and, of these, a smaller number have diagnostic abnormalities (Table 10.9).[54] The most common abnormality is ST depression, which is a result of myocardial ischaemia from reduced cardiac output and arterial pressure as well as increased right ventricular pressure. Radioactive pulmonary scanning remains the most frequently employed technique in the diagnosis of pulmonary embolism (Fig. 10.8). In a non-hypotensive patient with a normal chest radiogram, the perfusion scan is a useful screening technique, particularly when the perfusion defects approach a lobar pattern. The addition of a ventilation scan to give a combined ventilation–perfusion image enhances diagnostic accuracy, provided that there is no past history of pulmonary embolism and that one large or two moderate-size areas of ventilation–perfusion mismatch are present. Radiological interpretation of ventilation–perfusion scans is based on the probability of embolism. Low probability means subsegmental perfusion defects without a ventilation scan performed, or matched perfusion and ventilation defects. Moderate probability indicates multiple subsegmental perfusion defects with normal ventilation scans, or segmental perfusion defects without a ventilation scan performed. Intermediate probability signifies chronic obstructive pulmonary disease on chest radiographs or abnormal chest films

Table 10.8   Clinical manifestations of pulmonary embolism (n = 1000)

Symptoms	
Dyspnoea	77
Chest pain	63
Haemoptysis	26
Altered mental status	23
Dyspnoea, chest pain, haemoptysis	14
Signs	
Tachycardia	59
Recent fever	43
Rales	42
Tachypnoea	38
Leg oedema and tenderness	23
Elevated venous pressure	18
Shock	11
Accentuated P_2	11
Cyanosis	9
Pleural friction rub	8

Adapted from ref. 78

Table 10.9   Electrocardiographic and radiographic manifestations of pulmonary embolism (n = 1000)

Electrocardiographic changes after pulmonary embolism	
T-wave inversion	40
ST-segment depression	33
Right bundle branch (complete or incomplete)	16
Rhythm disturbances	11
$S_1Q_3T_3$	11
ST-segment elevation	9
P pulmonale	4
Chest radiography finding associated with pulmonary embolism	
Consolidation/infiltration	41
Diaphragmatic elevation	41
Pleural effusion	28
Distention of proximal pulmonary artery	23
Cardiomegaly	21
Atelectasis	20
Focal oligaemia	15

Adapted from ref. 78.

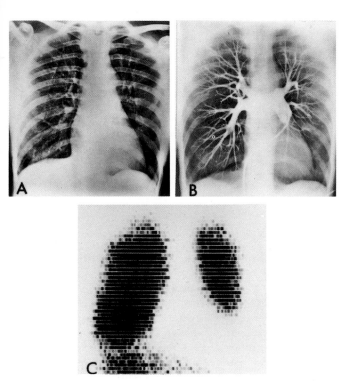

Fig. 10.7 Films from a patient with pulmonary embolism involving the left lower lobar pulmonary artery. (a) Slight diminution of the vascular markings to the lower lobe is noted compared with those in the right lower lobe of the plain chest film (Westermark's sign). (b) Pulmonary arteriogram illustrating occlusion of the left lower lobe pulmonary artery. (c) Pulmonary scan showing absence of perfusion of the left lower lobe.

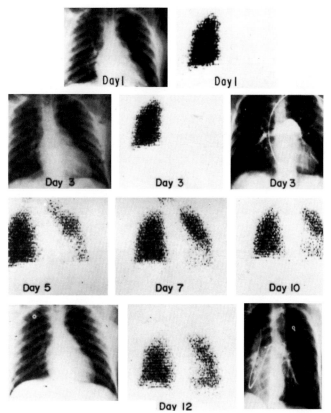

Fig. 10.8 Serial chest radiographs and scans following a massive pulmonary embolus to the left pulmonary artery in a 25-year-old woman after a pelvic operation. On the fifth postoperative day discomfort was noted in the left chest with dyspnoea. A plain chest radiograph taken on this day (day 1) showed diminished vascular markings (Westermark's sign). A radio-active pulmonary scan showed no evidence of pulmonary flow to the entire left lobe. Beginning on the third day after the embolus, the scan and the arteriogram both show evidence of flow to the left lung. In subsequent scans and pulmonary arteriograms resolution of the thrombus occurred with progressively increasing amounts of flow by the twelfth day. (Reproduced with permission from D.C. Sabiston Jr, Pulmonary embolism, *Textbook of surgery* (ed. D.C. Sabiston Jr) (14th edn), Chapter 50, Saunders, Philadelphia, PA, 1991.)

in regions of perfusion defects. High probability indicates segmental or greater perfusion defects with normal ventilation scans. High-probability scans occur in only a few patients and do not identify many who require arteriography and are subsequently found to have thromboembolism. The most definitive method of diagnosing pulmonary embolism is still the pulmonary arteriogram,[55] which allows a definition of the presence, size, and distribution of the pulmonary emboli. It has a mortality rate of 0.3–0.5 per cent. In most patients who survive the initial attack, the obstruction in the pulmonary arteries involves lobar or segmental branches (Fig. 10.7). The defect should remain constant on several successive films in the series. Blood flow may be sluggish, which is confirmed by pooling on the contrast medium in the artery above the obstruction after the venous phase of the arteriogram. When a pulmonary arteriogram is performed later in the course of an embolic event, contrast medium may pass around the obstruction causing delayed opacification of the artery distally. In some areas, the pattern may show avascular segments that represent unresolved thromboembolism.

Management

Prevention

Prophylaxis of DVT and pulmonary embolism is quite important.[52,56] Ideally, the method should be safe, effective, easily administered, inexpensive, simple to monitor, and acceptable to the patient. No method or combination of methods completely prevents throm-

boembolism. Primary prophylaxis is a necessary cost and quality-of-care requirement (Table 10.10 and 10.11). In considering DVT prophylaxis, the physician should consider the risk of thromboembolism, the potential benefit to the patient of the available modalities, and the related complications and their equivalent expenses (Table 10.4).[22] Prior to operation, attempts should be made to reduce any identifiable risk factors that a patient may have (Table 10.1).[18] Oral contraceptives increase the risk of DVT; they should be discontinued 4 weeks before operation and an alternative form of contraception recommended.

Simple interventions which reduce the risk of DVT include regular physical activity and elevation of the lower extremities for gravity drainage of venous return. Early ambulation and resumption of physical activity after operation or bed rest for any reason is strongly recommended. In the interim, elevation of the legs with flexion of the knees will cause a rapid run-off of the blood in the legs and thighs due to gravity (Fig. 10.9). Every patient should be encouraged to walk (a maximum of 5 min every hour), and distinction must be made between early ambulation and early sitting out of bed. Ambulation achieves movement of venous blood, while sitting

Table 10.10 Incidence of venous pulmonary embolism following general surgical procedures without prophylaxis

Endpoint	Incidence (%)
All DVT	25
Clinically detected DVT	9
Proximal DVT	7
All pulmonary emboli	1.6
Fatal pulmonary emboli	0.8

Adapted from ref. 16.

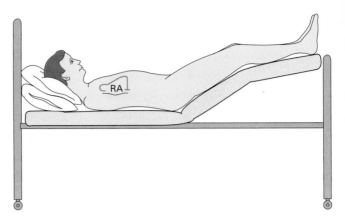

Fig. 10.9 Correct position for lower extremities in prophylaxis of pulmonary embolism. Note the additional break at the knees. It is important that the level of the veins in the lower extremities is above the mean level of the right atrium (RA).

Table 10.11 Prevention of venous thromboembolism in general surgery

Regimen	No. of patients	Incidence (%)	Relative risk reduction (%)
Controls	4310	25	–
Low-molecular-weight heparin	3637	4	86
Low-dose heparin	6882	8	68
Graduated compression stockings	300	9	63
Intermittent pneumatic compression	313	10	61

Adapted from ref. 16.

out provides no advantage to venous flow and induces vascular stagnation. It may often improve respiratory function. Graduated compression stockings (thigh length), which are often employed as prophylactic measures, are intended to increase flow in the venous system by reducing the lumen of the veins and increasing the pressure differential from foot to groin. These stockings must fit firmly and should be combined with physical activity for optimal utility.[57]

Some consider pneumatic compression devices to be an effective approach to stimulate the physiological calf muscle pump and counteract the venous pooling and stasis that occurs during and after surgical procedures.[16] Their use decreases stasis, promotes muscular activity, and increases venous blood flow. Pneumatic compression devices have a secondary effect of promoting increased systemic fibrinolytic activity. It is interesting that the effect of the compression devices on the fibrinolytic system is independent of the site of the device (i.e. on the upper or lower limb). Patients who develop DVT despite this therapy have a high incidence of an intrinsic defect in their fibrinolytic system that is not observed in patients who remain thrombus free.

Judicious use of a variety of pharmacological agents can significantly reduce the incidence of DVT. Low-dose subcutaneous heparin is the most widely used form of prophylactic anticoagulation and is associated with an overall reduction in the incidence of DVT from 25 to 8 per cent.[16] The incidence of pulmonary embolism and fatal pulmonary embolism showed similar reductions.[58] Low-dose heparin reduces the incidence of venous thromboembolism following major operations by two-thirds and reduces death from pulmonary embolism by 50 per cent. It is less effective following hip procedures and may be ineffective following operation on the knee.[59] Low-dose heparin has been the subject of 29 randomized clinical trials with 8000 general surgical patients. Meta-analyses show that low-dose heparin is an effective prophylactic measure against thromboembolism and does not increase the incidence of major haemorrhagic complications.[60] Low dose heparin is best given two hours preoperatively and then every 8 or 12 hours postoperatively at a dose of 5000 units subcutaneously. Low-dose heparin should not be used in patients undergoing procedures on the brain, spine, and eye.[59] Low-molecular-weight fractions of heparin have significantly better efficacy in preventing thromboembolism than unfractionated heparin.[61] These low-molecular-weight heparins have a longer half-life and thus, if begun preoperatively, dosage once daily is effective. However, when begun postoperatively twice-daily doses are significantly more effective. Compared low-dose heparin, low-molecular-weight heparin fractions have an equal efficacy following major general surgical procedures but appear more effective in preventing thromboembolic complications after operations on the hip and knee. The rates of major haemorrhagic complications remain the same as those for low-dose heparin.[62] There is a very serious complication of heparin therapy which deserves considerable emphasis as it can cause major complications. Heparin-associated thrombosis syndrome can cause catastrophic consequences and has renewed the concerns over the use of prophylactic heparin regimens.[63,64]

Oral anticoagulants such as warfarin given in doses which prolong the International Normalized Ratio (INR) to 2.0–3.0 are highly effective in preventing thromboembolism.[65] These compounds require long lead-in times, frequent monitoring of INR, and an increased risk of bleeding.[66] Manipulations of the therapeutic regimen to begin as an outpatient at low doses and increase to high doses after the window for surgically related haemorrhage has passed are now showing promise for the high-risk patients who have become the target of this therapy. Dextran is a glucose polymer which reduces plasma viscosity, alters platelet function, and decreases firbin polymerization. It is widely used in the prevention of thromboembolism after hip procedures, more often in Europe than in North America. Current data suggest that antiplatelet agents are not effective and do not provide sufficient protection for the high-risk patient.

In low-risk patients who undergoing minor or relatively short procedures, are less than 40, and have no other clinical risk factors, no specific prophylaxis is required. In low-risk patients undergoing lengthy procedures without defined risk factors, pneumatic compression devices, graduated compression stockings, and possibly low-dose heparin (every 12 h) are advisable. In medium-risk patients who are over 40 or have additional clinical risk factors and are undergoing any operative procedure, pneumatic compression devices, graduated compression stockings, and possibly low-dose heparin (every 12 h) are effective. In high-risk patients who are over 40 and have additional clinical risk factors, graduated compression stockings in combination with pneumatic compression devices, low-dose heparin, or low-molecular-weight heparin should be used. In the very high-risk patients (i.e. patients with four or more risk factors), a combination of pharmacological, compression stockings, and pneumatic compression devices should be used.

Therapy for deep vein thrombosis

The therapeutic goals in the management of DVT are to minimize the risk of pulmonary embolism, to limit propagation of the existing thrombus, and to facilitate resolution of the existing thrombus. Anticoagulation prevents the propagation of the original thrombus and the development of new thrombi, while the existing thrombus is lysed by naturally occurring fibrinolysis. In patients who are medically stable, the standard anticoagulant therapy for venous thromboembolism is a combination of continuous intravenous heparin followed by oral warfarin. This is combined with bed rest, elevation of the leg, and the application of light to medium elastic support stockings to reduce oedema. Two recent studies have demonstrated that outpatient administration of a combination of subcutaneous low-molecular-weight heparin followed by oral warfarin is as effective as the standard inpatient combination of continuous intravenous heparin followed by oral warfarin. These outpatient therapies are safe and will provide substantial cost containment for health care systems.[67,68]

Intravenous heparin has a rapid action and can be discontinued or its effects reversed rapidly with protamine sulphate should bleeding complications arise. Subcutaneous low-molecular-weight heparin has also been shown to be effective.[69] The anticoagulant activity of unfractionated heparin depends on its unique pentasaccharide configuration that binds to antithrombin III, allowing potentiation of the inhibition of thrombin and factor X_a by antithrombin III.[70] The major complication associated with heparin therapy is bleeding, thrombocytopenia with the heparin-induced thrombocytopenia syndrome, hypersensitivity, arterial thromboembolism (heparin associated thrombosis syndrome occurring 7–10 days after initiation of therapy), and osteoporosis (therapy extended for more than 6 months). The therapeutic range for heparin based on the activated partial thromboplastin time is a ratio of 1.5 to 2.5.[71] However, the incidence of bleeding with heparin correlates with the clinical risk of bleeding. Ninety-seven per cent of patients are therapeutic on heparin if a weight-based nomogram is followed (starting dose 80 U/kg bolus and 18 U/kg/h infusion) (Table 10.12).[72,73] Failure to exceed the lower limit of this range is associated with an unacceptably high risk of recurrent venous thromboembolism, whereas little association exists between supratherapeutic APTT and the risk of bleeding.

Table 10.12	Intravenous heparin protocol	

1	Initial heparin bolus (80 U/kg)		
2	Continuous heparin infusion (18 U/kg/h IV)		
3	APTT and platelet count prior to commencing infusion		
4	APTT 4 h after commencing infusion		
5	APTT 4–6 h after implementing a change in dosage		

APTT	Change (U/h)	Additional action
>45	+240	Repeat APTT in 4–6 h
46–54	+120	Repeat APTT in 4–6 h
55–85	No change	None
86–110	+120	Stop heparin for 1 h, repeat APTT 4–6 h after restarting heparin
>10	+240	Stop heparin for 1 h, repeat APTT 4–6 h after restarting heparin

6	APTT is performed once daily unless patient is subtherapeutic.		

Adapted from ref. 72.

Warfarin produces its anticoagulant effect by inhibiting the vitamin-K-dependent gamma carboxylation of coagulation factors II, VII, IX, and X. Warfarin also inhibits vitamin-K-dependent gamma carboxylation of proteins S and C.[66,74] Vitamin K antagonist therapy should be commenced as soon as the diagnosis is confirmed, provided that no contraindications exist. Vitamin K antagonists create a coagulation paradox by producing an anticoagulation effect due to multiple factor inhibition but a thrombogenic effect by impairing proteins C and S.[74] Therefore heparin and warfarin therapies should be overlapped by 4 to 5 days prior to discontinuation of the heparin in patients with thrombotic diseases. The complications with warfarin therapy are haemorrhage, skin necrosis, dermatitis, and teratogenicity. The peak effect of vitamin K antagonists does not occur until 36–72 h after drug administration. Warfarin is administered in a dose of 10 mg/day for the first 2 days. The daily dose thereafter is adjusted to the INR. Heparin may be discontinued on the fourth or fifth day after initiation of warfarin therapy provided that the INR is therapeutic (INR 2.0–3.0).[71] Daily INR is obtained until the patient has established a dosing regimen which achieves therapeutic anticoagulation. Thereafter the INR may be checked weekly for the duration of therapy. It is generally recommended that all patients with a first episode of venous thromboembolism receive therapy for 12 weeks.[73] The recurrence rate of thromboembolism following a 3-month treatment has been reported to be 4–7 per cent. Treatment with warfarin for more than 3 months is indicated for patients with recurrent venous thromboembolism or in patients in whom there is a continuing risk factor for venous thromboembolism. Patients should be followed for up for 3 years to ensure that there is no recurrent thromboembolic event. Discontinuation of warfarin therapy in patients with recurrent venous thromboembolism is associated with an approximately 20 per cent risk of recurrent venous thromboembolism during the following year and a 5 per cent risk of fatal pulmonary embolism. In patients with a continuing risk factor which is reversible, long-term therapy should usually be continued until the risk factor is reversed. Anticoagulant therapy should be continued indefinitely in patients with an irreversible risk factor.

Although anticoagulation is the management of choice for most patients, fibrinolytics have also been studied.[75] Fibrinolytics can completely lyse up to 70 per cent of existing thrombi, a feature that conventional anticoagulants lack. Routine use of fibrinolytic therapy has been made more difficult by bleeding complications, particularly in the postoperative and post traumatic patient. Fibrinolysis is most efficient in cases of recent non-adherent thrombus. The incidence of major clinical haemorrhage after fibrinolysis for DVT is between 6 and 30 per cent, a threefold increase compared with standard heparin therapy. Studies have shown that the action of fibrinolytics in DVT is incomplete. Long-term follow up shows only a marginal reduction in the incidence and severity of post-thrombotic limb syndromes.[76] Surgical extraction of venous thrombi has been almost completely discontinued because of a recurrence rate. Although venous thrombectomy has no role in the management of calf DVT, it may still have a role in the management of patients with extensive iliofemoral disease, in which limb loss is imminent, such as 'phlegmasia alba dolens'. In these patients, there are benefits to avoiding limb loss, preventing pulmonary embolism, and reducing the severity of post-thrombotic syndromes. The procedure should be performed early before the thrombus has had time to organize and should be directed at the iliofemoral veins. Adaptation of the principles of surgical embolectomy has been the addition of a temporary arteriovenous fistula to provide sustained rapid flow in the thrombectomized vein postoperatively. This adaptation appears to maintain the patency of the iliofemoral veins and produces a substantial reduction in eventual post-thrombotic syndrome.

Therapy for pulmonary emboli

The management of pulmonary embolism is threefold: (1) to support the cardiovascular system, (2) to prevent further emboli and thrombosis within the pulmonary vasculature, and (3) to identify and treat the source of the emboli. In controlled trials, therapy for DVT, or pulmonary embolism, 10 per cent of patients with a first episode and 20 per cent of patients with a recurrent episode develop a new event within 6 months of the initiation of anticoagulant therapy. It is most important to establish the diagnosis unequivocally prior to the initiation of therapy (Fig. 10.10).

The principal management of pulmonary embolism is anticoagulation. A continuous infusion of heparin should be instituted, preceded by bolus injection, as outlined previously (Table 10.12). The dose of heparin should be sufficient to maintain an APTT 1.5–2.5 times greater than the upper limit of normal. Duration of therapy is generally 5–10 days.[73] This approximates the time necessary for thrombi to become adherent to the venous wall. Oral warfarin therapy is begun as outlined previously and adjusted to maintain an INR of 2–3 for a period of 6 months.[73]

Current estimates are that no more than 10 per cent of patients with pulmonary embolism receive thrombolysis in the United States.[77] Greater application becomes apparent as recognition of the fact that pulmonary thrombolysis can now be applied within a 2-week time window via a peripheral vein. The National Institutes of Health Heart, Blood and Lung Institute conducted a national co-operative study which showed that urokinase combined with heparin therapy significantly accelerated the resolution of pulmonary thromboembolism at 24 h with an improvement in cardiovascular haemodynamics and pulmonary imaging.[78,79] Importantly, no significant differences were noted in the recurrence rate of pulmonary

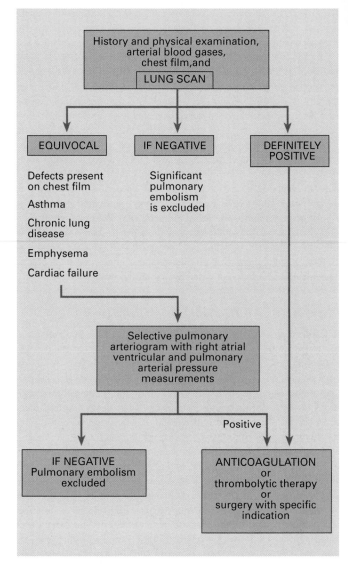

Fig. 10.10 A schematic outline of the plan to be followed in establishing the diagnosis of pulmonary embolism.

embolism or in the 2-week mortality. Bleeding was a major complication, occurring in 45 per cent of the patients. Other studies with streptokinase and tPA have indicated similar results.[79] recommended dosage for each of the thrombolytics is shown in Table 10.13. A study of intrapulmonary and intravenous administration of recombinant tPA indicates that pulmonary arterial infusion does not offer a significant benefit over the intravenous route and suggests that a prolonged infusion over 7 h (100 mg) is superior to a single infusion of 50 mg over 2 h. The incidence of haemorrhage is 5–10 per cent in patients with pulmonary embolism and 20 per cent in those who undergo pulmonary arteriography, many of which are catheter related. Contraindications to thrombolytic therapy can be divided into those which are firm and those which are relative (Table 10.14). Firm contraindications include internal bleeding (recent or active), recent neurosurgery or cranial trauma, and a history of a haemorrhagic stroke. Relative contraindications include a recent surgical procedure (within 7–10 days), cardiopulmonary resuscitation (within 7–10 days), and the presence of a coagulopathy.

Table 10.13 Recommended dosing for thrombolytic therapy	
Streptokinase	250 000 U IV over 30 min, then 100 000 U/h over 24 h (continue infusion for 24 h for pulmonary embolism and 48–72 h for DVT)
Urokinase	4400 U/kg IV over 10 mins then 4400 U/kg/h over 24 h (continue infusion for 24 h for pulmonary embolism and 48–72 h for DVT)
tPA	100 mg IV over 120 min

Table 10.14 Contraindications for thrombolysis
Major internal bleeding in previous 6 months
Intracranial or intraspinal disease
Operation or biopsy in the preceding 10 days
Hypertension (systolic BP >200 mmHg; diastolic BP >110 mmHg)
Active or infective endocarditis
Pericarditis
Aortic or cerebral aneurysm
Presence of a bleeding disorder

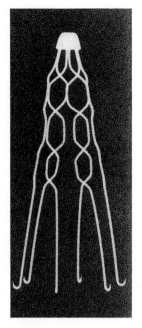

Fig. 10.11   Example of the Kim-Ray Greenfield filter.

Table 10.15 Indications for inferior vena cava filter
Recurrent thromboembolism despite adequate anticoagulation
DVT or thromboembolism in a patient with a contraindication to anticoagulation
Complication of anticoagulation that requires cessation of therapy
Recurrent pulmonary emboli with pulmonary hypertension and cor pulmonale
Immediately after pulmonary embolectomy for massive pulmonary embolus
Previous device or ligation failure with recurrent embolism
Patients with chronic pulmonary embolism syndrome (>50% of vascular occluded)
Propagating iliofemoral thrombosis despite anticoagulation
High-risk patient with a large free-floating iliofemoral thrombosis on venogram

In addition to the therapies which are directed at preventing pulmonary emboli and treating the venous thrombosis, alternative methods of preventing pulmonary emboli from lower-extremity venous thrombi are required for those patients who have contraindications to anticoagulation, suffer complications from anticoagulation therapy, or have recurrent pulmonary emboli on therapeutic anticoagulation.[80] Initial interruption of the vena cava was recommended but is seldom performed today. The procedure has a high mortality and morbidity and does not necessarily prevent subsequent embolism since evidence of recurrent pulmonary embolism is reported in as many as 20 per cent of patients after ligation. Several procedures designed to simplify caval interruption have been developed, with an emphasis on reducing postoperative morbidity and mortality. The most successful of these are the percutaneous inferior vena cava filters.[81,82] Inferior vena cava filters are mechanical intravascular devices inserted below the renal veins and are designed to prevent thrombi embolizing to the lungs (Fig. 10.11). Indications for the placement of these filters are shown in Table 10.15. The long-term patency rate is over 95 per cent. The recurrent thromboembolism rate after filter placement ranges from 2 to 4 per cent.[82] The basic filter is a cone-shaped stainless steel umbrella which causes minimal reduction in venous flow. It is fixed in place by hooks that grasp the wall of the inferior vena cava to prevent migration, and the filter becomes even more securely fixed when emboli become trapped. Cephalad or caudal filter migration is a serious complication (Fig. 10.12). Other complications associated with the devices include thrombosis at the site of insertion (25 per cent), misplacement (7 per cent), retroperitoneal haemorrhage, perforation of the duodenum or the ureter, and development of thrombosis

proximal to the umbrella producing recurrent emboli.[82,83] The filter may stimulate distal thrombosis in the vena cava and late occlusion may occur. Preliminary clinical experience with temporary inferior vena caval filters is encouraging and adds new dimensions to mechanical interventions to reduce pulmonary embolism.[84]

Anticoagulation therapy for pulmonary embolism is generally successful. The primary indications for emergent pulmonary embolectomy is refractory hypotension despite maximal resuscitation in a patient with proven embolism which is usually massive and definitely documented by either a pulmonary scan or a pulmonary arteriogram.[85] Transvenous embolectomy is seldom used.[86] When cardiovascular collapse is present the patient may be supported by

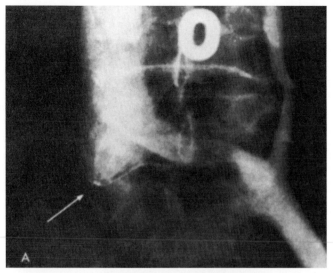

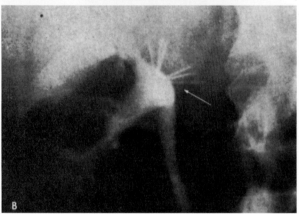

Fig. 10.12 (a) A venogram showing the umbrella filter in the right common iliac vein. (b) Radiograph of the abdomen demonstrating misplacement of the umbrella filter in the right renal vein. (From K. Mobin-Uddin, J.K. Trinkle, and L.R. Bryant, Present status of the inferior vena cava umbrella filter, *Surgery* 1971. Reproduced with permission from W.G. Wolfe and D.C. Sabiston Jr, *Major problems in clinical surgery*, Vol. 15, *Pulmonary embolism*, Saunders, Philadelphia, PA, 1980.)

partial cardiopulmonary bypass using the femoral vein and artery for immediate access. Embolectomy can then be performed by the open method on one or both pulmonary arteries (Fig. 10.13). Either a right or left anterior thoracotomy can be undertaken when there is proximal occlusion of one vessel. Patients with bilateral pulmonary emboli or with embolus of the main pulmonary artery generally require a median sternotomy and cardiopulmonary bypass. The mortality for open pulmonary embolectomy is approximately 40 per cent. One of the postoperative complications reported is massive endobronchial haemorrhage. Reperfusion pulmonary oedema after pulmonary thromboembolectomy has been described and is a serious complication requiring prolonged mechanical ventilation.

Sequelae

After a DVT, a limb that is adequately treated sometimes remains oedematous and uncomfortable for many months with slow improvement as the occluded veins are recanalized and collateral vessels enlarge. The two principal sequelae of DVT are post-phlebitic syndrome and pulmonary embolism. Thrombus within the deep veins may be completely lysed by the body's endogenous systems. More often, the thrombus becomes organized to produce a deformity of the vein, a fibrotic occlusion of the vein, or irreparable damage to the venous valves. This results in the inability of the vein to maintain a cephalad pumping mechanism, incompetence of the valves, and development of a collateral circulation. The culmination of these events is venous hypertension which manifests itself clinically as a post-thrombotic syndrome (see Chapter 6). A rarer complication of DVT is the development of septic deep venous thrombosis. The principal sequelae of pulmonary embolism are death, respiratory failure, pulmonary infarction, and chronic thromboembolic pulmonary hypertension.

Chronic pulmonary emboli and their management

Although most pulmonary emboli resolve spontaneously, a few patients have continued pathological evidence of emboli long-term. About 0.1–0.5 per cent of patients suffering acute pulmonary events progress to chronic thromboembolic pulmonary hypertension.[87,88] In chronic thromboembolic pulmonary hypertension, defective fibrinolysis may produce a cycle of incomplete lysis of pulmonary emboli, partial recanalization of obstructed pulmonary vasculature, and organization and fibrosis of retained thromboembolic and proximal thrombotic extension. However, studies of the fibrinolytic system have not demonstrated a consistent pattern of plasminogen activation or inhibition. The only identifiable thrombotic predisposition has been the presence of lupus anticoagulant in 10 per cent of these patients.[89] Less than 1 per cent of patients have antithrombin III, protein C, and protein S deficiencies.[88] The majority of patients present late in their disease. The preliminary asymptomatic period may range from months to years until progressive respiratory insufficiency, hypoxaemia, and right ventricular failure appear.[88] Initially, the gradual accumulation of these thromboemboli within the pulmonary arterial vasculature was considered part of the patho-physiology that produce chronic thromboembolic pulmonary hypertension. However, sequential perfusion scans are correlated with haemodynamic and symptomatic changes, and no new perfusion defects are found. The unchanging perfusion scans also make local extension unlikely. It appears that there are global changes in vessels with low pulmonary resistance which are similar to lesions found in pulmonary vasculature of congenital or acquired cardiac disease. These morphological findings are further supported by the recognition that the degree of chronic angiographic obstruction correlates poorly with the degree of pulmonary hypertension and the phenomenon of pulmonary steal which occurs after thromboembolectomy. There is now evidence to suggest that there are significant changes in endothelial NO synthase expression and function in patients with secondary pulmonary hypertension, suggesting an aetiology for the increasing degree of pulmonary hypertension with time.[90] Sufficient embolic occlusion leads to the loss of the normal regulatory/ compensatory patterns of the pulmonary vascular bed, and a patient at rest may have acceptable but high pulmonary pressures. On mild exercise, there is a marked increase in pulmonary arterial pressures with attendant effects on right heart function. In the majority of patients, it appears that recurrent events of local extension of thrombus are not the true pathophysiological cause of chronic

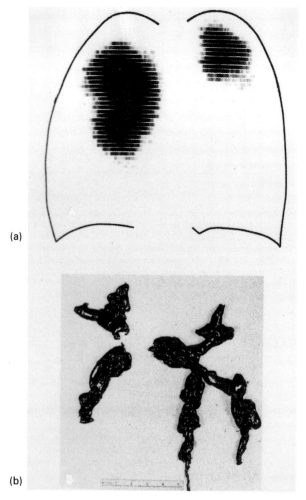

(a)

(b)

Fig. 10.13 Illustration from a patient with massive pulmonary embolism on the twelfth postoperative day following an orthopaedic operation and accompanied by intractable shock. (a) The pulmonary scan shows massive occlusion of the right lower and middle lobar pulmonary arteries as well as nearly all the pulmonary arterial circulation of the left lung. (b) Emboli removed from both pulmonary arteries at the time of pulmonary embolectomy.

thromboembolic pulmonary hypertension and that the changes are more likely to be a single massive and non-terminal embolic event which is frequently undiagnosed and untreated. Resolution of such thrombi are incomplete, which in turn begins a spiral of changes in the morphology and function of the pulmonary vasculature that culminates in the rapidly progressive deterioration in pulmonary and right heart function.

Patients with chronic thromboembolic pulmonary hypertension present with progressive respiratory insufficiency, hypoxaemia, and right ventricular failure.[88] They may also present with recurrent episodes of thrombophlebitis, haemoptysis, and chest pain. Physical findings include signs of pulmonary hypertension with evidence of right ventricular failure manifested by an increased P_2, a systolic murmur hepatomegaly, and an S_3 or S_4 gallop. A unique feature of these patients is the finding of flow murmurs over the lung fields owing to turbulent blood flow in partially occluded or recanalized pulmonary arteries. Chest radiographs show dilated pulmonary arteries and oligaemic lung fields in 50 per cent of patients. Right ventricular enlargement is present in about 66 per cent of patients and a pleural effusion in 33 per cent of patients. Arterial blood gases

on room air often show hypoxaemia with a P_aO_2 of 55–60 mmHg and a P_aCO_2 in the range of 30 mmHg. However, the P_aO_2 may be within normal limits, but will show a decrease on exercise but with a widened resting alveolar–arterial oxygen gradient. Electrocardiographic findings are consistent with cor pulmonale (P pulmonale, right axis deviation, and right ventricular hypertrophy). Twenty per cent of patients demonstrate a mild restrictive defect on pulmonary function testing and the majority show a reduction in diffusion capacity. Echocardiography shows right atrial and ventricular enlargement, tricuspid regurgitation, and elevated pulmonary artery pressures. Ventilation and perfusion scanning show at least one or more segmental or larger mismatches, confirming the presence of pulmonary emboli. The perfusion defects often match the areas of oligaemia in the plain chest radiograms and on the pulmonary arteriogram. Pulmonary arteriography in association with right heart catheterization allows documentation of the anatomical distribution of the emboli and the measurement of pulmonary arterial pressures.[91] The five distinct patterns on angiography are (1) pouch defects which refer to the concave appearance of organized thrombus within the vessel, (2) pulmonary artery webs or bands which refer to lines that traverse the lumen of a pulmonary vessel at a segmental or lobar level, (3) scalloping of the intimal surfaces, (4) abrupt narrowings of the major pulmonary vessels, and (5) obstruction of lobar and segmental vessels at their points of origin.[92] An important angiographic point that may differentiate chronic thromboembolic pulmonary hypertension from other diagnoses is that the patterns described are noted in both pulmonary vascular beds. Arteriography shows emboli in both lungs, with up to 75 per cent of pulmonary blood flow being obstructed. A thoracic aortogram to demonstrate the bronchial arterial circulation is necessary for preoperative evaluation prior to surgery.[93] Venography and/or MRI may confirm the presence of venous thrombosis in the lower extremities. Pulmonary angioscopy confirms the presence of thromboembolic obstruction and whether it is accessible to surgical intervention.[94] The normal pulmonary artery has a round or oval contour with a smooth pale glistening appearance of the intima and bright red blood (back-flow) filling the lumen. The features of organized chronic emboli on angioscopy consist of roughening or pitting of the intimal surface, bands, and webs across the lumen, pitted masses of chronic embolic material within the lumen, and partial recanalization.

Medical therapy for the chronic pulmonary emboli syndrome is unsatisfactory and the condition has a poor prognosis.[95] The natural history of chronic pulmonary embolism is related to the magnitude of the pulmonary arterial hypertension (Fig. 10.14). If the mean pulmonary artery pressure is greater than 30 mmHg, survival at 5 years is 30 per cent; pressures greater than 50 mmHg are associated with a 5-year survival rate of less than 10 per cent. The decision to proceed to pulmonary thromboembolectomy is based on several objective and subjective factors. First, the patient should have haemodynamic (pulmonary vascular resistance > 300 dyn/s/cm) and ventilatory impairment (high minute volumes) at rest or at exercise. Second, the thrombi must be accessible as determined by angiography or angioscopy. Third, the patient should not have significant co-morbid risk factors (coronary artery disease, renal impairment, parenchymal lung disease) which will adversely affect perioperative and long-term viability.

Pulmonary thromboembolectomy in patients with proximal pulmonary arterial obstruction is likely to produce a reduction in pulmonary hypertension with decreased respiratory insufficiency and an improvement in right-sided heart failure (Figs 10.15 and 10.16). Pulmonary artery embolectomy can be unilateral or bilateral.

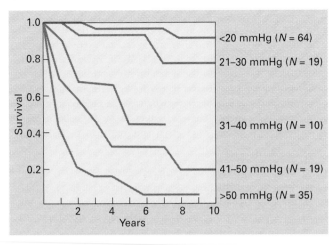

Fig. 10.14 Survival in patients with pulmonary hypertension resulting from chronic recurrent emboli. Groups of patients are compared at different mean pulmonary artery pressures. (Modified from M. Riedel, V. Stanek, J. Widimsky, *et al.*, Long term follow up of patients with pulmonary thromboembolism, *Chest*, **81**, 151, 1982. (Reproduced with permission from D.C. Sabiston Jr, Pulmonary embolism, *Textbook of surgery* (ed. D.C. Sabiston Jr) (14th edn), Chapter 50, Saunders, Philadelphia, PA, 1991.)

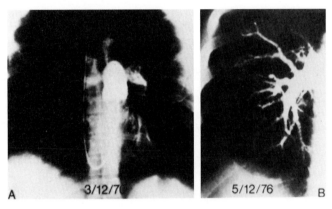

Fig. 10.15 (a) Pulmonary arteriogram in a patient before embolectomy. (b) Six years after right lower lobe embolectomy. Note the continued perfusion of the right lower lobe after embolectomy. (From W.R. Chitwood Jr, H.K. Lyerly, and D.C. Sabiston, Surgical management of chronic pulmonary embolism, *Ann Surg* **201**, 11, 1985. (Reproduced with permission from D.C. Sabiston Jr, Pulmonary embolism, *Textbook of surgery* (ed D.C. Sabiston Jr) (14th edn), Chapter 50, Saunders, Philadelphia, PA, 1991.)

Proximal embolectomy has been undertaken through a thoracotomy incision in the past, but nowadays a median sternotomy and cardiopulmonary bypass is recommended for both bilateral and main pulmonary artery lesions. Emboli are firmly attached to the artery wall and require meticulous dissection. Thus the procedure is more akin to a formal thromboendarterectomy than a thromboembolectomy. All distal emboli should be removed until there is adequate back-bleeding of bright red arterialized blood. Postoperative complications include right ventricular failure, haemorrhagic lung syndrome, and phrenic nerve palsy.[96] Thromboendarterectomy for chronic embolism generally decreases pulmonary artery pressures and increases P_aO_2 towards normal. In patients with proximal lesions, pulmonary thromboendarterectomy is likely to produce relief of respiratory insufficiency and reduction of pulmonary hypertension, and to improve right ventricular function (Fig. 10.16).

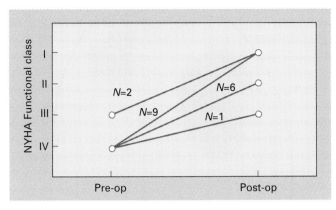

Fig. 10.16 Preoperative and postoperative functional class of 13 patients having a successful pulmonary embolectomy by New York Heart Association (NYHA) criteria. (From H.K. Lyerly and D.C. Sabiston, Chronic pulmonary embolism, *Surgery of the chest* (ed. D.C. Sabiston Jr and F.C. Spencer), Saunders, Philadelphia, PA, 1992.) (Reproduced with permission from D.C. Sabiston Jr, Pulmonary embolism, *Textbook of surgery* (ed. D.C. Sabiston) (14th edn), Saunders, Philadelphia, PA, 1991.)

References

1. Virchow, R. (1858). *Die Cellularpathologie in ihrer Begrudung auf physiologische und pathologische Gewebelehre.* Hirschwald, Berlin.
2. Laennec, R.T.H. (1819). *De l'auscultation mediate.* Brossen et Chaude, Paris.
3. Rokitansky, C. (1842–6). *Handbuch der pathologischen Anatomie. Handbuch der speciellen pathologischen Anatomie.* Vienna.
4. Cornheim, J.E. (1872). *Untersuchungen uber die embolischen processe.* Hirschwald, Berlin.
5. Viamonte, M. (1964). Selective bronchial arteriography in man. *Radiology*, **83**, 830.
6. Trendelenberg, F. (1908). Uber die operative behandlung der embolie der lungenarterie. *Arch. Klin. Chir.*, **86**, 686.
7. Sabiston, D.C., Jr (1983). Trendelenberg's classic work on the operative treatment of pulmonary embolism. *Ann. Thorac. Surg.*, **35**, 570–5.
8. Kirschner, M. (1924). Ein durch die Trendelenbergsche Operation geheilter Fall von Embolie der Arterien pulmonalis. *Arch. Klin. Chir.*, **133**, 312.
9. Sharp, E.H. (1962). Pulmonary embolectomy: successful removal of a massive pulmonary embolus with the support of cardiopulmonary bypass: a case report. *Ann. Surg.*, **156**, 1.
10. Carroll, D. (1950). Chronic obstruction of major pulmonary arteries. *Am. J. Med.*, **9**, 175.
11. Allison, P.R., Dunnill, M.S., and Marshall, R. (1960). Pulmonary embolism. *Thorax*, **15**, 273.
12. Daily, P.O., Dembitsky, W.P., Peterson, K.L., and Moser, K.M. (1987). Modification of techniques and early results of pulmonary thromboendarterectomy for chronic pulmonary embolism. *J. Thorac. Cardiovasc. Surg.*, **93**, 221–33.
13. Dalen, J.E. and Alpert, J.S. (1975). Natural history of pulmonary embolism. *Prog. Cardiovasc. Dis.*, **17**, 257–70.
14. Dismuke, S.E. and Wagner, E.H. (1986). Pulmonary embolism as a cause of death; the changing mortality in hospitalized patients. *J. Am. Med. Assoc.*, **255**, 2039–42.
15. Salzman, E.W. and Hirsh, J. (1994). The epidemiology, pathogenosis and natural history of venous thromboembolism. In: *Hemostasis and thrombosis* (ed. R.W. Colman, J. Hirsh V.J. Marder, and E.W. Salzman), pp. 1275–96. Lippincott, Philadelphia, PA.

16. Clagett, G.P., Anderson, F.A., Levine, M.N., *et al.* (1992). Prevention of venous thromboembolism. *Chest*, **102**, 391S–407S.

17. Anderson, F.A., Wheeler, H.B., Goldberg, R.J., *et al.* (1991). A population-based perspective of the hospital incidence and case fatality rates of deep venous thrombosisand pulmonary embolism. The Worcester DVT Study. *Arch. Intern. Med.*, **151**, 933–8.

18. Anderson, F.A. and Wheeler, H.B. (1992). Physician practices in the management of venous thromboembolism: a community-wide survey. *J. Vasc. Surg.*, **15**, 707–14.

19. Gillum, R.F. (1987). Pulmonary embolism and thrombophlebitis in the US: 1970–1985. *Am. Heart J.*, **114**, 1262–4.

20. Carson, J.L., Kelley, M.A., Duff, A., *et al.* (1992). The clinical course of pulmonary embolism. *New Engl. J. Med.*, **326**, 1240–5.

21. Browse, N.L. and Thomas, M.L. (1974). Source of nonlethal pulmonary emboli. *Lancet*, **i**, 258–9.

22. Wheeler, H.B., Anderson, F.A.J., Cardullo, P.A., *et al.* (1982). Suspected deep vein thrombosis: management by impedance plethysmography. *Arch. Surg.*, **117**, 1206–9.

23. Benotti, J.R. and Dalen, J.E. (1984). The natural history of pulmonary embolism. *Clin. Chest Med.*, **5**, 403–9.

24. Davies, M.G. and Hagen, P.-O. (1993). The vascular endothelium: a new horizon. *Ann. Surg.*, **218**, 593–609.

25. Eisenberg, P.R. (1991). Endothelial cell mediators of thrombosis and fibrinolysis: review in depth. *Coronary Artery Dis.*, **2**, 129–66.

26. Jaffe, E.A. (1992). Physiologic function of the normal endothelial cell. In *Vascular medicine* (ed. J. Loscalzo, M. Creagher, and V.) pp. 3–46. Little Brown, Boston, MA.

27. Seyer, J.M. and Kang, A.H. (1992). Connective tissues of the subendothelium. In: *Vascular medicine* (ed. J. Loscalz, M. Creagher, and V.J. Dzau), pp. 47–78. Little Brown, Boston, MA.

28. Clouse, L.H. and Comp, P.C. (1986). The regulation of hemostasis: the protein C system. *New Engl. J. Med.*, **314**, 1298–1304.

29. Gertler, J.P. and Abbott, W.M. (1992). Prothrombotic and fibrinolytic functions of normal and perturbed endothelium. *J. Surg. Res.*, **52**, 89–95.

30. Cosgriff, T.M., Bishop, D.T., Herrshgold, E.J., *et al.* (1983). Familial antithrombin III deficiency: its natural history, genetics, diagnosis and treatment. *Medicine*, **62**, 209.

31. Comp, P.C. and Esmon, C.T. (1984). Recurrent venous thromboembolism in patients with a partial deficiency of protein S. *New Engl. J. Med.*, **311**, 1525.

32. Ridkar, P.M., Hennekens, C.H., Lindpaintner, K., *et al.* (1995). Mutation of the gene coding for coagulation factor V and the risk of myocardial infarction, stroke and venous thrombosis in apparently healthy men. *New Engl. J. Med.*, **332**, 912–17.

33. Tollefsen, D.M. (1989). Antithrombotic deficiency. In: *The metabolic basis of inherited disease* (ed. C.R. Scriver, A.L. Beaudet, W.S. Sly, and D. Valle) (6th edn), pp. 2207–18. McGraw-Hill, New York.

34. Gorham, L.W. (1961). A study of pulmonary embolism, Parts I and II. *Arch. Intern. Med.*, **108**, 8, 189.

35. Sabiston, D.C., Jr and Wolfe, W.G. (1968). Experimental and clinical observations on the natural history of pulmonary embolism. *Ann. Surg.*, **168**, 1–15.

36. Burnett, W.E., Long, J.H., Norris, C., *et al.* (1949). The effect of pneumonectomy on pulmonary function. *J. Thorac. Surg.*, **18**, 569.

37. Brofman, B.L., Charms, B.L., Kohn, P.M., *et al.* (1957). Unilateral pulmonary artery occlusion in man. Control studies. *J. Thorac. Surg.*, **34**, 206.

38. Gurewich, V., Sasahara, A.A. and Stein, M. (1965). Pulmonary embolism, bronchoconstriction and response to heparin. In: *Pulmonary embolic disease* (ed. A.A. Sasahara and M. Stein), pp. 162–9. Grune and Stratton, New York.

39. Liu, S.-F. and Barnes, P.J. (1994). Role of endothelium in the control of pulmonary vascular tone. *Endothelium*, **2**, 11–33.

40. Browse, N. (1969). Deep vein thrombosis. Diagnosis. *Br. J. Med.*, **4**, 676–8.

41. Hull, R., Hirsh J., Sackett, D.L. and Stoddard, G. (1986). Cost effectiveness of clinical diagnosis, venography and non-invasive testing in patients with symptomatic deep vein thrombosis. *New Engl. J. Med.*, **314**, 823–8.

42. Hull, R., Hirsh, J., Sackett, D.L., *et al.* (1981). Clinical validity of a negative venogram in patients with clinically suspected venous thrombosis. *Circulation*, **64**, 622–5.

43. Appleman, P.T., DeJong, T.E., and Lampmann, L.E. (1987). Deep venous thrombosis of the leg: US findings. *Radiology*, **163**, 743–6.

44. Cronan, J.J. (1993). Venous thromboembolic disease. The role of ultrasound. *Radiology*, **186**, 619–30.

45. Glew, D., Cooper, T., Mitchelmore, A.E., *et al.* (1992). Impedance plethysmography and thromboembolic disease. *Br. J. Radiol.*, **65**, 306–8.

46. Huisman, M.V., Buller, H.R., Cate, J., and Vreeken, J. (1986). Serial impedence plethysmography for suspected deep venous thrombosis in outpatients. *New Engl. J. Med.*, **314**, 823–8.

47. Heijboer, H., Buller, H.R., Lensing, A.W.A., *et al.* (1993). A comparison of realtime compression ultrasonography with impedance plethysmography for the diagnosis of deep vein thrombosis in symptomatic outpatients. *New Engl. J. Med.*, **329**, 1365–9.

48. Gomes, A.S., Webber, M.M., and Buffkin, D. (1982). Contrast vs. radionuclide venography: a study of discrepancies and their possible significance. *Radiology*, **142**, 719–28.

49. Sandler, D.A., Duncan, J.S., Ward, P., *et al.* (1984). Diagnosis of deep vein thrombosis. Comparison of clinical evaluation, ultrasound, plethysmography and veoscan with X-ray venogram. *Lancet*, **ii**, 716–19.

50. Erdman, W.A., Jayson, H., Redman, H., *et al.* (1988). Deep venous thrombosis of the extremities: role of MR imaging in the diagnosis. *Radiology*, **174**, 425–31.

51. Millar, G.H. and Feied, C.F. (1995). Suspected pulmonary embolism. The difficulties of diagnostic evaluation. *Postgrad. Med.*, **97**, 51–8.

52. Goldhaber, S.Z. and Morpurgo, M. (1992). Diagnosis, treatment and prevention of pulmonary embolism: report of the WHO/International Society and Federation of Cardiology Task Force. *J. Am. Med. Assoc.*, **268**, 1727–33.

53. Westermark, N. (1938). On the roentgen diagnosis of lung embolism. *Acta Radiol.*, **19**, 357.

54. Littmann, D. (1965). Observations on the electrocardiographic changes in pulmonary embolism. In: *Pulmonary embolic disease* (ed. A.A. Sasahara and M. Stein), pp. 180–98. Grune and Stratton, New York.

55. Greenspan, R.N. (1994). Pulmonary angiography and the diagnosis of pulmonary embolism. *Prog. Cardiovasc. Dis.*, **37**, 93–105.

56. Anonymous (1986). Consensus Conference: Prevention of venous thrombosis and pulmonary embolism. *J. Am. Med. Assoc.*, **256**, 744–9.

57. Wells, P.S., Lensing, A.W.A., and Hirsh, J. (1994). Graduated compression stockings in the prevention of postoperative venous thromboembolism. *Arch. Intern. Med.*, **154**, 67–72.

58. Anonymous (1975). Prevention of fatal postoperative pulmonary embolism by low doses of heparin: an international multicenter trial. *Lancet*, **ii**, 45–51.

59. Collins, R., Scrimgeour, A., Yusuf, S., *et al.* (1988). Reduction in fatal pulmonary embolism and venous thrombosis by

perioperative administration of subcutaneous heparin. Overview of results of randomized trials in general orthpedic and urologic surgery. *New Engl. J. Med.*, **318**, 1162–73.

60. Clagett, C.P. and Reisch, J.S. (1988). Prevention of venous thrombosis in general surgical patients. Results of meta-analysis. *Ann. Surg.*, **208**, 227–40.

61. Cosmi, B. and Hirsh, J. (1994). Low molecular weight heparins. *Curr. Opin. Cardiol.*, **9**, 612–18.

62. Green, D., Hirsh, J., Heit, J., *et al.* (1994). Low molecular weight heparin: a critical analysis of clinical trials. *Pharmacol. Rev.*, **46**, 89–109.

63. Makhoul, R.G., Greenberg, C.S., and McCann, R.L. (1986). Heparin associated thrombocytopenia and thrombosis: a serious clinical problem and potential solution. *J. Vasc. Surg.*, **4**, 522–8.

64. Makhoul, R.G., Devine, D.V., Brenckman, W.D.J., *et al.* (1987). Evidence for the involvement of platelet glycoproteins other than GPIb in heparin-associated thrombocytopenia and thrombosis. *Thromb. Res.* **45**, 421–5.

65. Pinto, D.J. (1970). Controlled trial of an anticoagulant (warfarin sodium) in the prevention of venous thrombosis following hip surgery. *Br. J. Surg.*, **57**, 349–52.

66. Hirsh, J. (1991). Oral anticoagulant drugs. *New Engl. J. Med.*, **324**, 1865–75.

67. Levine, M., Gent, M., Hirsh, J., *et al.* (1996). A comparison of low molecular weight heparin administered primarily at home with unfractioned heparin administered in the hospital for proximal deep vein thrombosis. *New Engl. J. Med.*, **334**, 677–81.

68. Koopman, M.M.W., Prandoni, P., Piovella, F., *et al.* (1996). Treatment of venous thrombosis with intravenous unfractioned heparinadministered in hospital as compared with subcutaneous low molecular weight heparin administered at home. *New Engl. J. Med.*, **334**, 682–7.

69. Lensing, A.W., Prins, M.H., and Davidson, B.L. (1995). Treatment of deep venous thrombosis with low molecular weight heparins: a meta-analysis. *Arch. Intern. Med.*, **155**, 601–07.

70. Bjork, I. and Lindahl, U. (1982). Mechanism of the anticoagulant action of heparin. *Mol. Cell Biochem.*, **48**, 161–82.

71. Hyers, J.M., Hull, R.D., and Weg, J. (1992). Antithrombotic therapy for venous thromboembolic disease. *Chest*, **102**, 408S–25S.

72. Hull, R.D., Raskob, G.E., Rosenbloom, D.R., *et al.* (1992). Optimal therapeutic level of heparin therapy in patients with venous thrombosis. *Arch. Intern. Med.*, **152**, 1589–95.

73. Research Committee of the British Thoracic Society (1992). Optimum duration of anticoagulation for deep vein thrombosis and pulmonary embolism. *Lancet*, **340**, 873–6.

74. Freedman, M.D. (1992). Oral anticoagulants: pharmacodynamics, clinical indications and adverse effects. *J. Clin. Pharmacol.*, **32**, 196–209.

75. Sherry, S., Bell, W.R., Duckert, H., *et al.* (1980). Thrombolytic therapy in thrombosis: a National Institutes of Health Consensus Development Conference. *Ann. Intern. Med.*, **93**, 141–4.

76. Comerota, A.J. and Alderidge, S.C. (1993). Thrombolytic therapy for deep venous thrombosis: a clinical review. *Can. J. Surg.*, **36**, 359–64.

77. Goldhaber, S.E. (1995). Contemporary pulmonary embolism thrombolysis. *Chest*, **107**, 45S–51S.

78. Anonymous (1973). Urokinase Pulmonary Embolism Trial: a national co-operative study. *Circulation*, **470**, 1–108.

79. Levine, M.N. (1993). Thrombolytic therapy in acute pulmonary embolism. *Can. J. Cardiol.*, **9**, 158–9.

80. Greenfield, L.J. (1992). Evolution of venous interruption for pulmonary thromboembolism. *Arch. Surg.*, **127**, 622–26.

81. Greenfield, L.J. and Michna, B.A. (1988). Twelve year clinical experience with the Greenfield vena caval filter. *Surgery*, **104**, 706–12.

82. Becker, D.M., Philbrick, J.T., and Selby, J.B. (1992). Inferior vena cava filters: indications, safety, effectiveness. *Arch. Intern. Med.*, **152**, 1985–94.

83. Kniemeyer, H.W., Sandmann, W., Bach, D., *et al.* (1994). Complications following caval interruption. *Eur. J. Vasc. Surg.*, **8**, 617–21.

84. Millward, S.F., Bormanis, J., Burbridge, B.E., *et al.* (1994). Preliminary clinical experience with the Gunter temporary inferior vena cava filter. *J. Vasc. Intern. Radiol.*, **5**, 863–8.

85. Bloomfield, P., Boon, N.A. and DeBono D.P. (1988). Indications for pulmonary embolectomy. *Lancet*, **i**, 329–31.

86. Langhans, M.R.J. and Greenfield, L.J. (1986). Transvenous catheter embolectomy for life threatening pulmonary embolism. *Infect. Surg.*, **5**, 694–6.

87. Riedel, M., Staned, V., Widimsky, J., *et al.* (1982). Longterm follow up of patients with pulmonary thromboembolism. Late prognosis and evolution of hemodynamic and respiratory data. *Chest*, **81**, 151–8.

88. Moser, K.M., Auger, W.R., and Fedullo, P.F. (1990). Chronic major vessel thromboembolic pulmonary hypertension. *Circulation*, **81**, 1735.

89. Auger, W.R., Moser, K.M., Fedullo, P.F., *et al.* (1991). The association of heparin-induced thrombocytopenia and lupus anticoagulant inpatients with chronic thromboembolic pulmonary hypertension. *Am. Rev. Respir. Dis.*, **143**, A803–7.

90. Giaid, A. and Saleh, D. (1995). Reduced expression of endothelial nitric oxide synthase in the lungs of patients with pulmonary hypertension. *New Engl. J. Med.*, **333**, 214–21.

91. Nicod, P., Peterson, K., Levine, M., *et al.* (1987). Pulmonary angiography in severe chronic pulmonary hypertension. *Ann. Intern. Med.*, **107**, 565–8.

92. Auger, W.R., Fedullo, P.F., Moser, K.M., *et al.* (1992). Chronic major vessel thromboembolic pulmonary artery obstruction appearance at angiography. *Radiology*, **182**, 393–8.

93. Kauczor, H.U., Schwickert, H.C., Mayer, E., *et al.* (1994). Spiral CT of bronchial arteries in chronic thromboembolism. *J. Comput. Assisted Tomogr.*, **18**, 855–61.

94. Shure, D., Gregoratos, C., and Moser, K.M. (1985). Fiberoptic angioscopy; role in the diagnosis of chronic pulmonary arterial obstruction. *Ann. Intern. Med.*, **103**, 844–50.

95. McIntyre, K.M. and Sarahara, A.A. (1971). The hemodynamic response to pulmonary embolism in patients without prior cardiopulmonary disease. *Am. J. Cardiol.*, **28**, 288–94.

96. Couves, C.M., Makai, S.S., Sterris, L.P., *et al.* (1973). Hemorrhagic lung syndrome. *Ann. Thorac. Surg.*, **15**, 187–95.

97. Greenfield, L.J. (1993). Venous thrombosis and pulmonary thromboembolism. In: *Surgery: scientific principles and practice* (ed. L.J. Greenfield, M.W. Mulholland, K.T. Oldham, and G.B. Zelenoch), pp. 1764–78. Lippincott, Philadelphia, PA.

Bibliography to Part II

Goldhaber, S.Z. (ed.) (1985). *Pulmonary embolism and deep venous thrombosis*. Saunders, Philadelphia, PA.

Sabiston, D.C., Jr (1995). Pulmonary embolism. In: *Surgery of the chest* (ed. D.C. Sabiston Jr and F.C. Spencer), pp. 773–821.

Tapson, V.F., Fulkerson, W.J., and Saltzman, H.A. (1995). Venous thromboembolism. *Clin. Chest Med.*, **16**, 229–338.

Part III

The swollen limb and lymphatic problems

Peter Mortimer

11 The swollen limb and lymphatic problems

Introduction

The lymphatic system should be considered as part of the peripheral cardiovascular system interlinking closely with the blood circulation at its origins, through the interstitial space, and at its drainage point, the thoracic duct. To a large extent the anatomy of lymphatics parallels that of the veins, and the two systems show many similarities in structure and function. Fluid and cellular exchange between blood and lymph can occur at points along the drainage route, particularly within the lymph nodes.

The lymphatic system comprises the lymph, the lymphatic vessels, the lymph nodes, and other organs containing lymphoid tissue, particularly the spleen and bone marrow. Although not a true circulation like the blood vascular system, the lymphatic vessels provide an important 'limb' of the microcirculation in most tissues, and with the blood vessels cater for the constant recirculation of protein and cells. Through its own specialist cell, the lymphocyte, a close relationship exists between the peripheral lymphatic system, the blood circulation, and the spleen and liver. Therefore, while lymph drainage serves a predominantly 'plumbing' role, the lymphatic system does possess important immunological responsibilities. The lymphatic vessels are essential for the continual drainage of both plasma proteins and lymph-borne cells from the body tissues. If this drainage ceases, death will ensue.

The embryonic origin of the lymphatic system remains uncertain, but its close development with the venous system is not in doubt. The first lymphatics to be observed lie close to veins as lymph sacs (jugular, iliac, retroperitoneal, and cisterna chyli). These sacs arise from nearby major veins. Whether subsequent growth is by endothelial budding in a centrifugal direction or by lymphatic vessels arising from mesenchymal spaces is still not clear. It is the continued failure to this day of positive identification of lymphatics by an endothelial marker which prevents clarification. Nevertheless, despite the similarities with veins and the difficulties distinguishing a blood vessel from a lymphatic in a histopathological section, it is interesting to note that lymphatic capillaries anastomose with other lymphatic vessels but never with blood capillaries. Therefore they recognize a difference!

The importance of the lymphatic system has not been truly recognized, largely because of a lack of reliable and sensitive investigatory methods. As a result it is still not possible to measure, for example, limb lymph flow or lymphatic contractility in humans except in very extenuating (and invasive) circumstances. This means that we are far from fully understanding the pathogenesis of most

forms of lymphoedema or indeed the role of the lymphatic in many disease states.

It is important when dealing with peripheral vascular disorders, particularly in the presence of oedema, to 'think lymphatic', otherwise the full pathophysiology of the condition confronting the clinician is unlikely to be appreciated. A good example is when unilateral leg lymphoedema first presents with a sudden onset of swelling. It is frequently (and understandably) diagnosed as a deep vein thrombosis, but once thrombosis has been excluded a careful search for clinical signs of lymphatic insufficiency should suggest lymphoedema and the diagnosis can then be confirmed by lymphoscintigraphy. What frequently happens is that the patient is discharged without a satisfactory diagnosis and the opportunity for early treatment is lost. A good understanding of the lymphatic system is essential for the venous specialist.

The swollen limb

Swelling of the lower limb can have many different underlying causes. While the most common cause will be oedema, expansion of all or part of a limb may be the result of an increase in any tissue component (e.g. muscle, fat, blood, etc.). Further consideration should be given to whether swelling is acute or chronic, symmetrical or asymmetrical, localized or generalized, or congenital or acquired, if the underlying mechanism is to be fully understood. Limb swelling is usually a manifestation of chronic oedema arising from venous or lymphatic disease, and here we consider only swelling of vascular or lymphatic origin. Possible causes of limb swelling are listed in Table 11.1.

Normal anatomy and physiology of lymphatics

Anatomy

Lymphatic or lymph vessels constitute many of the vessels of the body and, although fewer in number than blood vessels, are potentially larger in size at capillary level. Lymphatic vessels are essentially of two types: (1) smaller non-contractile initial lymphatics (previously called terminal lymphatics) which commence or 'initiate' the drainage process within the tissues, and (2) larger contractile

Table 11.1   Causes of a swollen limb

Congenital

Vascular

  Haemangioma

  Venous angioma (diffuse phlebectasia)

  Klippel–Trenaunay syndrome

  Parkes–Weber syndrome

  Maffucci's syndrome

Lymphatic

  Lymphoedema

  Lymphangioma

Other

  Fat hypertrophy

  Congenital lipomatosis

  Plexiform neurofibroma

  Proteus syndrome

  Muscle hamartoma

  Gigantism

  Hemihypertrophy

Acquired

Vascular

  Deep vein thrombosis

  Post-thrombotic syndrome

  Chronic venous insufficiency

  Venous outflow obstruction (e.g. inferior vena cava obstruction)

  Thrombophlebitis

  Venous injury (e.g. intravenous drug abuse)

  Cockett's syndrome

  Idiopathic oedema of women

  Acute arterial ischaemia

Lymphatic

  Lymphoedema

    Tumours (e.g. Kaposi's sarcoma, infiltrative cancer)

    Cancer treatment

    Filariasis

    Podoconiosis

  Armchair legs

  Trauma

  Reconstructive surgery (e.g. coronary artery bypass graft, femoropopliteal bypass)

  Factitial lymphoedema (e.g. Secretan's syndrome)

  Reflux sympathetic dystrophy

  Pretibial myxoedema

Inflammatory

  Cellulitis/erysipelas

  Varicose eczema/lipodermatosclerosis (also venous)

  Asteototic dermatitis

  Psoriasis

Table 11.1   Continued

Musculoskeletal

  Arthritis

  Joint effusion/haemarthrosis

  Ruptured Baker's cyst

  Haematoma

  Torn gastrocnemius muscle

  Pathological fracture

  Achilles tendonitis

  Myositis ossificans

Tumours

  Sarcoma

  Liposarcoma

  Leiomyosarcoma

  Angiosarcoma

  Lymphangiosarcoma

  Malignant fibrous histiocytoma

  Osteosarcoma

lymphatic collectors or trunks into which the initial lymphatics drain. Afferent collectors drain to lymph nodes and efferent collectors drain from lymph nodes.

The skin in the lower limb is most richly endowed with initial lymphatics. Here lymphatic capillaries originate as blind-ending endothelial-lined tubes in the superficial dermis from where, via a network of intercommunicating vessels, lymph drains through a series of enlarging precollectors until it enters the contractile collecting vessels within the subcutaneous compartment.

The initial lymphatics in the skin are arranged in loosely constructed polygonal meshes (Fig. 11.1) which are located high in the dermis just below the superficial blood vascular plexus. Territories of skin are drained by these meshes into vertically draining precollectors (Fig. 11.2) and hence into the deeper collectors. A series of valves ensure that flow is unidirectional. The capacity of initial lymphatics for dilatation is such that the valves can readily become incompetent. In such circumstances, i.e. obstruction to deeper lymphatic routes, retrograde flow of lymph results in 'dermal backflow' as witnessed on both conventional X-ray lymphography and lymphoscintigraphy (see later). The cutaneous initial lymphatic network provides collateralization by which lymph can escape to other (more) normally draining areas.

The anatomy of initial lymphatics is not so well documented elsewhere in the lower limb as it is in the skin. The subcutaneous compartment appears relatively devoid of initial lymphatics. Indeed, it is difficult to identify lymphatic capillaries within fat. Lymphatics are identifiable within the fascia, but are difficult to find within muscle or bone. Paradoxically, however, lymphangiomatous malformations can occur within muscle and bone, suggesting that lymphatics do exist there or can infiltrate.

The lymphatics of the leg, like the main veins, are divided into superficial and deep systems by the deep fascia. Anastomoses between superficial and deep lymphatic systems (except via a lymph node) do not occur in the lower limb. Moreover, the lymphatic

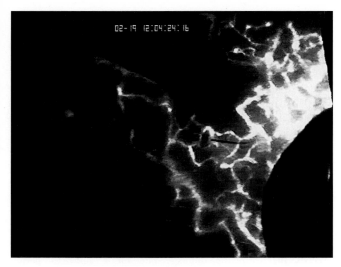

Fig. 11.1 Polygonal network of superficial dermal lymphatics demonstrated following injection of FITC-dextran and observed through a fluorescence microscope (fluorescence microlymphography).

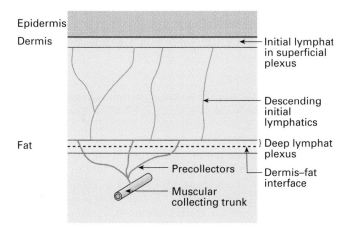

Fig. 11.2 Anatomy of initial lymphatics, descending precollectors, and muscular collecting trunks.

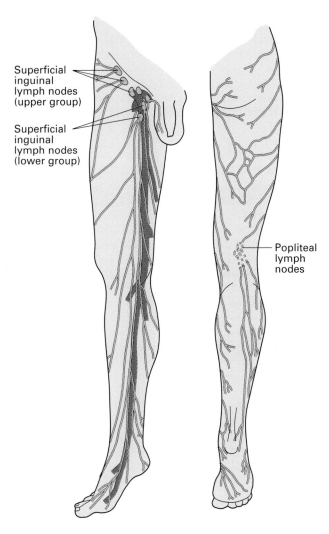

Fig. 11.3 The lymphatic drainage of the lower limb superficial to the fascia: (a) antero medial bundle); (b) superficial lateral bundle.

system is strictly regional in character. Most of the superficial (suprafascial, epifascial) compartment is drained by the **anterome-dial group of collecting trunks** which drain to the groin follow-ing the course of the long saphenous vein. One or two collecting trunks start from the medial half of the dorsum of the foot and persist as single trunks to the groin. From the lateral half of the dorsum of the foot a further one or two trunks run proximally on the front of the leg and join those previously described just below the knee. Anything from seven to 12 trunks drain to the groin via the anteromedial route. One or two collecting trunks arise from the lateral aspect of the heel close to the short saphenous vein and form the **superficial lateral group** which generally drain to the popliteal fossa. Therefore the greater part of the lymph from the skin and subcutaneous tissues of the leg drains via the superficial anterome-dial group of lymphatics (Fig. 11.3).

The **deep system** of lymphatics drains the joints, fascial planes, muscles, and bone. The lymph-collecting trunks run in close prox-imity to the main deep blood vessels. Connections between the deep and superficial lymphatics are rare.

Purpose of lymphatics

Lymphatics are primarily concerned with draining materials from the tissue spaces which cannot return to the blood stream directly. Colloids, and particularly protein, fall into this category as do many cells (extravasated red cells, macrophages, lymphocytes, and of course malignant cells). Bacterial and other micro-organisms are channelled through lymphatics, presumably as a protective mechan-ism to prevent noxious agents from directly entering the blood stream. Presumably this failure to 'police' infection is the reason why cellulitis and erysipelas can be such a recurrent problem with lymphoedema. Similarly, inorganic matter such as carbon and silica is removed by the lymphatics (as witnessed by the black pulmonary lymph nodes in coalminers).

Under normal circumstances water acts predominantly as a solvent or vehicle for the colloids, cells, and particulate matter which can only be drained via the lymph route. Nevertheless, lym-phatics also serve as an 'overflow pipe' to drain excess interstitial fluid. It is important to understand this role of the lymphatic acting as a 'safety valve' or buffer against fluid overload because it incrimi-nates the lymphatic system in some way in every form of oedema.

Physiology of lymphatic function

Lymph differs very little from interstitial fluid, and the process of lymph drainage starts at the point of net plasma filtration from the blood stream. From there three interdependent steps occur: (i) transport of fluid and other materials (prelymph) across the interstitial space and into initial lymphatics, (ii) movement of lymph through the network of non-contractile initial lymphatics, and (iii) active pumping of lymph through the series of contractile collecting trunks.

Initial lymphatics act as simple passive conduits which respond to changes in pressure around them generated by local massaging of tissues by arterial pulsation, external pressure, movements, and, in particular, intermittent striated muscle contractions. More proximal (central) lymph flow is almost certainly influenced by breathing. Initial lymphatics are supported by connective tissue fibrils, particularly elastin, which distend the lymphatic vessel lumen with the slightest rise of interstitial pressure. Tension in the fibrils opens the large junctions between endothelial cells and so permits entry of macromolecules. It is the intermittent nature of the pressure changes that generates initial lymphatic flow. Lymphatic vessels are closely valved right down to the initial lymphatics, with the valves directing flow centripetally (Fig. 11.4).

The collecting trunks consist of intervalve segments or lymphangions which act like independent lymph hearts in series. The stimulus to lymphatic contraction is the filling and distension of the lymphangions. Their behaviour is akin to the inotropic and chronotropic actions of the heart. While lymphatic pumping is largely dependent on the supply of lymph to the collectors, it is probably also true to say that it creates a 'suction force' which influences initial lymphatic flow. Contractions in the human leg have been measured at 10–15 per minute. The frequency and stroke volume of the lymphangion increase with lymph volume.

Lower-limb drainage is extremely low at rest with the legs supine. Passive movements and massage will generate some lymph flow, but the most potent stimulus to flow is weight bearing and in particular activation of the calf muscle pumps during walking. It is likely to be a sudden increase in lymphatic preload (lymphatic filling) from muscle use with a consequent increase in intrinsic pumping (contractility) rather than passive squeezing of lymphatics by the muscles (as happens with the veins) which generates lymph drainage in the leg.

Oedema

Oedema is an excess of interstitial fluid. Interstitial fluid volume must increase by over 100 per cent before oedema is clinically detectable. Oedema develops when the capillary filtration rate exceeds the lymphatic drainage rate for a sufficient period. Understanding oedema should be a relatively straightforward process if it is considered from physiological principles, but unfortunately it tends to be 'pigeon-holed' according to the underlying medical condition (e.g. heart failure, nephrotic syndrome, venous oedema). All oedema, whatever the cause, results from an imbalance between capillary filtration and lymph drainage:

$$\frac{\mathrm{d}v}{\mathrm{d}t} = \mathcal{J}_\mathrm{v} - \mathcal{J}_\mathrm{L}$$

where $\mathrm{d}v/\mathrm{d}t$ is the rate of swelling, $\mathcal{J}_\mathrm{v}$ is the net capillary filtration rate, and $\mathcal{J}_\mathrm{L}$ is the lymph flow.

Therefore it follows that the pathogenesis of any oedema involves either a high filtration rate or a low lymph flow or a combination of the two. Elevation of capillary pressure is usually secondary to chronic elevation of venous pressure caused by heart failure, fluid overload, or deep vein thrombosis. Reduced plasma colloid osmotic pressure (e.g. hypoproteinaemia) raises net filtration rate and consequently lymph flow (if permitted). Changes in capillary permeability (e.g. inflammation) increase the escape of protein into the interstitium and water follows osmotically. Impairment of lymph drainage results in the accumulation of predominantly protein and water in the interstitial space because lymph is the sole route for returning escaped protein to the plasma.

Most oedemas arise from increased capillary filtration overwhelming lymph drainage. To some extent, therefore, any oedema incriminates the lymphatic through its failure to keep up with demand. However, lymphoedema is oedema arising principally from a failure of lymph drainage.

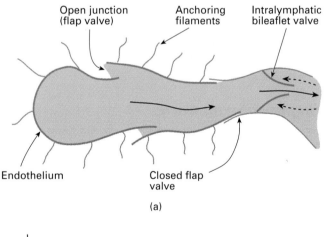

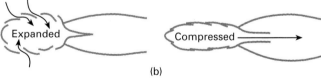

Fig. 11.4   (a) Simplified model of an initial lymphatic showing two flaps valve which permit entry into the lymphatic and the bileaflet valve which controls the direction of flow within the lymphatic. (b) Expansion (filling) and compression (emptying of initial lymphatic. Flap valves open during expansion because the pressure within the lumen falls below the pressure in the adjacent interstitium.

Lymphoedema

Pathophysiology

Lymphatics may fail for a number of reasons. First, there may be an intrinsic abnormality of the lymph-conducting pathways. Such cases are referred to as **primary lymphoedemas**, and in practice this simply means that no identifiable outside cause can be found. **Secondary lymphoedemas** are those due to some factor originating outside the lymph system, such as surgical removal of lymph nodes, radiotherapy, or a severe infection. Physiologically

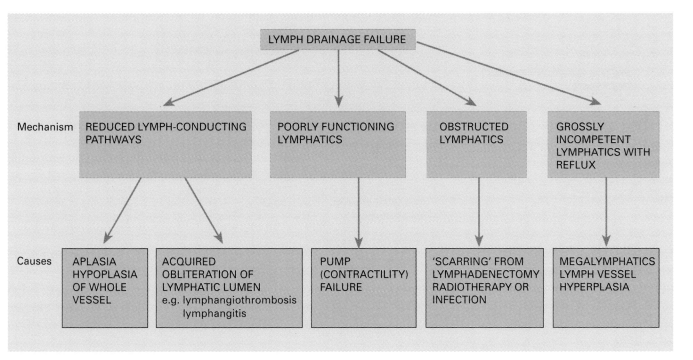

Fig. 11.5   Possible (theoretical) causes of lymphoedema

there are only a limited number of ways that lymphatics can fail. They may be reduced in number, obliterated, obstructed, or simply fail to function. A lack of sensitive methods for investigation makes it difficult to distinguish between these mechanisms (Fig. 11.5).

A reduction in lymphatics may be total aplasia, such as the absence of skin lymphatics in Milroy's disease, or partial hypoplasia which is more often the case. In the most common form of primary lymphoedema—that presenting at or soon after puberty with distal leg swelling—lymphangiograms usually demonstrate a reduction in size and number of peripheral leg lymphatic collectors. It is often assumed that the lymphatics have been abnormal since birth, but it is always possible that the lymph vessels have undergone an accelerated atrophy or ageing process. Therefore the congenitally determined abnormality may not be an underdevelopment of lymphatics from birth but rather a failure of growth or regeneration following damage or injury. This would explain the latent period before swelling manifests, particularly in those forms presenting later in life (lymphoedema tarda). In fact, we do not know and these possibilities are speculative.

An obliterative process, where there is permanent obliteration of the lymphatic lumen and consequently of the vessel itself, probably develops through lymphangiothrombosis or lymphangitis in the same way as for veins. Like blood, lymph will clot, but not so readily. Unfortunately, there is no clinical investigation for lymph thrombosis.

The contractility of the lymphatic collecting trunks may fail. Unfortunately, there is no clinical investigation to confirm this.

Lymph drainage routes may become obstructed as a result of scarring or fibrosis of the tissues; this is most commonly seen in the treatment of cancer, following lymphadenectomy with or without radiotherapy. The longer a surgical scar the less likely it is that successful reanastomosis of damaged lymphatics will occur. Nevertheless,

such is the regenerative power of lymphatics that lymphoedema is avoided in the majority of patients.

Megalymphatics cause lymphoedema of the lower limbs by virtue of gross incompetence of the valves. Enormous dilatation of the lymphatic collectors results in rapid reflux due to gravitational forces. Megalymphatics can be associated with chylous reflux.

Classification of clinical types

Figure 11.6 shows the clinical classification of lymphoedemas.

Primary lymphoedema

Truly congenital (connatal) lymphoedema, which present at or within, a few hours of birth, is rare (Fig. 11.7). The cause is presumed to be aplasia of collecting lymphatics. Miraculously swelling can improve or remit spontaneously. This is often the case in lymphoedema associated with genetic syndromes such as Turner's and Noonan's syndromes. Generally, swelling persists but there is remarkably little physical disability. Growth and development remain normal.

In 1892 Milroy described a large family pedigree where the onset of lymphoedema was at or soon after birth. Nonne described a similar family at the same time, and so the condition bears both their names. Unfortunately, many clinicians consider Milroy's disease (Fig. 11.7) to be synonymous with primary lymphoedema. This is incorrect, as Milroy's disease must be familial by definition (Fig. 11.8). Familial lymphoedema with onset during childhood or puberty at the latest is known as Meige's syndrome.

More numerous than the familial forms are the sporadic cases which do not bear eponymous names but are simply referred to as primary lymphoedema. Distal hypoplasia of the leg lymphatics is the most common cause of primary lymphoedema (Fig. 11.9). Oedema begins in the foot and ankle extending proximally. The

Fig. 11.6   Classification of primary lymphoedema

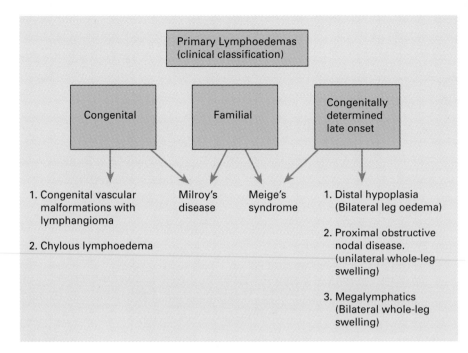

Fig. 11.7   Congenital lymphoedema

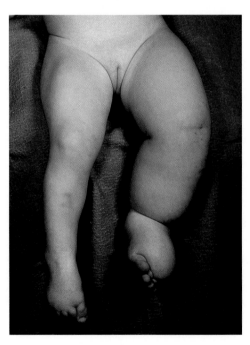

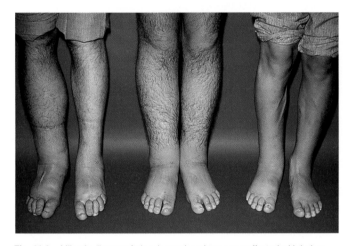

Fig. 11.8   Milroy's disease: father (centre) and two sons affected with below knee swelling.

onset is often at puberty and females are predominantly affected. The oedema is usually bilateral but asymmetrical, with minimal if any swelling above the knee.

Lymphoedema of the proximal obstructive type manifests with sudden onset of unilateral whole-leg swelling (Fig. 11.10). It is of paramount importance to exclude pelvic causes of venous or lymphatic obstruction (e.g. tumour, thrombosis). Lymphatic studies of these cases have demonstrated sclerosis and atrophy of the inguinofemoral nodes, but no cause has been identified. Whole-leg swelling, which is sometimes bilateral, can be a manifestation of

megalymphatics. Here, grossly dilated (varicose) lymphatics with valvular incompetence give rise to lymph, and sometimes chylous, reflux.

Lymphoedema may be the predominant manifestation of a congenital vascular syndrome (e.g. Klippel–Trenaunay syndrome). In such patients malformed lymphatics coexist with an aberrant venous system, and therefore oedema may result from both increased capillary filtration and poor lymph drainage. Limb swelling may be the presenting and major manifestation of congenital lymphatic malformations (e.g. cavernous lymphangioma).

Secondary lymphoedema

Damage to lymph-conducting pathways may occur secondary to any number of causes originating outside the lymphatic system. In the United Kingdom surgical removal or radiation (or both) of lymph

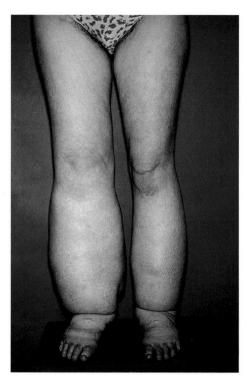

Fig. 11.9   Primary lymphoedema due to distal hypoplasia of the leg lymphatics.

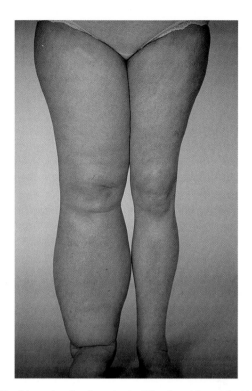

Fig. 11.10   Primary lymphoedema due to obliteration of the proximal lymph nodes and vessels.

nodes as a necessary part of cancer treatment probably makes up the largest group. The most common cancers in which treatment gives rise to lower-limb swelling are melanoma, sarcoma, and pelvic tumours, including cervix, uterus, and prostate. It is noteworthy that cancer of the pelvis and infiltrating sarcomas can present with lymphoedema, and recurrent tumours should always be considered as a cause of limb swelling, particularly if associated with pain. Full staging investigations should always be undertaken in such circumstances.

Trauma to lymphatics either from elective surgery or by accident usually needs to be extensive to induce lymphoedema. Indeed, the experimental production of lymphoedema is extremely difficult owing to the extremely efficient regenerative powers of lymphatics. It is probably the failure of lymphatics to regenerate and reanastomose satisfactorily through scarred or irradiated tissue which is responsible for lymphoedema following cancer treatment. Trauma to the lower limb, such as a degloving injury, will produce widespread scarring. Swelling frequently occurs distal to the lesion (Fig. 11.11).

Filariasis is probably the most common cause of lymphoedema worldwide. It results from infection with a nematode worm (usually *Wucheria bancrofti*) and is transmitted by mosquitoes, which introduce microfilariae into the skin. These larvae migrate to the lymphatics where they mature into adult worms. Progressive and permanent damage to the infested lymphatics causes lymphoedema. Filariasis should be considered in any patient with lymphoedema who has travelled or lived in an endemic area, and a filarial complement fixation test should be performed.

In the author's view lymphangitis or cellulitis only cause lymphoedema when the lymphatics are already perilously vulnerable. In other words, lymphatic insufficiency pre-exists. Indeed, the lymphatic insufficiency may even predispose to the first inflammatory

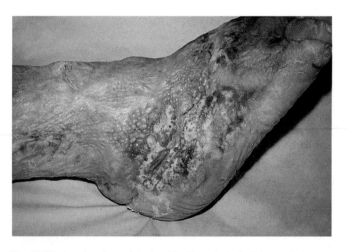

Fig. 11.11   Lymphoedema of the foot following a degloving injury to the leg. Scarring prevents much swelling but skin changes of lymphoedema prevail.

episode. Any patient suffering recurrent lymphangitis/cellulitis in the same leg is likely to have impaired lymph drainage. Proving which came first—the cellulitis or the lymphatic insufficiency—is difficult. Recurrent inflammatory episodes (cellulitis/lymphangitis) are not only debilitating for the patient but frequently lead to a stepwise deterioration in swelling.

Podoconiosis is a form of endemic lymphoedema caused by particles of silica dust which penetrate the feet during barefoot walking. The microparticles are taken up by the lymphatics and cause lymphatic damage.

Clinical diagnosis

Lymphoedema differs from other oedemas (in which increased capillary filtration is the major factor) in that cells, proteins, lipids, and debris accumulate. This results in a 'solid' as well as a 'fluid' component to the swelling, thus giving many lymphoedemas a 'brawny' texture. Pitting (displacement of interstitial fluid by surface pressure) occurs in most patients, and many early forms of lymphoedema will pit readily.

History

The clinical diagnosis of leg lymphoedema depends on the history and on changes in the skin and subcutaneous tissue. Lymphoedema does not usually respond to elevation or diuretics, except in the early stages or when it is compounded by increased capillary filtration. Chronic oedema that does not reduce significantly after overnight elevation is likely to be lymphatic in origin.

The symptoms accompanying uncomplicated lymphoedema are few. Swelling frequently develops rapidly (e.g. overnight). In the distal hypoplastic type one ankle may swell. Pain may feature initially, prompting diagnoses including deep vein thrombosis and soft tissue injury. Oedema is often intermittent before becoming permanent and painless, although discomfort, aching, and tightness are common symptoms. Eventually both legs swell. In proximal obstructive lymphoedema swelling usually develops in the thigh and progresses distally. Functional impairment is slight and the major difficulty is the disfigurement, particularly in relation to clothes and footwear.

Clinical signs

Although most swelling occurs in the subcutaneous layer, the skin exhibits most changes. It becomes thicker, as demonstrated by the Kaposi–Stemmer sign (a failure to pick up or pinch a fold of skin at the base of the second toe) (Fig. 11.12). Skin creases become enhanced and a warty texture (hyperkeratosis) develops; such skin changes are termed 'elephantiasis'. As dermal lymph stasis progresses, elephantiasis becomes more marked. Dilatation of upper dermal lymphatics with consequent organization and fibrosis gives rise to papillomatosis (Fig. 11.13). Lymphangiomas also represent

bulging upper dermal lymphatics, but they appear similar to blisters on the skin surface. They are soft and easily compressible, and for some reason do not possess the surrounding fibrosis of the less compressible papillomas.

Truncal and genital lymphoedema

It is important to remember that the ilio-inguinal nodes drain lymph from the adjoining quadrant of the trunk as well as the lower limb on that side. Close examination will often reveal oedema of the abdominal wall on the affected side, which can be a source of concern and discomfort as the patient is usually aware of its presence. Genital lymphoedema can occur when pelvic lymph drainage is compromised, as is the case after treatment for cancer of the cervix, uterus, or prostate. Lymphoedema of the male external genitalia can occur as a primary event. In such cases it suggests impairment of local skin and subcutaneous initial lymphatics because of the bilateral drainage routes for collecting vessels. Recurrent cellulitis frequently coexists, as may swelling of one or both legs.

Complications of lymphoedema

Lymphatic insufficiency has three major consequences:

- swelling (oedema)
- a predisposition to infection, in particular cellulitis
- the uncommon complication of malignancy arising within the lymphoedema (e.g. Stewart–Treves syndrome).

Swelling leads to discomfort, limb heaviness, reduced mobility, and impaired function. The size and weight of the affected limbs sometimes produces secondary complications (e.g. musculoskeletal problems). Psychological handicap also occurs as a result of the disfigurement. In a recent case–control study comparing breast cancer patients with and without swelling, significant increases in depression and psychosocial maladjustment to illness were found in the group with lymphoedema. The difficulty in finding clothes or shoes to fit creates social problems. Poor footwear will further compound the swelling by discouraging a normal gait and sufficient exercise.

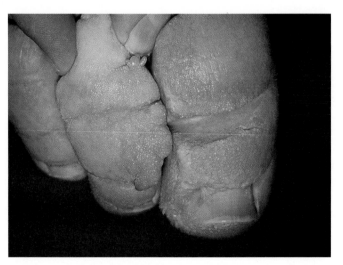

Fig. 11.12 The Kaposi–Stemmer sign. A failure to pinch a fold of skin at the base of the second toe, because of thickened skin and subcutaneous tissue, indicates lymphoedema.

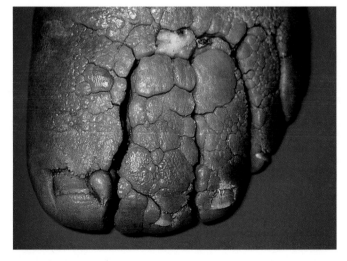

Fig. 11.13 Dilatation of upper dermal lymphatics with consequent organization and fibrosis gives rise to papillomatosis.

Cellulitis: recurrent inflammatory episodes are a characteristic complication of poor lymph drainage. These episodes can be frequent and debilitating and impair lymph drainage further, leading to progressive infection and swelling. The bacterial aetiology of such cases has been questioned, although many infections, including fungal, are more common in patients with lymphoedema. Failure of local immune mechanisms to contain a bacterial, probably streptococcal, antigen seems likely.

Malignancy: there is a small but significant risk of the development of malignancy as a result of impaired lymph drainage. Lymphangiosarcoma (Stewart–Treves syndrome) is the best-known malignancy, but other tumours have been reported including basal cell carcinoma, squamous cell carcinoma, melanoma, and malignant fibrous histiocytoma.

Investigation

Unlike the many methods available for investigating the venous system, there are just two that are widely available for the lymphatic system: radiocontrast X-ray lymphangiography and lymphoscintigraphy (isotope lymphography). Other methods such as computed tomography (CT) and magnetic resonance imaging (MRI) are included in the discussion because of their value in investigating the swollen limb.

Direct contrast X-ray lymphography (lymphangiography)

Lymphography implies imaging of lymph nodes, whereas lymphangiography implies imaging of lymphatic vessels. Lymphography is still used as a staging investigation for cancer, but is applied less often to confirm lymphoedema since the advent of lymphoscintigraphy. It is still of value to define anatomy prior to consideration of surgery as well as classifying the different types of primary lymphoedema.

The technique involves first the interstitial subcutaneous injection of a vital dye (e.g. patent blue violet) to visualize the lymphatic for cannulation. The oily contrast medium Lipiodol is then administered directly into a peripheral lymphatic, usually on the dorsum of the foot. A lymphangiogram is easy to perform when the lymphatics are normal and the feet are not swollen. In the presence of oedema the technique is difficult and better success can be achieved under general anaesthetic. The failure to opacify subcutaneous collectors with the vital dye and the persistence of the dye in the tissues for days afterwards are sufficient evidence for a diagnosis of lymphoedema. If there is lymphatic obstruction, the dye will often flow retrogradely into the dermal network, so-called 'dermal backflow'. A normal lymphangiogram will usually opacify five to 15 collectors, each measuring approximately 1 mm in diameter as they approach the lowermost inguinal lymph nodes. Lymphangiography is not without hazard. Anaphylaxis to the contrast medium can occur, as can pulmonary oil embolism if too much Lipiodol is administered. There is some concern that the oily material can damage the lymphatics and so exacerbate lymphoedema.

Indirect lymphography (lymphangiography)

Indirect lymphography involves the intracutaneous injection of a water-soluble contrast medium. The contrast medium is administered with an infusion pump over a period of 10 min to create a depot of approximately 3 ml. Intradermal and subcutaneous lymphatics can be opacified by X-ray using the mammography film method, sometimes as far as the first lymph node. The advantages over conventional lymphography are the convenience of the interstitial injection without recourse to direct access into lymphatics and the application to multiple sites. The disadvantages are discomfort from the depot and rather limited visualization of lymph collectors.

Lymphoscintigraphy (isotope lymphography)

The essential function of the lymphatic system is to return to the vascular compartment proteins and colloids that are too large to re-enter directly. Lymphoscintigraphy utilizes this principle so that the dynamics of lymph flow, as depicted by the tracer uptake, transit via lymphatic vessels, and trapping in regional nodes, can be studied using a scintiscanner or a gamma camera with a large field of view (Fig. 11.14). Labelled protein or colloid is injected subcutaneously into the first web space of each foot. Measurement of transit times and time–activity curves calculated from regions of interest over vessels or nodes permit quantitative analysis of lymph drainage. Quantitative lymphosintigraphy is now the investigation of choice for identifying chronic oedema of lymphatic origin. Measurement of tracer uptake at the inguinofemoral nodes at a specified time following a standardized exercise routine will discriminate lymphoedema from oedema of non-lymphatic origin. The main lymph drainage routes can be seen, but not individual lymphatic collectors as in lymphangiography. Poor clearance from the depot suggests distal hypoplasia, while dermal backflow indicates proximal obstruction (Fig. 11.15).

Fluorescence microlymphangiography

Fluorescence microlymphangiography enables the superficial lymphatic network of the skin to be seen under the vital microscope by means of fluorescing macromolecules (FITC-Dextran, Sigma) which, when injected subepidermally, are taken up by the initial lymphatics. Information regarding the morphology of the superficial lymphatic network can be recorded on video. It is possible to distinguish between Milroy's disease and other forms of primary lymphoedema because of the total aplasia of initial lymphatics in the former. Obstructed lymphatics result in 'dermal backflow' and an extensive network can be visualized. In advanced venous disease, damaged gaiter skin lymphatics have been demonstrated using this methodology. It remains predominantly a research tool.

Imaging using computed tomography and magnetic resonance imaging

CT of lymphoedematous limbs demonstrates a characteristic 'honeycomb' pattern in the subcutaneous department which other oedemas do not. CT not only provides information through the cross-sectional area of volume change to a limb, but identifies the compartment in which that change takes place. Whereas in post-thrombotic syndrome the muscle compartment deep to the fascia is enlarged, in lymphoedema it is unchanged or may even show some reduction in size. Thickening of the skin is also a characteristic feature of lymphoedema, although it is not diagnostic.

MRI may be more suitable than CT because of its ability to detect water and the lack of radiation. Preliminary results have shown features similar to that reported with CT. The length of time taken to perform the examination is a disadvantage, but this should improve as software is developed.

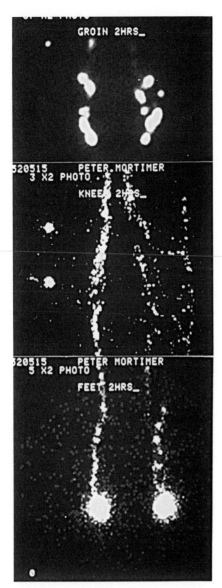

Fig. 11.14 Lymphoscintigraphy. Lymph drainage from each foot to the ilioinguinal nodes is demonstrated. A collateral drainage can be seen in the left thigh.

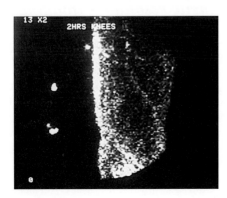

Fig. 11.15 Dermal backflow of tracer seen on lymphoscintigraphy owing to proximal lymphatic obstruction.

Differential diagnosis of the swollen limb

A clinical approach to the diagnosis of a swollen limb which considers causes of excessive capillary filtration versus poor lymph drainage will reveal that both components frequently coexist (Fig. 11.16). Indeed, even in classical lymphoedema there is evidence that with time tissue blood flow is increased and increased flow will result in higher capillary filtration. As a result swelling will deteriorate, but not because of any further reduction in lymph drainage. A similar but reverse problem exists with venous disease where oedema is assumed to be simply 'venous oedema' (see also Chapter 2).

'Venous' oedema
Chronic venous insufficiency

Why is it that clinical oedema does not manifest in many cases of chronic venous insufficiency? The massive downflow in superficial or deep veins increases venous, and therefore capillary, pressure and so filtration must increase. The margin of safety against any oedema is due to three buffering factors: changes in interstitial pressure, interstitial colloid osmotic pressure, and lymph flow. It is likely that increases in lymph flow prevent oedema, provided that the compensation capacity exists within the lymphatic system. This suggests that the development of clinical oedema is as much a failure of lymph drainage to compensate for increased filtration as it is due solely to overwhelming filtration.

It must be remembered that expansion of the venous pool in the leg due to dilatation of veins will also contribute to an increase in limb girth independent of oedema (see also Chapters 4 and 6).

Venous ulceration

Oedema is generally present. At first it is reversible and markedly affected by gravity. With time clinical features of lymphoedema begin to appear, including the characteristic skin changes of hyperkeratosis and papillomatosis particularly in the sub- and retromalleolar regions and the lateral border of the foot. Damaged dermal and subcutaneous lymphatic networks have been demonstrated using fluorescence microlymphography. A study using lymphoscintigraphy to assess lymph drainage in the legs of patients with chronic venous ulcers demonstrated significantly reduced drainage in ulcerated compared with non-ulcerated legs (Fig. 11.17). This suggests that lymphoedema is a contributing factor to the leg swelling associated with venous ulcers. This is not altogether surprising because an open wound with heavy bacterial colonization is likely to give rise to lymphatic damage. To what extent the lymphoedema compromises wound healing is not clear but it will certainly produce more permanent oedema and predispose to infection (cellulitis/lymphangitis) which will make treatment more difficult (see also Chapter 9).

Post-thrombotic syndrome

It is difficult to separate clinically cases of chronic deep venous insufficiency due to deep vein thrombosis from those due to congenital venous disorders. In many cases the 'post-thrombotic' or 'post-phlebitic' syndrome (see also Chapter 6) develops not from a single thrombotic episode but from a series of attacks involving both superficial and deep thrombophlebitis. Indeed, it is more than likely that lymphangitis/lymphangiothrombosis is an acompanying process, although there is no proof of this. Oedema is arguably the most common manifestation of the syndrome. While swelling is confined

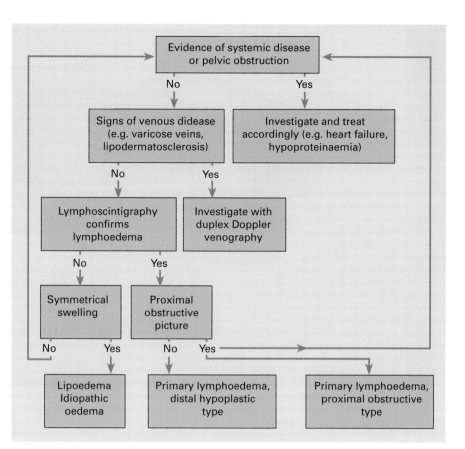

Fig. 11.16 Clinical algorithm for evaluating chronic lower limb swelling.

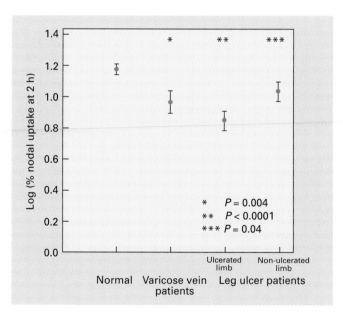

Fig. 11.17 Measured nodal uptake on lymphoscintigraphy indicates reduced lymph drainage in patients with venous disease.

in the main to the superficial compartment, it may occur deep to the fascia. This can be visualized on CT. Most pundits believe the oedema of post-thrombotic syndrome to be solely venous but, as previously discussed, it is likely to be compound, i.e. venous and lymphatic.

Superficial vein incompetence

Oedema can accompany simple varicose veins, but it is usually limited to the foot and ankle and readily dissipates overnight. Nevertheless, the underlying mechanisms are the same as for all forms of chronic venous insufficiency.

Armchair legs

This syndrome, which is also known as elephantiasis nostras verrucosis, refers to the syndrome whereby patients who sit in a chair day and night with their legs dependent develop bilateral leg oedema. No pre-existing or structural abnormalities of veins or lymphatics are present initially, but the immobility results in minimal lymph drainage and 'functional lymphoedema' ensues compounded by increased capillary filtration from dependency of the limb. The clinical picture is ultimately indistinguishable from classical lymphoedema (Fig. 11.18). Indeed, it is likely that structural changes within lymphatics occur with time, particularly if lymphangitis/cellulitis supervenes. Patients predisposed to this syndrome include those suffering cardiac or respiratory failure who cannot lie flat, those paralysed from strokes or spinal damage including spina bifida, and those with arthritis, particularly rheumatoid arthritis. Indeed, rheumatoid arthritis can be associated with genuine lymphoedema as has been demonstrated by upper-limb involvement and confirmed by quantitative lymphoscintigraphy.

Intravenous drug abuse

Repeat intravenous administration of drugs for recreational use or by addicts results in vein injury and thrombosis. Frequent attacks of infection from the use of dirty needles will damage lymphatics. The

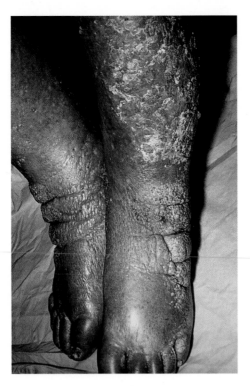

Fig. 11.18   Armchair legs (elephantiasis notras) arises from sitting day and night in a chair.

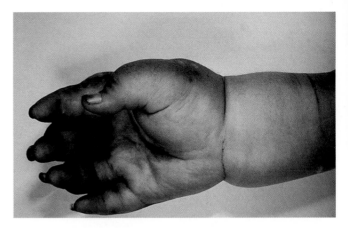

Fig. 11.19   Factitial lymphoedema (Secretan's syndrome) due to repeated application of a limb tourniquet.

combination of venous and lymphatic insufficiency can lead to chronic limb swelling.

Congenital vascular syndromes

The Klippel–Trenaunay and Parkes-Weber syndromes also cause limb enlargement. Klippel–Trenaunay syndrome is occasionally associated with lymphoedema where it may be the predominant feature. In most cases limb enlargement is due to a combination of soft tissue overgrowth and expansion of the venous pool due to the many aberrant dilated veins. In Parkes-Weber syndrome increased blood flow results from multiple arteriovenous anastomoses. Overgrowth of all tissue components leads to limb enlargement (see Chapter 8).

Other forms of chronic oedema

Oedema following vascular surgery

Transient oedema not uncommonly follows reconstructive surgery such as femeropopliteal bypass and harvesting of the superficial veins for coronary artery bypass graft. In both circumstances there is evidence that lymphatic damage contributes to the formation of oedema. Rarely, oedema can be permanent, indicating lymphoedema.

Factitial lymphoedema

Chronic limb oedema arising for psychological reasons include Secretan's syndrome and hysterical immobility. Repeated application of a constricting tourniquet as an act of self-mutilation (Secretan's syndrome) will eventually result in chronic swelling. Quantitative lymphoscintigraphy reveals permanently impaired lymph drainage. The clue to the diagnosis is evidence of tourniquet application at the root of the limb such as circumferential erythema or pigmentation and fat atrophy (Fig. 11.19).

Reflex sympathetic dystrophy (Sudek's atrophy, causalgia)

This poorly understood condition manifests with pain and oedema with loss of function, usually following an injury or surgery. With lack of use atrophy and demineralization of the bone occur. The diagnosis is clinical.

Lipoedema (lipidosis, lipodystrophy)

Lipoedema, in which a 'fatty' non-pitting swelling is confined to the legs, thighs, and hips, is frequently misdiagnosed as lymphoedema. It is peculiar to females and is usually dismissed as a variant of normality in women with large legs and hourglass figures. Onset is usually at puberty. Characteristic inverse shouldering occurs above the ankle because of sparing of the foot (Fig. 11.20). The skin is soft and is not thickened or hyperkeratotic as in lymphoedema. The tissues are often tender and bruise easily. Lipoedema can coexist with morbid obesity, but is clinically distinct as dieting characteristically results in weight loss from everywhere but the affected parts. In time pitting oedema can appear, particularly in the foot, possibly as the result of poor lymph drainage which has been shown by quantitative lymphoscintigraphy to be marginally impaired.

Plexiform neurofibroma

Elephantiasis neurofibromatosa is a diffuse neurofibromatosis of nerve trunks associated with overgrowth of the subcutaneous tissue and of the skin, producing considerable enlargement of that region.

Management

Lymphoedema represents endstage failure of lymph drainage, and is essentially irreversible and incurable. Treatment is difficult because of the presence of the 'solid' component in the swelling. In addition, most of the underlying causes are irreversible.

Since it is a non-fatal condition and the treatment has shortcomings and difficulties, most patients are told to learn to live with it. This is neither necessary nor acceptable. Although the condition is incurable, much can still be achieved to improve quality of life.

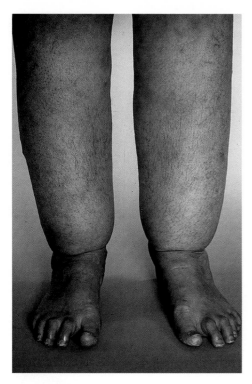

Fig. 11.20 Lipoedema (lipidosis, lipodystrophy) is frequently mistaken for lymphoedema.

Indeed, improvements in the strategy for lymphoedema care and the development of dedicated lymphoedema clinics have prompted the National Health Service Executive to insist that lymphoedema treatment is an essential component of rehabilitation following cancer therapy.

In the United Kingdom lymphoedema has traditionally been managed as follows:

- conservative treatment
- reduction operations
- attempting to re-establish lymph drainage (e.g. vessel transplantation).

Surgery provides long-lasting benefit in only a few patients, and is generally considered no better than conservative treatment.

There are two problems that must be overcome in lymphoedema—the predisposition to infections and the swelling.

Prevention of infection

Prevention of infection, particularly lymphangitis/cellulitis, is crucial to the control of lymphoedema. Prophylactic penicillin is effective in most patients. Care of the skin, good hygiene, control of tinea pedis, and good antisepsis following abrasions and minor wounds are important. Administration of antibiotics at the time of an attack of cellulitis must be prompt; otherwise they do not significantly influence the course of the illness. The only effective treatment is penicillin V (500 mg daily) prophylactically for an indefinite period. On an empirical basis, the author recommends treatment for 2 years, but if recurrent attacks recommence, lifelong prophylaxis may be necessary. Control of the oedema may help to reduce antibiotic requirements.

Control of skin changes

The skin changes in elephantiasis are not only unsightly but lead to problems including infection, odour, lymph leakage (lymphorrhoea), restricted movement, and poor wound healing. Such problems can be particularly marked in patients who have undergone reducing operations where scarring and fibrosis have become excessive. Tinea pedis (athlete's foot) is almost invariable because of the tightly packed swollen toes, and these circumstances are not improved by elastic hosiery. Unfortunately, modern antifungal creams macerate skin further and therefore old-fashioned half-strength Whitfield's ointment, applied regularly each night, is preferable. For deep cracks and crevices where bacteria readily colonize regular toilet is necessary followed by an antiseptic drying agent (e.g. Castillani's paint) applied with a cotton bud. Areas which constantly seep lymph should respond to sustained compression, but where this is not possible simple cautery or CO_2 laser therapy will often discourage leakage, if only for a short period. Warty changes (hyperkeratosis) can often be improved through the application of 5 per cent salicylic acid ointment, but the best treatment to reverse elephantiasis-type skin changes is long-term compression (hosiery or bandage).

Physical treatment to reduce swelling

Therapy aims to control lymph formation (capillary filtration) and improve lymph drainage through existing lymphatics and collateral routes by applying normal physiological processes which stimulate lymph flow.

Exercise is crucial to lymph drainage. Dynamic muscle contractions (isotonic exercises) encourage both passive (movement of lymph along tissue planes or through non-contractile lymphatics) and active (increased contractility and therefore propulsion of lymph within contractile lymphatics) phases of lymph drainage. Overexertion and excessive static exercise (isometric, e.g. gripping) increase blood flow and therefore tend to increase oedema.

External support (hosiery) complements the exercise programme. Support garments (below-knee or full-length stockings, half or full tights) are not designed to 'squeeze' oedema, but to act as a counterforce to striated muscle contractions and so generate greater interstitial pressure changes. They have the additional benefit of limiting capillary filtration (and thereby lymph load) by opposing capillary pressure. Treatment of lymphoedema requires hosiery of the highest compression strength (>40 mmHg), and double hoses may be required occasionally. Most garments last no more than 6 months (less in an active young patient). Two garments (or pairs) should be provided, one to wear and one for the wash. Prescription is possible only through a hospital; general practitioners can prescribe only stockings of classes I–III and not higher-compression stockings or sleeves. Close collaboration is advised between the clinician, the fitter, and the surgical appliance officer to ensure patient comfort, compliance, and continued improvement.

Manual lymphatic drainage therapy is a form of massage which is an accepted component of lymphoedema treatment in continental Europe. Gentle tissue movement through surface massage is a stimulus to lymph flow. The principle of manual lymphatic damage is to stimulate lymph flow in more proximal normally draining lymph node areas and so 'siphon' or 'milk' lymph from the congested region. It is intended as a downstream siphon to complement the upstream muscular pumps. Manual lymphatic drainage probably has little or no effect when used on its own.

Other conservative treatments

Pneumatic compression therapy (intermittent/sequential pneumatic compression) is employed widely. It softens and reduces limb volume during treatment, but it is doubtful that there is any long-term benefit compared with hosiery (plus exercise) alone. An inflatable boot or legging is connected to a motor-driven pump and lymph is displaced towards the root of the limb; this can result in increased truncal and genital swelling. If hosiery is not fitted immediately after compression therapy, the limb reswells readily.

Multilayer bandaging can be used for compression therapy in limb reduction. Layers of strong non-elastic (short stretch) bandages are applied to generate a high pressure during muscular contractions but low pressure at rest. The use of foam helps to distribute pressure more evenly and protect the skin (Fig. 11.21). The strategic positioning of rubber pads 'irons out' pockets of swelling and restores shape so that, subsequently, hosiery fits better and is more effective at maintaining volume reduction. However, multilayer bandaging is a skill which takes time to learn and should not be undertaken by any professional without appropriate training.

Drug therapy is generally disappointing. Diuretics remain the most commonly used treatment because most doctors consider oedema to be an indication for such drugs. However, diuretics alone have very little benefit in lymphoedema because their main action is to limit capillary filtration by reducing circulating blood volume. Improvement with diuretics suggests that the predominant cause of the oedema is not lymphatic.

Rutosides have been advocated for use in lymphoedema, and a recent placebo-controlled trial of benzopyrones (not licensed for use in the United Kingdom) showed benefit in a variety of forms of lymphoedema; however, experience with the use of rutosides in doses of up to 3 g daily for at least 6 months suggests that the clinical effect is minimal.

Surgery

Surgery has a limited role in the management of lymphoedema. It is of value in a few patients in whom, even after conservative treatment, the size and weight of a limb inhibit its use or interfere with mobility. Surgery involves either removing excessive tissue or bypassing local lymphatic defects (Box 11.1 and Figs. 11.26–11.28). Lifelong non-surgical measures must be continued postoperatively.

Reduction operations remove a longitudinal ellipse of skin and the underlying abnormal subcutaneous tissue down to the deep fascia. Undercutting of the skin allows removal of additional tissue. This procedure is preferred to circumferential excision and skin grafting or the addition of in-rolling of one of the skin flaps (which is often followed by troublesome dermal sinuses). Two or three ellipses may be required for each circumference; the operations are separated by 3–6 months. Procedures involving surgery both above and below the knee or elbow are usually undertaken one region at a time, because blood loss can be extensive.

Bypass operations: if the lymphoedema results from excision of or damage to a local group of lymph nodes (e.g. in the axilla, inguinal, or iliac regions), the area can be bridged with omentum or an isolated and opened-out segment of gut. Other procedures to bypass obstructed areas include lymphovenous anastomoses and drawing cut dilated distal lymphatics into the lumen of a vein. These procedures are not routine practice in the United Kingdom.

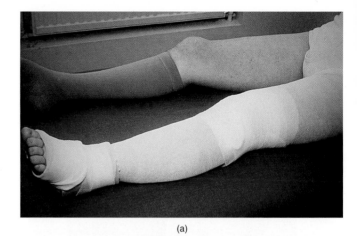

(a)

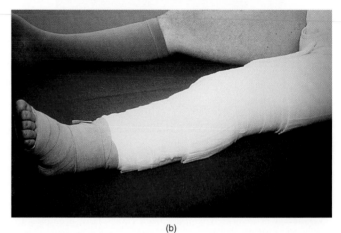

(b)

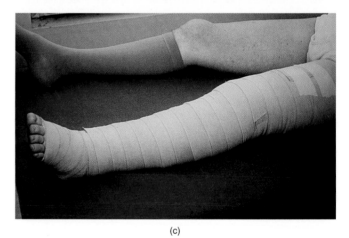

(c)

Fig. 11.21   Multilayer bandaging is used to reduce volume and reshape the limb ready for hosiery.

Provision of care

The best results are obtained with an interdisciplinary approach to care. Improvement will be gained only by implementing all measures known to improve lymph drainage and to control excessive capillary filtration. The philosophy of care is to transfer the responsibility for treatment to the patient. Once started, treatment must be maintained, otherwise deterioration will occur; lymphoedema will progress, particularly in the lower limb, unless controlled.

Posture and limb positioning are important. Any dependent limb will tend to swell as a result of increased intravascular hydrostatic pressure. Elevation just above heart level is adequate; extreme elevation is unnecessary and probably unwise unless venous hypertension coexists.

Many patients with lymphoedema are overweight because of morbid obesity as well as fluid retention. Excessive weight gain is likely to impair lymph drainage in the same way as it impairs venous drainage, and obesity reduces mobility (and therefore exercise). Control of weight through appropriate dieting is desirable; in combination with physical treatment, it may be sufficient to resolve oedema completely in some patients.

Close monitoring of limb volume is necessary to assess the progress of treatment. Subjective improvement is important for the patient. Objective measurement of swelling must be undertaken to evaluate treatment regimens and to ensure that appropriate hosiery is fitted. In most patients, physical treatment can improve the quality of life considerably. Enabling patients to understand their condition and know what they can do for themselves is central; only then can a high level of motivation and compliance with treatment be generated.

Lymphatic disorders

Identification of lymphatic vessels

The lymphatic system has been poorly characterized compared with blood vessels. One of the major problems has been the histopathological identification of lymphatics in tissues. At present the only certain way of distinguishing a lymphatic from a blood vessel is by electron microscopy. Lymphatics have wide open junctions which ultrastructurally are characteristic. Until a positive marker for lymphatic vessels in routine tissue sections is available, the role of lymphatics in determining or contributing to the pathology of disease is likely to remain obscure. The development of vascular biology has led to the introduction of vascular markers, initially those of endothelium-binding lectins (*Ulex europaeus*), and later those of more specific polyclonal antibodies (e.g. against von Willibrand factor/factor VIII related antigen and angiotensin-converting enzyme) and monoclonal antibodies against endothelial specific antigens (e.g. EN-4 and PAL-E). Unfortunately, none are positive for lymphatic endothelium only, and therefore a positive lymphatic marker still does not exist. PAL-E monoclonal antibody emerges as the only label that is consistently negative in lymphatics, but it is strongly positive for blood venules and small veins which are the vessels most likely to be mistaken for lymphatics. However, results are dependent on fixation methods.

Congenital lymphatic malformations

Like the venous system, the lymphatic system is subject to many minor aberrations. Surgeons are only too well aware of the individual differences in position and number of regional lymph nodes and territories drained, which is a significant problem in cancer management. Because of the similar ontology between veins and lymphatics, it is not surprising that the two can coexist. Also, it is not unusual to find blood within a pure lymphatic malformation such as lymphangioma circumscriptum.

Generally speaking, lymphatics may be absent (aplasia), reduced (hypoplasia), or increased (hyperplasia). Congenital hyperplasia of lymph vessels may occur in isolation without other anomalies being present, for example circumscribed hyperplasia of lymph vessels of extremities found fortuitously by lymphography or at post mortem.

Simple sustained dilatation of lymphatic vessels is referred to as **lymphangiectasia**, but when lymphatics are distended to tumour-like proportions the term **lymphangioma** is preferable. Congenital lymphangiomas, like angiomas, are best classified as hamartomatous malformations. They consist of dilated lymph channels of various sizes lined with normal lymphatic endothelium. The majority of lymphatic malformations arise in infancy, but some may not manifest clinically until later in life. Although congenital, they do not appear genetic as familial cases do not seem to occur.

Lymphangioma circumscriptum

Lymphangioma circumscriptum is a term best reserved for a lymphatic malformation which is localized to an area of skin, subcutaneous tissue, and sometimes muscle. Clinically, the condition manifests with fluid-filled vesicles which bulge on the skin surface (Fig. 11.22). The vesicles may be well defined and discrete, or grouped into structures resembling frog-spawn. The lymphangiomas may be translucent when the overlying epidermis is very thin, or they may vary in colour from red to blue-black when containing blood, as frequently happens. Alternatively, the surface of the lymphangiomas may appear extremely warty and the lesions may be mistaken for warts. There may or may not be swelling of the underlying tissues. This occurrence will depend on the size of the enlarged anastomosing lymphatic channels beneath the skin. The term 'circumscriptum' may be misleading in many cases because there may be an extensive deeper component to the malformation which is not clinically apparent. Indeed, simple surgical excision of the visible lymphangioma will frequently result in further development of surface vesicles, indicating a more widespread subcutaneous malformation. It has been postulated that the original malformation

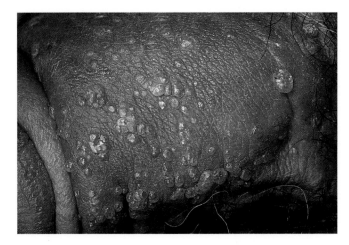

Fig. 11.22 Lymphangioma: Dilatation of upper-dermal lymphatics to produce fluid-filled vesicles or blisters on the skin.

arises from deep contractile lymphatics which are malformed and not in continuity with the normal lymph-conducting pathways. Consequently, tissue drainage into these abnormal lymphatics results in their gradual dilatation into lymphatic cisterns, contraction of which results in retrograde flow into the initial lymphatics of the skin. Only by identifying the limits of the subcutaneous cisterns before subsequent wide excision will there be any chance of cure.

Lymphangioma circumscriptum may present at any age but is usually noted at birth or appears during childhood. The most common sites are the axillary folds, shoulders, flanks, proximal parts of the limbs, and perineum. Frequently the vesicles are filled with fresh or altered blood, but how the blood gets there is a mystery. Lymphangioma circumscriptum may or may not be associated with lymphoedema of the lower limb. The presence of limb swelling suggests an extensive underlying lymphatic abnormality. Lymph weeping (lymphorrhoea) from one or more surface vesicles is common and is likely to increase the risk of infection.

Diffuse lymphangioma (deep cavernous lymphangioma)

There is no clear distinction between lymphangioma circumscriptum and diffuse lymphangioma. The difference depends solely on the extent of the malformation. Diffuse lymphangioma usually gives rise to ill-defined swelling, sometimes involving large areas of a limb. The swelling may be due to either lymphoedema (tissue oedema) or gross dilatation of abnormal lymphatic channels (lymphangioma) or both. Surface pressure with a digit will result in an indentation, but a cavernous lymphangioma will rapidly refill unlike pitting oedema where it takes many seconds for the interstitial fluid to redistribute when the pressure is released. Surface lymphangiomas are the result of dermal backflow. In diffuse lymphangiomas the vesicles are more widely distributed, indicating the more extensive nature of the underlying malformation. The presence of chylous lymphorrhoea indicates retrograde flow from the cysterna chyli (Fig. 11.23). The thigh is the most common site affected. Diffuse lymphangioma may not manifest with any surface vesicles.

Diffuse lymphangiomas, although present from birth, may go unnoticed for many years and only manifest when disturbed by accidental injury, surgery, or infection. Bleeding into a lymphangioma may be a cause of sudden pain. Swelling may or may not be apparent and, understandably, the diagnosis may be missed.

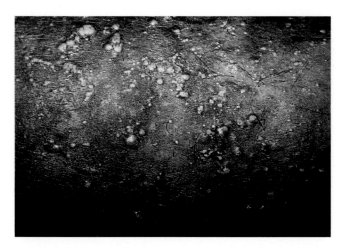

Fig. 11.23 Chylous lymphangioma: milky fluid seen within skin lymphangiomas on the leg.

Cystic hygroma

Lymphangiomas with a few large cyst-like cavities containing clear lymph are called cystic hygromas (a hygroma is a moist or watery tumour). Most occur in the neck, but they frequently extend into the upper mediastinum. To all intents and purposes cystic hygromas are no different from cavernous lymphangiomas but, structurally, hygromas have larger cystic spaces. The term tends to be reserved for those congenital lymph malformations which appear at birth or in infancy. They usually occur in the neck, presumably arising from an embryonic jugular lymph sac, whereas lymphangiomas derive from more peripheral lymph vessels. Exceptionally, a cystic hygroma occurs in the groin, presumably from an embryonic iliac lymph sac.

Acquired lymphatic abnormalities
'Seroma' (lymphocoele, lymphocyst)

Following lymphadenectomy, it is not unusual for a localized swelling containing clear fluid to develop. This is often referred to as a 'seroma', but the fluid is not serum but lymph which has drained from the cut ends of the lymphatic collectors and fills the space originally occupied by the nodes. Aspirated fluid is indistinguishable from lymph. Repeat aspiration is often necessary until a collateral lymph drainage forms. A 'seroma' may herald the onset of lymphoedema if alternative drainage routes are not established.

Acquired lymphangiomas (lymphangiectasia)

Acquired or secondary lymphangiomas arise following damage to previously normal deep lymphatic vessels. The mechanism by which they form is identical with that for congenitally determined lymphangiomas, namely obstruction to drainage leads to back-pressure and dermal backflow with subsequent dilatation of upper-dermal lymphatics. Acquired lymphangiomas are not true neoplasms or hamartomas but represent simple dilatation (lymphangiectasia) of surface lymphatics. Lower-limb lesions usually arise in association with lymphoedema following ilio-inguinal block dissection or pelvic surgery and radiotherapy for gynaecological cancer.

Their clinical appearance may vary greatly, ranging from clear fluid-filled blisters to smooth flesh-coloured nodules (Fig. 11.24). Histologically, the latter show oedematous polypoid nodules within which are dilated lymphatics. Lesions may be solitary but scattered throughout a lymphoedematous limb or they may be grouped as seen in lymphangioma circumscriptum.

Lymphangiomas of the vulva are described following cancer treatment, tuberculous inguinal lymphadenitis, and genital involvement with Crohn's disease. Clinically, the most common lesions are circumscribed groups of tense thin-walled vesicles. However, a hyperkeratotic appearance may make distinction from viral wart's difficult (Fig. 11.25). Recognition and appropriate treatment of vulval lymphangiomas is important primarily because the lesions may act as portals of entry for infection. In addition, persistent leakage of lymphatic fluid may be mistaken for urinary incontinence.

Treatment of acquired lymphangiomas is essentially reduction of underlying lymphoedema and control of infection. This may be relatively straightforward on the leg, but not so easy on the genitalia where compression is not possible. Simple excision may prove successful, particularly as tightening of the labial skin will discourage recurrence.

Acquired lymphangiomas may be widespread and problematic in palliative circumstances where advanced cancer produces profound oedema of the lower limbs, genitalia, and lower trunk. In these

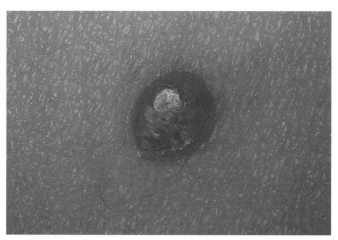

Fig. 11.24 Acquired lymphangioma: a lymphangiomatous nodule on a lymphoedematous leg following ilio-inguinal node dissection for melanoma.

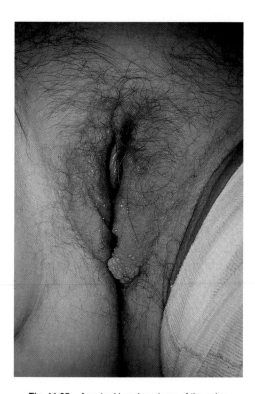

Fig. 11.25 Acquired lymphangioma of the vulva.

circumstances widespread lymphangiomas weep copious lymph. Opposing intralymphatic pressure with equivalent surface compression is the only way of controlling the lymphorrhoea unless the lymphatic obstruction can be relieved.

Lymphatic tumours
Acquired progressive lymphangioma

This benign tumour differs from simple acquired lymphangioma by its clinical behaviour and histopathology. Acquired progressive lymphangioma presents as reddish or bruise-like plaques which are usually located on the abdominal wall, thigh, or calf. Typically, the condition affects young adolescents but may also arise in adults. It is usually localized and flat and grows slowly. It is considered to originate from lymphatic endothelium, and the histopathological appearance can mimic a low-grade sarcoma or Kaposi's sarcoma. Anastomosing dilated channels, with a tendency to dissect the collagen bundles, are lined by swollen endothelial cells but without cellular atypia.

Lymphangiomatosis

Deep cavernous or diffuse lymphangiomas that slowly progress due to an intrinsic proliferative process, as opposed to extension due solely to raised hydrostatic pressure, are termed lymphangiomatosis. Histologically, it is impossible to distinguish from simple lymphangioma (lymphangiectasia). The diagnosis is based on the slow progression and infiltration of surrounding structures including bone.

Maffuci's syndrome is diffuse haemolymphangiomatosis accompanied by severe widespread deformities of bone and cartilage. On lymphography, the lymphangiomas do not appear to communicate with the main lymphatic pathways and often possess both blood vascular and lymphatic elements. Hard nodules arising from the bones develop simultaneously with the cutaneous vascular swellings particularly on the fingers and toes. Pathologically, these are enchondromas which are radiologically translucent. Deformity may be gross and slowly uniting pathological fractures are common. The disease has a high potential for malignancy, including lymphangiosarcoma.

Lymphangiosarcoma

This is a rare but well-recognized complication of any chronic lymphoedema irrespective of cause. Red-brown or purple discoloration, like a bruise, appears in the skin of the lymphoedematous limb. Nodules or raised plaques may appear later. As the tumours proliferate, the oedema may increase and the older lesions ulcerate. The tumour metastasizes early and has a poor prognosis.

The tumour is best described in the upper limb following breast cancer treatment (Stewart–Treves syndrome), but it is well reported in the lower limb in association with lymphoedema, usually of many years duration.

Radical amputation may offer hope of cure if performed early enough.

Kaposi's sarcoma

There is increasing evidence that Kaposi's sarcoma may arise from lymphatic rather than vascular endothelium, although its origins may lie with a primitive cell capable of either differentiation. Histologically, the earliest stages of the disease show jagged proliferations of capillaries extending out from the normal capillaries in the mid-dermis. As the lesion develops, a network of spindle cells and large vascular spaces will be seen with characteristic thin-walled 'back-to-back' capillaries.

The classical form of the disease, as described by Kaposi, presents with dark blue or purple lesions, usually on the feet. Initially they may be flat, and when they become tumid pressure may produce partial blanching to reveal a brown tinge from extravasated blood. Individual tumours enlarge to a diameter of 10–30 mm and stop growing, whereupon adjacent areas fuse to form a plaque or tumour. New lesions appear proximally alongside a superficial vessel (?vein or ? lymphatic). Unlike lymphangiosarcoma, lymphoedema is rarely evident at the time that the first lesions appear, but otherwise the morphology is similar. However, Kaposi's sarcoma is characteristically multifocal and in time symmetrical, affecting both lower limbs. In prolonged venous hypertension of the lower legs, nodules with a close resemblance to Kaposi's sarcoma may develop; however, they differ, in lack of progression and spindle cell proliferation is not seen histopathologically (pseudo-Kaposi's sarcoma).

Brawny oedema resembling lymphoedema develops with advanced Kaposi's sarcoma. Oedema is often the first sign of the African type of Kaposi's sarcoma, with lymph nodes as the main tissue involved.

Kaposi's sarcoma associated with immunodeficiency, whether induced by HIV or not, produces subtle lesions that are often widely scattered and quite dissimilar from the classical type.

Where a small area is involved, excision or radiotherapy can be used. Superficial radiotherapy is rapid and effective, and is the treatment of choice for the majority of patients with nodular disease of the extremities.

Lymphangitis

Acute lymphangitis

In theory, the lymphatic system has evolved in man as a host defence mechanism. Noxious agents and predators such as bacteria, if not dealt with at the point of entry to the host, access the lymphatic system. Lymphatic vessels, together with adjoining lymph nodes, effectively act as the second line of defence, with the aim of preventing further onward spread and so limiting systemic involvement. In some circumstances the inflammatory response may be profound, perhaps due to a heavy infection load, and an overt lymphangitis or lymphandenitis or both arise. Lymphangitis represents inflammation of the lymphatic collectors and is clinically seen as tender red streaks up the limb corresponding to the inflamed vessels. Oedema is so often an accompanying feature in the lower limb that red streaks, such as are seen with lymphangitis of the arm, are rarely seen. A more diffuse erythema is seen extending up the medial side of the leg and thigh. Distinction from an ascending cellulitis becomes difficult.

Infection is usually limited by the lymph nodes, and in the lower limb lymphadenitis may give rise to painful swelling in the groin. Occasionally, infection bypasses a group of lymph nodes and affects those at a higher level. Constitutional upset can be severe and is the greater the more proximally the infection has extended.

Lymphangitis may occur without any demonstrable inflammation or be recurrent, for example following relapsing herpes simplex infection. Permanent obliteration of lymphatic collectors may follow severe or recurrent lymphangitis. In those cases where reserve lymphatic capacity is limited, permanent swelling (lymphoedema) can result.

Recurrent acute inflammatory episodes (recurrent cellulitis)

Where lymphatic insufficiency exists and the local lymphoid tissue/lymphatic system fails in its host defence duty, recurrent infection can occur. Clinically this manifests as recurrent cellulitis/erysipelas. Indeed, any patient who presents with recurrent attacks of cellulitis in one leg almost certainly has a compromised lymph drainage in that leg whether or not overt lymphoedema is present. In most cases, however, subtle signs of lymphoedema are evident, particularly in the skin over the toes and forefoot. Because there is no localization of infection by the lymphatics, the first sign of illness may be constitutional upset with fever, rigors, or vomiting. Only later may redness and tenderness appear in the leg and the diagnosis become clear.

No lymphangitis, as witnessed by red streaks up the leg, is seen because presumably the infection, uncontrolled by the lymphatic system, has spread through tissue planes (cellulitis) with rapid dissemination into the circulation.

Treatment for recurrent cellulitis should first address predisposing factors such as tinea pedis, foot dermatitis, leg ulcers, etc. If no portal of entry or cause can be identified, long-term prophylactic antibiotics may be necessary if the debilitating attacks are to be controlled.

Lymphangiothrombosis

Lymph is capable of clotting, but the circumstances in which this happens and the pathological effect of lymph thrombosis, are totally unknown. Extrapolating from venous thrombosis suggests that lymph thrombosis is likely to impair the function of lymphatic valves and the contractility of lymph collecting vessels.

Mondor's disease is alleged to be a superficial thrombophlebitis of the breast and chest wall. A similar process, whereby cords or threads like violin strings extend down the inner arm, is frequently seen following axillary lymphadenectomy. The manner in which the cords 'bowstring' across the axilla with the arm abducted, their diameter, and the fact that the cords can snap between finger and thumb suggest that lymph thrombosis may be more likely than phebothrombosis or thrombophlebitis. An equivalent condition may well exist in the lower limb but be mistaken for thrombophlebitis.

Chylous reflux

Chyle is a 'milky lymph' which flows from the lacteals of the gut through the cisterna chyli and then through the thoracic duct. Appearance of chylous lymphangiomas is the most common method of presentation in the lower limbs. Milky vesicles draining chyle may manifest in the skin at any point from toe to genitalia and are nearly always associated with lymphoedema.

Lymphoedema, usually of one leg, develops early in life and subsequently chylous lymphangiomas appear. It is not uncommon for a haemangioma to be present either on the limb or the adjoining quadrant of the trunk. In most cases the condition tends to progress with increasing oedema and more chylous lymphangiomas. This may be because the downforce of lymph/chyle gradually undermines the function of more distal lymphatic valves.

For chyle to appear in the leg it must reflux either from the point that the cisterna chyli joins the retroperitonal lymphatics or through fistulas adjoining the cisterna chyli with pelvic lymphatics. Lymphography always shows incompetent megalymphatics, i.e. large varicose main lymph trunks in which the valves are absent or totally incompetent. No obstruction is identified except in the thoracic duct in some cases.

The early age of onset, the association with congenital vascular anomalies such as the cutaneous angiomas, and the demonstration of aberrant lymph pathways in the abdomen all suggest an embryological fault in development.

Treatment of chylous reflux into the lower limb is by surgery, as no conservative or medical treatment offers any hope of cure. A low-fat diet will help alleviate symptoms by reducing the leakage of chyle. Surgical manoeuvres include(a) ligation of incompetent abdominal pathways and (b) ligation of lymphatics in the groin or lumbar region. Once the reflux is controlled, standard physical therapy measures should contain the lymphoedema.

Box 11.1 Relief of lymphoedema in the lower limbs by surgical means: *selective surgical procedures when all else fails*

Surgery does not offer any easy cure of lymphoedema in the lower limbs and should only be used for severe states that cannot be controlled by conservative treatment.

The two main categories of surgical treatment are, reconstruction of impeded lymphatics, and reduction in the bulk of the limb. When lymphoedema is due to a local obstruction to lymphatic return, with distended but open lymph vessels beneath it, there is an opportunity for this to be relieved by reconstructive surgery. It may be possible for these vessels to be connected in some fashion to normally drained lymphatics above the obstruction, or to be entered directly into a vein to drain there. However, lymphatic restoration of this sort is often not possible, and then a very different form of surgery, reduction in the bulk of the limb by excision of a mass lymphoedematous tissue, may be the only way to bring relief.

Indications for considering surgery are: excessive size, weight and bulk of the limb; pain; repeated severe attacks of cellulitis; malignant change (lymphangiosarcoma).

Localized obstruction of inguinal or iliac lymphatics

This may be caused by a primary state of proximal lymphatic hypoplasia, or by secondary states due to injury, infection, involvement of nodes by malignancy, previous surgery (for example, block dissection of glands) or radiation. There are several possible procedures:

1. *By-passing a block in the lymph system to re-establish lymphatic continuity*

   A tissue graft containing lymphatics is used as a bridge to connect patent lymphatics below the block with healthy iliac or para-aortic lymphatics above the block. An appropriate length of tissue containing lymphatics is removed from a normal area elsewhere, such as the arm, and is used as a free graft, anastomosed by microsurgery to lymphatics above and below the block. (Baumeister 1981). This is a highly skilled and prolonged procedure with uncertain success but may have potential for development.

2. *Providing an alternative outlet through a pedicle of tissue that is well provided with lymphatics and has good proximal drainage*

   A pedicle flap of skin, subcutaneous tissue, and lymphatics is raised from the arm and inlaid as a bridge from upper thigh to the axillary drainage area by a staged procedure (Gillies and Fraser 1935). This extensive operation has not proved sufficiently effective to justify its use.

   A pedicle of omentum (Goldsmith 1967), mesentery (Pugnaire 1968), or isolated small intestine (Kinmonth *et al.* 1978) is used as bridge between limb and visceral lymphatics. Omentum contains too few lymphatics and mesentery alone does not prove satisfactory. **However, small intestine (ileum) is liberally supplied with lymphatics and an isolated portion can be readily mobilized to reach patent lymphatics or nodes in the inguinal region. This offers the best prospect of successfully improving lymph drainage from the limb. (Fig. 11.26)**

   > **The enteromesenteric bridge.** (Kinmonth *et al.* 1978). Careful selection is essential. Indications: distress caused by lymphoedema in a lower limb which is not relieved adequately by conservative measures. It is only appropriate when there is a localized obstruction in the inguinal, iliac, or lower aortic lymphatics (for example, in congenital proximal hypoplasia or following surgery to inguinal lymph glands), but there must be open, distended lymphatics, and healthy lymph nodes below this level, to which the new lymphatic outlet can be attached. The ileum to be used must be known to have good normal lymph drainage to cisterna chyli and thoracic duct. A segment of ileum, about 5 cm long, together with the associated mesentery containing its vascular and lymphatic supply, is carefully separated as a pedicle. The remaining ileum is re-anastomosed and its mesentery sutured.

   > The ileal segment is now opened along its length and the mucosal layer removed so that the submucosal lymphatics are exposed. A tunnel, if necessary under the inguinal ligament, is prepared down to the lymph nodes which are to be used below the block, and the pedicle drawn through this. The raw enteric surface is now sutured to the afferent (collector) portions of two or more healthy nodes that have been suitably bisected. Following the operation, compression by bandage or stocking is continued to minimize oedema.

   > A good to moderate long-term improvement can be expected in about 50 per cent of patients. Studies by lymphangiogram have confirmed that the two sets of lymphatics connect well, with a good flow of lymph through the new pathway and onwards to the cisterna chyli.

3. *Providing a new outlet, locally into a vein, for lymphatics or nodes below the obstruction*

   The cut face of lymph glands is anastomosed into the side of a vein (Nielubowicz and Olszewski 1968). Again this is only suitable when lymphatics and nodes are open below a lymphatic block. In essence, several carefully chosen lymph glands are bisected and the afferent cut face of each is anastomosed to a side opening in a good sized vein nearby (Fig. 11.27(b)); alternatively the gland substance is shelled out and the raw capsule is joined to the vein opening. This can give an excellent initial result but the lymphovenous anastomosis tends to close off within a year or two. However, this operation is not too difficult and can bring valuable short-term relief in a patient with lymphoedema from malignant infiltration of inguinal or iliac lymph glands. Alternatively, lymph vessels may be anastomosed or implanted into a vein (Degni 1978). Again, this only applies when lymphatics are open beneath blocked lymph nodes. It may be done in one of several ways. Single lymphatics may be divided and their cut afferent ends

Continued

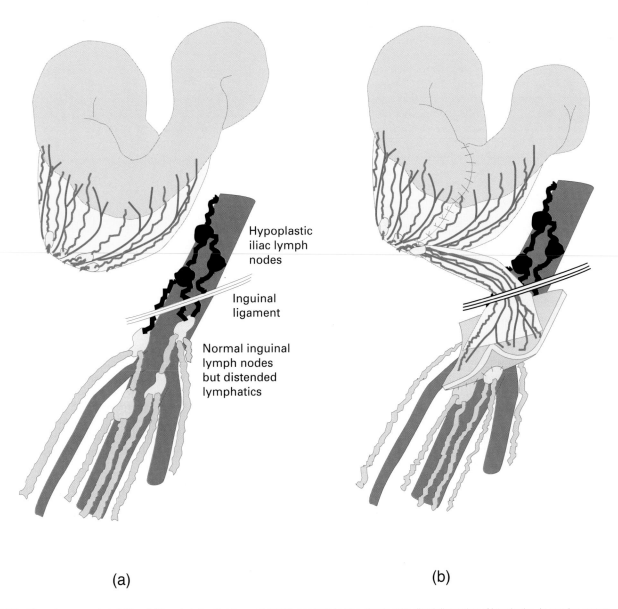

(a)   (b)

Fig. 11.26 The enteromesenteric bridge. (a) Local obstruction from proximal hypoplasia in iliac glands, with distal distension of lymphatics, is causing severe lymphoedema. (b) A 5 cm segment of ileum is mobilized together with a pedicle of its vascular and lymphatic supply. The bowel segment is opened along its length and the mucosa removed to expose underlying lymphatics. Normal lymph nodes below the obstruction are bisected and the cut face of each afferent portion sutured against the raw submucosal layer.

Box 11.1 *Continued*

implanted separately into a convenient vein, or a group of lymphatics may be divided and fed into the vein through a single opening (Fig. 11.27(c)). Special needles are available to simplify this and the operation can be performed quite quickly. The unwanted cut ends of the lymphatics above are ligated to prevent seepage through them causing a collection of lymph. Successful results with these techniques have been reported but there is uncertainty about their longevity, but again, they may be valuable in malignant lymphatic obstruction.

Yet another, and even more exacting, method is by microsurgery anastomosing individual lymphatics end to end with a small veins of similar size (O'Brien 1979). This is very time consuming and the results have not been sufficiently encouraging for it to be generally adopted as yet.

Note on megalymphatics with reflux of lymph. It is important to be aware that in about 3 per cent of lower limbs with lymphoedema this is due to megalymphatics which allow heavy reflux. This usually occurs only on one side, with massive enlargement of lymphatics which have no valves and lack propulsive movement, in effect, a state of 'lymphatic varicosis'. It often extends up to the cisterna chyli, and chylous reflux from here may travel lower down the limb. The various manifestations of this are described in the main text but it is referred to here because it will not benefit from any of the surgical procedures so far described, but appropriate surgery, ligation of selected megalymphatics, may have a useful part to play. However, this does require considerable understanding of the varieties and extent of lymph reflux, and the likely response in any particular case. Like all surgery to relieve lymphoedema, it is best left to a specialist who has experience in this field.

If lymph reflux is the cause of lymphoedema it should be minimized by carefully selected ligation before considering any operation of surgical reduction in the bulk of a limb, since otherwise lymph fistulas may be a problem afterwards. Fortunately this form of lymphoedema can usually be controlled by conservative means so that surgery is seldom necessary.

Reduction of bulk by surgical excision
The restoration of lymph return by surgical means is very limited and can only help a few patients. In the majority, relief has to rely on conservative measures, but in some their distress and disability is so great that a drastic surgical excision of a large mass of oedematous tissue has to be considered. It can be a valuable solution when a massive limb virtually immobilizes the patient, to which may be added pain and illness from repeated infection in the skin crevices causing cellulitis and lymphangitis. The result is not cosmetically pleasing but the relief it brings makes this acceptable. Many procedures have been suggested but two are generally regarded as the most effective (Figs. 11.28(a) and 11.28(b)).

Sistrunk's operation (Sistrunk 1918). Here a broad ellipse of skin, together with a massive wedge of subcutaneous tissue and a strip of deep fascia are taken away from the full length of the one aspect of the limb. The skin edges are then sutured together and a firm bandage applied. When this has healed and two or three months later, the procedure is repeated on the opposite face of the limb and may be repeated yet again after this if need be. This is a major operation requiring a limb with a good set of arteries and veins, and of course, a patient who is fit enough. It is essentially an operation for disability and should not be used, for example, in a young woman who is mostly worried about appearance.

Charles' operation (Charles 1912). Similar cautions apply. This operation was originally suggested for the massive limb of filariasis but can be equally suitable for other conditions, such as congenital distal hypoplasia. Filariasis can, of course, be arrested by chemotherapy with diethylcarbamazine (DEC) but the lymphoedema and all its problems remain so that surgical reduction of a huge limb is still necessary. It is particularly suitable where the skin is deeply creviced and prone to repeated infections. The skin and subcutaneous tissues from ankle to knee are completely removed circumferentially, often with an area of deep fascia as well, but with preservation of periosteum. Skin coverage is then restored by split skin grafts. The knee and lower thigh require skilful shaping to avoid an abrupt change in girth, and healing may not be easy. The final result is a slender leg with irregular outline below the knee, but free from the miseries of a heavy limb and recurring cellulitis.

General comment on aftercare: continuing care by compression bandaging or stocking, with elevation whenever possible, is essential to maintain the benefits after any of the procedures described above. A true cure is seldom achieved but the condition can be much easier to control.

Note on operations, now largely abandoned, attempting drainage to the sub-fascial deep layer
The muscle compartment under the deep fascia is not involved in the lymphoedematous process because it has its own independent lymphatic system without any connection to the superficial layers. Many attempts by a variety of operations have been made to create lymphatic connection between the two compartments but none has succeeded. Thompson's operation (1962) is one example. This had a considerable vogue in the 1970s, but eventually it was realized that the benefits were in fact due to reduction in bulk by excision of

Continued

Box 11.1   *Continued*

subcutaneous tissue and the efficient use of compression bandaging, rather than from improved lymph drainage. In this operation two extensive skin flaps were raised on the leg, the underlying mass of subcutaneous tissue excised and a long incision made in the deep fascia. The outer aspect of one skin flap was denuded with a dermatome to limit the growth of hair, and was then rolled inwards to be inserted deeply between the muscles in the hope of establishing connection with the lymphatics there. The other skin flap was used to restore skin coverage by suturing it to the surface of the inrolled flap, and firm bandaging applied. The initial reduction in size was usually pleasing but the swelling gradually reasserted itself, and, as might be expected, hair growing in the buried skin could cause troublesome infection and pilonidal sinuses. Studies to assess whether lymph drainage to the deep layers was ever achieved all failed to demonstrate this. This operation and similar ones have no advantage over the simple principle of reduction by surgical excision and maintaining the benefits by compression bandaging.

See Appendix (p. 235) for a historical summary of surgical procedures attempting relief of lymphoedema and references to their original description.

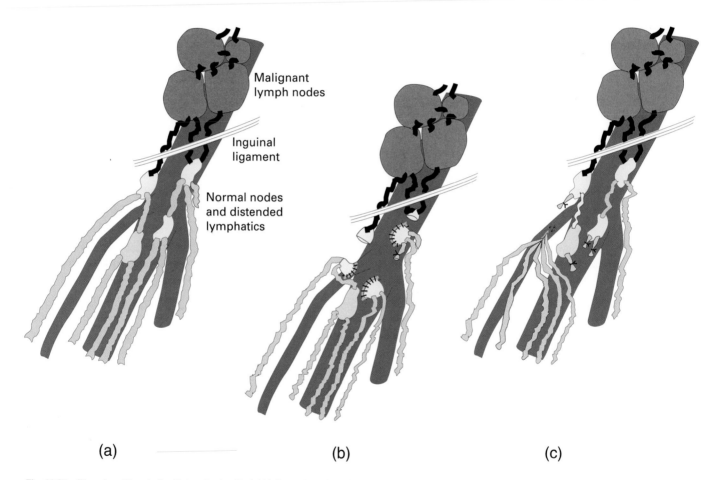

Malignant
lymph nodes

Inguinal
ligament

Normal nodes
and distended
lymphatics

(a)   (b)   (c)

Fig. 11.27   Diversion of lymph directly to veins locally. (a) Malignant invasion of iliac lymph glands is causing severe secondary lymphoedema. Short term relief may be helpful. (b) Lymphadeno-venous shunt. Inguinal lymph glands below the obstruction are bisected and the cut face of each afferent portion is anastomosed to side openings in neighbouring veins. (c) Lymphatico-venous shunt. A group of distended lymphatic vessels are divided and the distal ends (afferent) fed into a neighbouring vein, each is held in place by a suture. The proximal ends are ligated to prevent a collection of lymph by back-seepage.

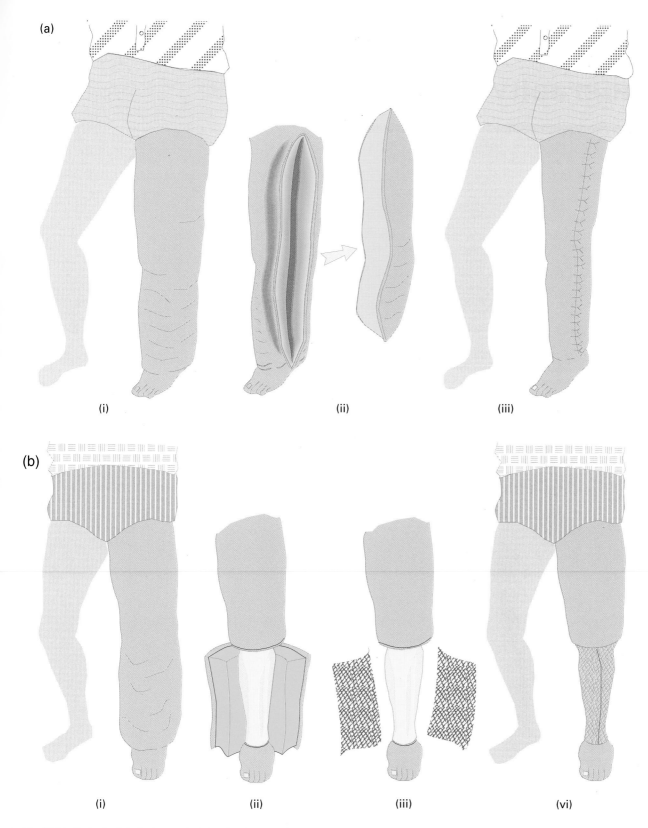

Fig. 11.28 Reduction in bulk of a massively lymphoedematous limb by surgical excision. (a) Sistrunk's operation. (i) Massive lymphoedema caused by distal lymphatic hyoplasia. (ii) A generous ellipse of skin and underlying oedematous subcutaneous tissue is excised as a wedge down the length of the limb. A strip of fascia may also be taken but the value of this is debatable. (iii) The skin edges are then sutured and a firm bandage applied. This procedure can be repeated once or twice more at intervals of a few months to other aspects of the limb. (b) Charles' operation. (i) Severe secondary lymphoedema from filariasis is present. (ii) The skin and oedematous subcutaneous tissue is entirely removed from knee to foot. Deep fascia need not be removed and periosteum is preserved. (iii) Split skin grafts are applied to the muscles and periosteum. (iv) The final result has an inelegant shape but gives effective relief.

Following these procedures, firm compression by bandaging or stocking, and elevation whenever possible, must be continued indefinitely to maintain the benefits.

Bibliography to Part III

Browse, N.L. (1986). *A colour atlas of reducing operations for lymphoedema of the lower limb*. Vol. 39, Single surgical procedures. Wolfe Medical, London.

Browse, N.L. and Stewart, G. (1985). Lymphoedema: pathophysiology and classification. *J. Cardiovasc. Surg.*, **6**, 91–106.

Foldi, M. and Casley-Smith, J.R. (1983). *Lymphangiology*. Schattauer, Stuttgart.

Johnson, H.G. and Pflug, J. (1975). *The swollen leg*. Heinemann, London.

Kinmonth, J.B. (1982). *The lymphatics*. Arnold, London.

Levick, J.R. (1995). *An introduction to cardiovascular physiology* (2nd edn). Butterworth Heinemann, London.

Mortimer, P.S. (1990). Investigation and management of lymphoedema. *Vasc. Med. Rev.*, **1**, 1–20.

Roddie, I.C. (1990). Lymph transport mechanisms in peripheral lymphatics. *News Physiol. Sci.*, **5**, 85–9.

Stewart, G., Grant, J., Croft, D.N., and Browse, N.L. (1985). Isotope lymphography: a new method of investigating the role of lymphatics. *Br. J. Surg.*, **72**, 906–9.

Yoffey, J.M. and Courtice, J.M. (1970). *Lymphatics, lymph and the lymphomyeloid complex*. Academic Press, New York.

Appendix: Historical review on surgery for lymphoedema

Surgical procedures attempting to treat lymphoedema

Attempted regeneration or restoration of lymphatics

- Handley (1908). Insertion of silk threads. No success.

- Walther (1919). Rubber tubes buried in subcutaneous tissue. No success.

- Baumeister (1981). A tissue graft containing healthy lymphatics is taken from elsewhere and anastomosed by microsurgery to good lymphatics above block to patent lymphatics below it (transplantation). Limited success at best.

Attempts to utilize good lymphatics beneath deep fascia

- Lanz or Lang (1911). Exposed deep fascia and bone, raised periosteum, and trephined holes into bone; onto which periosteal flaps were laid.

- Kondoleon (1912). Excision of subcutaneous fat and deep fascia with skin flaps laid onto exposed muscle

- Sistrunk (1918). See Bulk reducing procedures below

- Homans (1936). See Bulk reducing procedures below

- Macey (1940). Skin grafts laid onto deep fascia. At later stage subcutaneous fat and skin removed, exposing previous skin grafts.

- Thompson (1962). Wide excision of subcutaneous tissue, with one skin flap buried between muscles beneath deep fascia.

Comment: the main benefit of these procedures is not from improved lymph drainage, but from massive reduction in bulk and compression maintained indefinitely afterwards,

By providing an alternative outlet by-passing area of lymphatic obstruction

Using a skin bridge containing lymphatics

- Gillies and Fraser (1935). A pedicle flap of skin, subcutaneous tissue, and lymphatics from the arm was inlaid in stages from upper thigh to the axillary drainage area. It was not sufficiently successful and is no longer attempted.

Using abdominal structures and their lymphatics

- Goldsmith (1967). A pedicle of omentum was used in the hope of providing new lymphatic drainage. Insufficient lymphatics in omentum.

- Pugnaire (1968). A bridge of intestinal mesentery was used to bring new lymphatics to healthy lymphatics in lower limb, but it was found to be much better to include the lymphatic bed in sub-mucosal layer of gut.

- Kinmonth (1978). A bridge of isolated small intestine, with mucosa removed, is used to bring new lymphatics to patent lymphatics in lower limb below a lymphatic obstruction. The intestinal lymphatics must be normal. Good results in about 50% of carefully selected patients. Is recommended when all criteria favourable.

By providing an outlet into a vein for lymphatics and nodes below an obstruction

- Nielubowicz and Olszewski (1968). Cut face of collector (afferent) half of lymph nodes anastomosed to vein, or substance of node removed before anastomosis of capsule to vein. Can give initial success but tends to cease functioning within a year or two, but is useful to relieve lymphoedema caused by malignancy.

- Degni (1978). Insertion of one, or a group, of lymphatics into a vein through its side. Reported successes but uncertain longevity.

- O'Brien (1979). Direct end to end anastomosis of lymphatic to a small vein by microsurgery. Limited success and uncertain longevity

- Campisi (1991). A graft of small vein into which the divided ends of lymphatics above and below the block are laid in the hope that a new lymphatic connection will be formed. No success yet reported; has yet to be evaluated.

Comment: The full potential of microsurgery has probably not yet been developed.

Bulk reducing procedures

- Charles (1912). Extensive removal of skin and subcutaneous tissue down to, and often including, deep fascia. Skin coverage is restored with split skin grafts laid on to muscle. Recommended in filariasis (after treatment with diethylcarbamazine) or other massive lymphoedema causing distress to patient.

- Sistrunk (1918). Extensive removal, down length of limb on one aspect, of a large wedge of skin and subcutaneous tissue, often including a strip of deep fascia. The skin edges are then sutured together and firm bandage applied. Repeated on other aspects later. Recommended for massive lymphoedema not controlled by conservative treatment and causing distress.

- Homans (1936). Extensive removal of subcutaneous tissue through double skin slaps, which are then laid onto the bared muscle and bone. Is effective but necrosis of skin flaps can be troublesome.

- Thompson (1962). Extensive removal of subcutaneous tissue, leaving two skin flaps, one of which has surface layer of skin and hair follicles removed with a dermatome, and then buried between muscles under deep fascia. The other skin flap used to close exposed area. Only limited success and hairgrowth in the buried skin may cause problems by infection and pilonidal sinuses. It is not recommended.

Ligation of megalymphatics

This is only appropriate in a minority (3%) of patients when oedema is caused by enlarged, valveless, noncontractile lymphatics allowing reflux of lymph (may be chylous) to a lower limb (lymphatic varicosis). Most cases are controlled by conservative means. The lymphatics in abdomen and thorax are commonly also involved and provide pitfalls for ill-considered surgery.

Knowledgeable ligation of carefully selected megalymphatics can bring benefit if conservative treatment is not sufficient. This should always precede surgical bulk reduction (seldom necessary) in these patients to minimize the problem of subsequent lymph fistulas.

The effect of sympathectomy

- Telford and Simmons (1938). Lumbar sympathectomy tried in five cases of lower limb lymphoedema without any lasting benefit. Not considered to be of any value for lymphoedema and not recommended.

Comment: Many of the above have long been abandoned as ineffective. However, the Kinmonth enteromesenteric bridge is effective in a highly selected group which have a localized obstruction in

lymphatics in the inguinal or iliac region. There must be patent lymphatics below and healthy nodes onto which an isolated portion of opened ileum, with mucosa removed, is sutured. The lymph drainage from the portion of gut must be known to be good and not also involved in lymphatic abnormality.

The more recent operations of lymph node or lymphatic vessel to vein shunts do offer some prospect of success but tend to cease functioning within a year or two, but may be useful in malignant obstruction. The operations by microsurgery anastomosing individual lymphatics to healthy grafted lymphatics or to small veins give hope for future development but at the moment require difficult and prolonged surgery by an expert in this field and the outcome is uncertain.

Otherwise, surgery can only offer a bulk reducing procedure; Sistrunk or Charles operations are probably the best for most circumstances. *Indications*: Massive size and weight; pain; repeated infection; malignant change (lymphosarcoma).

'The surgical treatment of lymphoedema has been more ingenious and varied than successful'. (Aird, 1949) The same is true today!

References

Aird, I. (1949). *Companion of surgical studies*. Livingstone, Edinburgh.

Baumeister, R.G.H., Seifert, J., Wiebeke, B., and Hahn D. (1981) Experimental basis and first application of clinical lymph vessel transplantation in secondary lymphedema. *World J. Surg.*, 5, 401.

Campisi, C. (1991). Use of autologous interposition vein graft in management of lymphedema: preliminary experimental and clinical observations. *Lymphology*, 24, 71–6.

Charles, H. (1912). In: *A system of treatment* (ed. A. Latham and T.C. English), Churchill, London.

Degni, U. (1978) New technique of lymphaticovenous anastomosis for the treatment of lymphedema. *J. Cardivasc. Surg.*, 19, 577.

Gillies and Fraser (1935). *Br. Med. J.*, 1, 96.

Goldsmith, H.S., De los Santos, R., and Beattie, G.J. (1967). Relief of chronic lymphoedema by omental transportation. *Ann. Surg.*, 166, 573–85.

Handley, W.S. (1908). Lymphangioplasty. *Lancet*, 1, 785.

Homans, J. (1936). Treatment of elephantiasis of legs. *New Eng. J. Med.*, 215, 1099.

Kinmonth, J.B., Hurst, P.A., Edwards, J.M. and Rutt, D.L. (1978). Relief of lymph obstruction by use of a bridge of mesentery and ileum. *Br. J. Surg.*, 65, 829–33.

Kinmonth, J.B. (1982). *The lymphatics: surgery, lymphography and diseases of the chyle and lymph systems*. Edward Arnold: London.

Kondoleon (1912). *Munchn. med. Woch.*, 1, 525.

Lanz (1911). *Zentralbl. f. Chir.*, 38, 153.

Macey (1940). *Proc. Staff. Meet. Mayo. Clin.*, 15, 49.

Nielubowicz, J., Olszewski, W. (1968). Surgical lymphaticovenous shunts. *Br. J. Surg.*, 55, 40.

O'Brien, B.M. (1977). Micro lymphatico-venous surgery for obstructive lymphoedema. *Aust. N.Z. J. Surg.*, 47, 284.

Pugnaire, M. de R. (1968). Linfangioplastia mesenterica en el tratamiento de las elefantiasis de las membros inferiores. *Angiologia*, 20, 146–52.

Sistrunk, W.E. (1918). Modification of the operation for elephatiasis. *J.A.M.A.*, 71, 800.

Telford and Simmons (1938). *Br. J. Surg.*, 25, 771.

Thompson, N. (1962). Surgical treatment of chronic lymphoedema in the lower limb. *Br. Med. J.*, 2, 1566–69.

Walther (1919). *Bull. acad. med. de Paris*, 82, 262.

Appendix: Emergency reference in case of anaphylactic shock or accidental intra-arterial injection of sclerosant

Two rare dangers are possible with sclerotherapy

Anaphylaxis

Distinguish between: *simple fainting or syncope*. Preceded by restlessness and sweating. Particularly likely if patient is standing or sitting upright. It occurs just before or during insertion of needle, often before injection of sclerosant, and is accompanied by a slow pulse. Recovers within a minute or two on lying patient down.

Anaphylaxis. Occurs a few minutes after injection. Patient shows pallor, rapid, faint pulse, difficulty in breathing, possibly nausea, and vomiting. Does not recover on lying patient flat but may progressively deteriorate.

The dangers of anaphylaxis are threefold—hypotension, bronchospasm and angioedema, which may affect the larynx and therefore require intubation or even trachiotomy. Urticaria or erythema may appear (see article on anaphylaxis in the British National Formulary).

Mainstays of treatment are:

- Lie patient flat

- Intramuscular adrenalin (1 ml amp of 1:1000 adrenalin) (1 mg/ml)

- Oxygen

- Repeat adrenalin if necessary

- Give antihistamine slowly intravenously or by IV drip (chlorpheniramine maleate 10 mg in 1 ml amp)

- Set up IV drip to give colloid (plasma) or saline

- Give hydrocortisone slowly IV to prevent return of symptoms as adrenalin wears off (100 mg)

- Be prepared to intubate (alert anaesthetist—have laryngoscope, endothracheal tube, and suction ready) or even trachiotomy

- Bronchospasm can be severe, if necessary, use salbutamol by nebulizer or intravenously

- Admit to hospital and ascertain the cause of anaphylaxis and, if it is the sclerosant, make sure the patient knows and will ensure that he/she does not have it ever again.

Note: Always enquire about allergies before sclerotherapy.

Accidental intra-arterial injection of sclerosant

This is signalled by great pain and pallor in the extremity. **Injection must cease immediately** but the situation may already be beyond redemption depending on dose and concentration. Never use more than 0.5 ml of 3% sclerosant at any single site but even this can cause severe damage if misplaced into an artery.

If accidental injection does occur

If the needle is still in, give 500 units heparin intra-arterially. Then remove needle from artery and continue heparin therapy by intravenous drip. Encourage vasodilatation by 'physiological' sympathectomy, that is, by warming the whole body (but not the affected limb-ischaemic tissue is easily damaged by direct heat). Do not risk sympathectomy by surgery or by injection for fear of anticoagulants causing added complication from haemorrhage. **Consult urgently with arterial specialist**.

Other possible measures:

- Dextran

- Cortisone (predenisolone 250 mg)

- Ancrod (Arvin) defibrinogenation

- Fibrinolysis by streptokinase

- Platelet disaggregation by prostacylcin

Note: **This is a potential disaster which can lead to peripheral gangrene and possible loss of a limb** and must be avoided at all costs:

- Always be aware of this possibility

- Avoid injection near the ankle where substantial arteries are near the surface and easily entered

- **Never inject blindly**. The target vein must always be identified by one of the following means:

Watching needle point enter a vein just under the skin
Always confirm location of needle in a vein by sucking back dark venous blood—abandon immediately if blood is bright red or is pulsatile, and reposition the needle elsewhere

If there is pain distally whilst injecting sclerosant stop immediately. Suck back to test for possible entry into an artery. *Do not proceed* if there is any suggestion of this.

If injecting into a relatively deep vein, the needle should be guided by ultrasonography (echosclerotherapy) and the veins response watched on the video screen. This requires skill and experience.

Appendix: Useful additional information

Therapeutic and diagnostic equipment

Sequential intermittent pneumatic compression systems for the limb

Indications: lymphoedema, chronic venous insufficiency with ulcer. Firms supplying these include:

Centromed Ltd
Unit 8
St Johns Court
Ashford Business Park
Sevington Ashford
Kent TN24 0S
UK
Tel: +44(0)1233 500551
Fax: +44(0)1233 500551
(This firm also manufacture a range of pneumatic devices for positioning patients)

Huntleigh Healthcare
310-312 Dallow Road
Luton
Bedfordshire LU1 1TD
UK
Tel: +44(0)1582 413104
Fax: +44(0)1582 459100

Kendall Healthcare Products Co.
15 Hampshire Street
Mansfield
MA 02048
USA
Tel: (001) 508 2618000
Fax: (001) 508 2618556

The Kendall Company (UK) Ltd
2 Elmwood
Chineham Business Park
Crockford Lane
Basingstoke
Hampshire RG24 8WG
UK
Tel: +44(0)1256 708880
Fax: +44(0)1256 708071

Impulse system (pneumatic compression) to foot

Indications: to promote venous return in an immobilized limb and prevention of post-operative deep vein thrombosis. Is under trial for use in critical ischaemia of foot. Manufactured and supplied by:

Novamedix Services Ltd
Viscount Court
South Way
Walworth
Andover
Hants SP10 5NW
UK
Tel: +44(0) 1264 334212
Fax: +44(0) 1264 334007

Intavent Orthofix Ltd
5 Burney Court
Cordwallis Park
Maidenhead
Berks FL6 7BZ
UK
Tel: +44 (0)1628 594500

Diagnostic equipment

Huntleigh Diagnostics
35 Portmanmoor Road
Cardiff CF2 2HB
UK
Tel: +44(0)1222 485885
Fax: +44(0)1222 492520
Supply a range of Doppler diagnostic equipment suitable for veins and arteries, including models giving computer analysis of findings.

PMS (Instruments) Ltd.
Waldeck House
Waldeck Road
Maidenhead
Berkshire SL6 8BR
UK
Tel: +44(0) 1628 773233
Fax: +44(0) 1628 770562

Supply a full range of equipment for venous diagnostic work, including, Doppler, plethysmographic, and ultrasonic imaging with colour scanning.

Vincent Medical Ltd
85 Sussex Place
Slough
Berks SL1 1NN
UK
Tel: +44(0) 1753 692055
Fax: +44(0) 1753 521757
Supply a range of Doppler diagnostic equipment with computer analysis and printout of findings. Also supply Photoderm high intensity light equipment for treatment of benign vascular lesions.

Medasonics
47233 Fremont Blvd
Fremont, CA 94538
USA
Tel: (001)800 227 8076
Supply a full range of ultrasonic diagnostic and imaging systems.

Liquid crystal thermography

Novamedix Services Ltd
Viscount Court
South Way
Walworth
Andover
Hants SP10 5NW
UK
Tel: +44(0) 1264 334212
Fax: +44(0) 1264 334007

Furniture for elevation of limbs

Elevation of the lower limbs plays a fundamental part in the management of chronic venous insufficiency and in lymphoedema. To obtain maximum benefit from this the limbs must be raised well above the level of the heart. But remember that a good arterial supply is essential when any elevation above the horizontal is used.

High elevation

Many reclining chairs are advertised, raising the legs horizontally but although these will bring substantial benefit to the patient with chronic venous insufficiency or lymphoedema it will be much less than it could be. However, there are a few recliners offering truly high elevation, with the limbs well above the level of the heart, as is required in the management of longstanding problems of recurring ulceration due to post-thrombotic syndrome, to primary deep vein valve deficiency, or in severe lymphoedema. A good example of such a chair is illustrated in Fig. A.1 and is supplied by:

Anatomia (BackSaver)
28 Wigmore Street
London W1
UK
Tel: +44(0) 800 374604

BackSaver Products Company
53 Jeffrey Avenue
Holliston

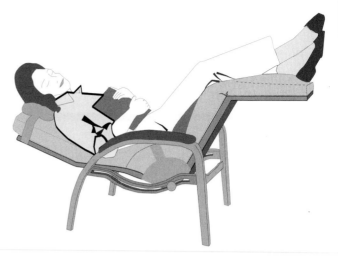

Fig. A1

Massachusetts, MA 01746
USA
Tel: (001) 508 429 5940
Fax: (001) 508 429 8698

Even with this excellent design some extra advantage for the patient with a severe problem can be provided by a wedge-shaped pillow raising the feet a few inches higher. The chair is available in different sizes to accommodate the height of the patient; the size chosen should ensure that the heels are supported by the leg-rest so that the weight of the limbs does not fall entirely on the calf muscles.

Moderate elevation

An example of a recliner giving elevation nearly up to heart level but providing comfort with good appearance, is supplied by:

Everstyle
91 South End
Croydon CRO 1BG
UK
Tel: +44 (0) 181 7605178
Fax: +44 (0) 181 6886581

Chairs in this category can give greater elevation if shaped pillows under the feet and legs are used, or by raising the front legs of the chair an inch or two (more than this can cause the chair to tilt over backwards). With any recliner the heels should be supported by the leg-rest to prevent prolonged weight falling on the calf muscles. (see also Centromed Ltd, given above under Pneumatic Compression Systems, for patient positioning aids).

Cosmetic masking and camouflage creams (concealers) to disguise vascular blemishes

Most of the well known cosmetic firms supply these, including: Pan-Stik by Max Factor and Perfect Covering Concealer by Elizabeth Arden.

High intensity light treatment for benign vascular lesions

ESC Inc
100 Crescent Rd
Needham, Ma 02194
USA
Fax: 001 (617) 444 8812

Compression sclerotherapy

For Fibro-Vein (sodium tetradecyl sulphate) sclerosant (formerly STD) and all requirements for compression sclerotherapy:

STD Pharmaceutical Products Ltd
Fields Yard
Plough Lane
Hereford HR4 0EL
UK
Tel: +44 (0) 1432 353684
Fax: +44 (0) 1432 342383
E-mail address: enquiries@stdpharm.co.uk
Addresses of distributors in various countries available on request.

Fibro-Vein comes in four strengths: 3%—for major veins (25G × 5/8 in needle); 1%—for lesser veins (27G × 1/2 in needle); 0.5%—for minor veins and medium venules (27 or 30G × 1/2 in needle); 0.2% for telangiectasis and minor venules (30G × 1/2 needle with a microsclerotherapay needle set).

Also supplied: the full range of Medi elastic support, the Medi Valet (to assist easy application of an elastic stocking), and computer software for patient records.

Aethoxysklerol or Sclerovein (polidocanol) is an alternative sclerosant that is widely used in Europe and in USA but is not yet fully licensed in UK. It comes in a range of dilutions and is used in similar fashion to that described above.

Notes on the treatment of venous ulcer and the materials used

Principles in treatment of venous ulcer

- Be sure of the cause. Is it venous? If it is arterial, venous treatment can be very harmful. Make sure a systemic factor such as diabetes is not present.

- The most important factor in treatment is reduction of venous pressure by elevation of the limb.

- If the ulcer is due to superficial vein incompetence, elastic support is usually effective and will allow ambulatory treatment. If deep vein insufficiency is the cause, either post-thrombotic or from inborn deficiency of valves, external support is far less effective but can minimize regression when ambulation is allowed. The most effective form of support is by inelastic external containment (for example, by a paste bandage—see below).

- Provision of favourable environment for the ulcer (see below).

Factors impeding healing of the ulcer

- Infection with pathogenic organisms, particularly staphylococcus aureus, beta haemolytic streptococcus, and anaerobic organisms.

- Presence of necrotic tissue. This harbours pathogens, and prevents formation of granulation tissue and epithelial ingrowth. Debridement is the most effective method of treatment but desloughing agents may be helpful. Occlusive hydrocolloid or gel is believed to promote separation of slough.

- Use of topical steroids. These may delay or prevent healing and should not be used on the ulcer itself. However, they may be used sparingly to control changes in the surrounding skin.

- Antiseptics or antibiotics, many of which may interfere with healing or cause allergic reactions. Normal saline is safest for cleansing an ulcer surface.

- Ischaemia in the limb (usually caused by atherosclerosis—absent ankle (Doppler) pulses and/or blanching on elevation of foot).

- Poor general background state. Diabetes, anaemia, nutritional, and vitamin deficiencies or any systemic disease may prevent healing.

Properties the ideal dressing should have

- Impermeable to infection from outside.

- Provides or preserves a moist environment.

- Absorbs excess exudate and bonds with it so that maceration of surrounding skin does not occur.

- Does not become adherent and is easily removed, taking debris with it, but not stripping away recent epithelial regrowth.

- Requires changing relatively infrequently, perhaps every few days.

- Discourages the growth of bacteria.

- Encourages formation of granulation tissue and epithelial ingrowth.

- Reduces odour (activated charcoal can be used in severe cases).

- Does not contain any additives likely to harm the tissues or causes sensitivity reactions.

These features are largely achieved by the following materials (with examples in brackets): hydrocolloids (Granuflex), hydrogels (Geliperm, Scherisorb, Opragel), and calcium alginate (Kalostat, Sorbisan). These materials may come as films, pads, gels, pastes, or beads and are recommended as first choice in treating venous ulcers. They interact with the ulcer surface and bind with its exudate. Some may form quantities of thick turbid fluid which has a strong odour and is mistaken for pus, but this is part of the process and is harmless. Patients may need reassuring on this.

A considerable range of other products are available for the treatment of ulcers and are listed in MIMS and similar collective indexes issued regularly by the pharmaceutical manufacturers. They may be classified in the following categories (examples given in brackets):

- Non- or low-adherent dressings. Some adherence may occur by exudate setting in perforations. Main shortcoming is failure to absorb exudate thus causing skin maceration. In an ischaemic ulcer they allow excessive drying which is most undesirable. (Melolin, N.A. dressing.)

- Semipermeable films. Suitable for shallow relatively clean ulcers or wounds. (Opsite, Tegaderm)

- Hydrogels. Recommended (see comments above)

- Hydrocolloids Recommended (″   ″   ″)

- Calcium, alginate. Recommended (″   ″   ″)

- Foams. Suitable for flat wounds with heavy exudate. (Allevyn, Lycofoam)

- Odour-absorbent dressings (deodorizers). Activated charcoal (Actisorb) is effective in absorbing odour.

- Paste bandages (and see below). These bandages are impregnated with paste which sets after application to form an inelastic shell or container. This is their most important feature when used for venous ulcer but many are impregnated with medical ingredients which bring little benefit to the ulcer. Moreover, such medicaments can be an active source of sensitivity and reaction by the skin, notoriously sensitive in the venous ulcer patient, and this possibility should always be borne in mind so that the type of bandage can changed without delay if skin reaction occurs. The fewer the ingredients the better and a simple zinc oxide paste (for example Viscopaste or Zincaband) is safest. If there are doubts, patch testing with the material in question applied to the skin of the arm or back can be used.

- Paraffin tulle (non-medicated) dressings. Can stick painfully and should not be used. If medicated, particularly with antibiotics, hypersensitivity is likely to be a problem.

- Topical antibiotics. The skin around venous ulcer is very prone to sensitivity reactions and generally speaking antibiotics used locally are best avoided. When a pathogen requires control by an antibiotic it is best administered systematically for a limited period.

- Antibacterial agents and antiseptics. Again, beware of sensitivity reactions locally or chemical damage that may impede cells involved in the healing process.

- Desloughing agents. These can help separation of slough but physical debridement with pointed scissors or a knife is much more effective and usually to be preferred. (Aserbine, Debrisan, Varidase)

- Dyes. May be used when surrounding skin becomes macerated but are unsightly and obscure the state of the skin. (Gentian violet, Brilliant green).

- Miscellaneous applications (Normasol—saline for wound irrigation).

Dressings and bandages

Paste bandage

This can be the most effective means for healing a venous ulcer apart from a policy of continuous elevation. Its success is due to its mechanical properties rather than the medicaments it may include (see above). It may be applied directly over an ulcer or with an absorbent dressing covering it and will conform easily to the contour of the leg. It is applied to the foot and up to the knee without including the toes. The main virtue is that it sets into a firm shell which provides an ideal inelastic container around the leg. The bandage should be applied without tension whilst the limb is elevated and the veins are empty. When the patient stands the bandage will then prevent the veins from over-distending and this improves the effectiveness of the damaged venous pumping mechanism. Because the pressure under the bandage can never exceed that of the veins, free upward flow is not impeded and when the leg is raised and external support is not required there is not any residual elastic compression that may reduce blood flow. Experience amply confirms that the principle of inelastic external containment is the most effective way of healing or preventing recurrence in a venous ulcer but at the same time allowing some degree of ambulation.

A paste bandage cannot easily be applied by the patient and usually will require renewing by a nurse every week or two (depending on the state of the ulcer). It is still necessary for the patient to take every opportunity, certainly overnight, to elevate the limb. When the ulcer has healed precautions must be still taken to prevent its recurrence, using an elastic stocking by day, with elevation whenever possible and at night.

Methods for keeping a dressing in place

A dressing over an ulcer may be kept in place by the following means (examples given in brackets);

- Cotton bandage

- Cotton conforming bandage (Crinx and Kling). To apply and stay in place without pressure

- Cotton crepe bandage (Elastocrepe). Conforms and stays in place well. Gives moderate pressure but tends to slacken within a few hours

- Cotton tubular bandage (Tubegauze). Is used as a covering layer without giving any pressure

All the above materials are non allergenic and are suitable for use when allergic skin reaction is a problem.

Adhesive tapes, films, bandages, and garments

The old problem of skin maceration under adhesive materials has been largely overcome by a range of porous and semipermeable materials which allow ventilation and evaporation of excess moisture. Moreover, care has been taken to reduce the likelihood of skin reaction in the hypersensitive skin of chronic venous insufficiency by avoiding the chief offenders such as rubber in adhesives or backing material. Nevertheless care has to be taken to avoid possible allergens (see Box 9.4, Chapter 9). The first two categories given below seldom cause reaction but can damage the skin surface if stripped off too roughly.

- Permeable non-woven synthetic surgical adhesive tape (Micropore).

- Semipermeable adhesive film dressings; usually polyurethane or polyvinychloide (Opsite, Bioclusive). They may be used to cover an ulcer (usually in combination with a hydrocolloid, or applied directly to relieve pain in a raw surface, for example, the donor site of a skin graft. They may be left in place for many days but if stretched on or forcibly removed may tear away the surface layer of the skin.

- Elastic adhesive bandage (Elastoplast, Lestreflex). These combine moderate to strong elastic compression with strong adhesion. Lestreflex is said to be 'hypoallergenic' but Elastoplast contains rubber in the adhesive to which a significant number of patients show a strong skin reaction within a few days. Warning of this is given by severe itching and the bandage should then be removed without delay, and the remnants of the adhesive sponged off with a suitable solvent (Zoff). For this reason elastic adhesive bandage should not be applied directly to the skin but instead a layer of cotton crepe bandage is first evenly applied and the adhesive elastic bandage is then placed over this, as a crossply, to give a strong inelastic container, closely shaped to the leg. This may be left in place for several weeks if necessary and seldom causes skin reaction. Used in this way between the ankle and the knee it gives suitable support for venous problems and following sclerotherapy.

- Cohesive (self-adherent bandages). These bandages adhere to themselves but not to skin or clothing. Coban 3M is a semi-synthetic material of moderate elasticity that follows the shape of the limb easily to form a firm resilient container suitable for the leg. It requires some skill to give a suitable degree of compression and to avoid rolling of the top edge, or creasing, to form a narrow band cutting in painfully. For this reason it should not be used to cross the ankle or knee joints. They are a valuable adjunct and have a variety of uses including sclerotherapy or for temporary application during this and other procedures. Another material with similar qualities is a cotton fabric coated with latex rubber (Tensoplus). Both these types of bandage may be left in place for several weeks and are well accepted by the skin. If an ulcer is present this should be covered by a dressing capable of absorbing exudate.

- Elastic webbing (red or blue line bandages). These are strongly elasticated and, in conjunction with a suitable dressing over an ulcer can be used to give sustained strong compression if required. However, they are unwieldy and do require skilful application because it is all too easy to apply excessive and painful pressure by being unaware of the cumulative effect of successive turns. If it is applied when the leg is elevated to empty the veins and is laid on with minimal tension it is possible to achieve the effect of an inelastic container that resists the overfilling of veins when the patient stands. Some patients learn to use them successfully in this way.

- Elastic compression bandages. Various designs that facilitate regulation of the tension used are available. One good example is the Thuasne two-way stretch bandage (Biflex), which has a series of rectangles printed along its length which becomes square when elongated by 30%. This allows pressure to be graduated evenly up the limb as it is applied. Again it may be applied over a dressing on an ulcer and is commonly used in the ambulatory treatment of venous ulcer.

- Short or limited stretch bandages. These bandages can only be stretched a short distance and then reach their limit of elasticity. They are designed to prevent excessive tension and once applied at near-maximal stretch will resist distension of the veins under them. In this way cumulative elastic recoil with added turns is avoided but a strong encasement around the leg is formed.

- Lightweight elastic stockings and elasticated tubular bandage (Tubigrip). These are often a neat and convenient way of supporting a dressing over an active ulcer which is too painful for a strong stocking to be used, and where repeated soiling by exudate may be problem. Elasticated tubular bandage is a good alternative and may be used in double thickness if extra compression is required.

The manufacturers of the various categories of products referred to in this Appendix have made considerable effort to meet the requirements of the medical profession and have contributed many improvements in materials and methods. Although a number of named examples have been given above there are many excellent alternatives that have not been mentioned. The full range may be found in the proprietary pharmaceutical compendiums widely circulated in most countries.

Elastic stockings
These are well listed in the manufacturers literature and in most countries regulations are laid down to ensure conformity to good standards and varying strengths (for example, the Drug Tariff of the National Health Service of UK) and these are summarized in Box 6.3, Chapter 6. Most manufacturers are careful to ensure that graduated compression is given by a stocking, that is, a lessening of elastic compression up the length of the limb, to match the hydrostatic pressure in the veins up the limb when standing, and ensuring the upper part of the stocking never exerts a constricting effect.

Keeping up-to-date

Phlebology has become an actively progressive subject with many workers constantly seeking to improve our understanding and methods of diagnosis and treatment. The best way of keeping up-to-date is through one of the excellent specialized journals available, and by belonging to a venous society. Some examples are given below.

Journals
In English
Phlebology Published quarterly by Springer Editors: P.D. Coleridge Smith, UK and L. Norgren, Sweden. The official Journal of the Venous Forum of the Royal Society of Medicine (UK), Societas Phlebologica Scandinavica, and Members of the Union Internationale de Phlebologie. It is devoted to venous disease and closely related topics. Contains original articles, reviews, reports on society meetings, correspondence, announcements of forthcoming meetings, and summaries in English of selected papers from other venous journal.

Dermatologic Surgery Editor: Dr.Ronald Moy, USA. Every three months the North American Society of Phlebology devotes a number of this journal to phlebology. Available in Europe from Elsevier Science, PO Box 211, Amsterdam, The Netherlands.

Scope on Phlebology and Lymphology Published quarterly. Editor: Prof. Lars Norgen. Contains editorials, reviews (many by invitation), and abstracts. Published by PMSI Bugamor B.V., The Netherlands, and distributed on behalf of Beiersdorf Jobst.

In French
Phlebologie Editor in Chief: Andre Davy.

In German
Phlebologie (Germany) Editors in Chief: Prof. Dr. U. Schulz-Ehrenburg and R. Zundler.

Venous societies
The list below gives only a few well-known examples. Many vascular societies mainly concerned with arterial or cardiac topics also include sessions on phlebology and lymphology. Meetings of

societies likely to interest phlebologists are announced well in advance in most of the venous journals given above.

The American Venous Forum
13 Elm Street
Manchester, MA 01944 USA
Tel: 001(508) 526 8330
Fax: 001(508) 526 4018

The North American Society of Phlebology
930 N. Meacham
Schaumburg, IL 60173-496
USA

The Venous Forum of the Royal Society of Medicine (U.K.)
The Societe Francaise de Phlebologie (France)
Societas Phlebolgica Scandinavica (Scandinavia)
German Society of Phlebology
The Hellenic Phlebological Society (Greece)
The Polish Phlebological Society
Japanese Society of Phlebology

A look ahead

What of the future? The opportunities ahead are great! One real need is to continue improving the accuracy and detail of diagnosis. Ultrasound imaging of the lower limb venous system is still at an early stage and capable of considerable development to give a complete moving picture of venous flow in a limb during a cycle of exercise in the upright position. Another great need is the development of means to replace veins and valves damaged beyond repair. There is little doubt that genetic bioengineering will be able to produce valved grafts of veins, immunologically acceptable to the patient, in the foreseeable future—but not yet a topic in this present book! Phlebology has become a dynamic subject, probing the future with a range of stimulating possibilities ahead. But, here we must content ourselves with what is attainable at the moment.

Index

Page numbers in *italics* indicate figures and tables.